BARBARA O'NEILL'S LOST BOOK OF NATURAL REMEDIES

A Better You Everyday Publications

Email: info@abetteryoueveryday.com

Disclaimer

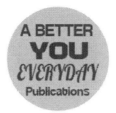

A Better You
Everyday Publications

info@abetteryoueveryday.com

www.abetteryoueveryday.com

Printed or published to the highest ethical standard.

Barbara O'Neill's Book of Natural Remedies

Discover 400+ Antibiotic Formulas, Herbal Remedies for Common Ailments, Superfoods, Anti-Inflammatory Dishes, Gut-Healing Protocols, Mindfulness, Vibrational Healing, and Ancestral Traditions for Complete Wellness.

By

Margaret Willowbrook

USA 2024

Table Of
Contents

ℱOREWORD

Welcome, dear reader, to a journey where the age-old wisdom of nature's healing powers is revealed through the pages of Barbara O'Neill's Lost Book of Natural Remedies. This book is a heartfelt invitation to explore and rediscover the profound benefits that come from living in harmony with the earth.

Drawing inspiration from renowned healers like Barbara O'Neill and Dr. Sebi, my purpose in writing this book has been shaped by my lifelong dedication to studying and sharing the natural solutions that our beautiful planet offers so freely. These solutions are not just alternatives to modern medicine; they are a call to return to a life of balance and wellness.

Each chapter of this compendium is carefully crafted to offer you not just knowledge, but practical wisdom that can be applied to everyday life. From homemade antibiotics to healing foods and from mindfulness practices to reconnecting with the rhythms of nature, this book spans a comprehensive spectrum of holistic well-being.

My hope is that you will find not only useful remedies and recipes within these pages but also a source of comfort and inspiration that encourages you to embrace a healthier, more sustainable lifestyle. Let this book serve as your guide in discovering the healing virtues hidden in plants and the natural world around us.

With warmth and kindness,

Margaret Willowbrook

ℐNTRODUCTION

Welcome to "Barbara O'Neill's Lost Book of Natural Remedies," a comprehensive guide that serves as a bridge between the timeless wisdom of nature and the health needs of today. Inspired by the teachings of Barbara O'Neill and Dr. Sebi, this book is a testament to the healing power of the natural world and an invitation to explore its restorative potential.

This book spans an extensive range of topics, each part meticulously crafted to guide you through the many facets of herbal medicine and holistic well-being.

What You Will Discover

■ **Homemade Antibiotics (Part I):**

Discover how to create natural antibiotics, from Garlic and Honey Tonic to Olive Leaf Extract Capsules, to combat infections without relying on synthetic drugs.

■ **Herbal Remedies for Various Ailments (Part II):**

Explore over 40 herbal solutions, such as Chamomile Tea for digestion and Ginkgo Biloba Tincture for improved memory and circulation.

■ **Remedies for Respiratory Issues (Part III):**

Find relief for respiratory ailments with remedies like Eucalyptus and Mint Steam Inhalation and Pine Needle Tea for bronchitis.

■ **Digestive Remedies (Part IV):**

Address digestive issues with natural solutions like Fennel and Ginger Tea for gas and Aloe Vera Juice for gut healing.

Pain and Inflammation Remedies (Part V):

Learn about natural pain relievers and anti-inflammatory solutions, including Willow Bark Tea for pain relief and Turmeric Gummies for inflammation.

Women's Health Remedies (Part VI):

Discover herbal care tailored for women's health, from Red Raspberry Leaf Tea for fertility to Evening Primrose Oil for breast health.

Immune-Boosting Remedies (Part VII):

Strengthen your immune system with powerful herbal and food-based remedies like Elderberry Syrup and Astragalus Root Decoction.

Nutrient-Dense Superfoods (Part VIII):

Integrate superfoods into your diet with recipes like Kale and Quinoa Salad and Spirulina Smoothie for enhanced nutrition.

Anti-Inflammatory Dishes (Part IX):

Enjoy healing recipes that reduce inflammation, such as Turmeric and Ginger Latte and Beet and Avocado Salad.

Gut-Healing Recipes (Part X):

Support your gut health with nourishing foods like Bone Broth and Probiotic Cashew Cheese.

Detoxifying Drinks and Smoothies (Part XI):

Cleanse and rejuvenate with detoxifying beverages like Green Detox Smoothie and Dandelion Root Tea.

Mindfulness and Stress Management (Part XII):

Embrace practices to reduce stress and enhance mindfulness, including Deep Breathing Exercises and Guided Meditation Scripts.

Exercise and Movement (Part XIII):

Incorporate physical activity into your routine with guides like the Gentle Yoga Flow Sequence and Low-Impact Cardio Routines.

- **Sustainable Living Practices (Part XIV):**

  Adopt eco-friendly lifestyle changes with tips on composting, organic gardening, and reducing plastic use.

- **Glossary of Common Herbs and Their Uses (Part XV):**

  A comprehensive glossary to help you understand the properties and applications of herbs like Aloe Vera, Ashwagandha, and Turmeric.

- **Vibrational Healing and Energy Medicine (Part XVII):**

  Dive into the subtle energies of the body with techniques like crystal healing, sound therapy, and Reiki.

- **Addressing Common Ailments Naturally (Part XVII):**

  Find herbal and lifestyle solutions for common health issues, from colds and flu to arthritis and joint pain.

This book is your guide to embracing a healthier, more balanced lifestyle through the power of natural remedies. Whether you are just beginning your journey or are an experienced practitioner, these pages will inspire, educate, and empower you to live in harmony with nature.

Join me on this transformative journey as we rediscover the lost wisdom of natural remedies and learn to harness the healing power of the earth.

With heartfelt warmth,

Margaret Willowbrook

Barbara O'Neill: A Journey Through Nature's Healing Path.

Barbara O'Neill, a revered figure in the field of natural health and wellness, has lived a life dedicated to unlocking the healing secrets of nature. Born in the picturesque landscapes of Australia, Barbara's early fascination with the natural world blossomed into a lifelong pursuit of knowledge and healing.

From her early years, Barbara exhibited a profound connection with the healing plants and herbs that surrounded her childhood home. This connection deepened as she pursued formal education in the health sciences, earning qualifications that positioned her as a respected naturopath and nutritionist. Her work is deeply influenced by her belief in the body's intrinsic ability to heal itself, a principle she has championed through her educational endeavors and public engagements.

Barbara's family life has been a cornerstone of her journey. Married to Michael O'Neill, she has found in him not just a partner but a collaborator in her mission to promote natural health. Together, they have raised their children with the same principles of wellness and balance that Barbara advocates publicly. Her family's support has been instrumental in her ability to reach out and touch the lives of thousands.

Professionally, Barbara's career has been marked by a series of pioneering initiatives. She founded the Misty Mountain Health Retreat, a sanctuary where individuals from all walks of life come to restore their health through natural methods. Here, Barbara applies her extensive knowledge of diet, exercise, and herbal remedies to help her guests rediscover their health.

Barbara O'Neill's philosophy extends beyond individual health. She is an advocate for sustainable living, teaching people how to grow their own food and reduce their environmental footprint. Her work in this area reflects her deep respect for the earth and her commitment to leaving a positive legacy for future generations.

In her writings and teachings, Barbara often refers to the wisdom of other natural health pioneers, such as Dr. Sebi, whose work on alkaline diets and herbal medicine has influenced her approach. Her dedication to learning and sharing has made her a beloved figure among those seeking a holistic path to wellness.

Barbara's journey is not just about healing the body but also about nurturing the spirit and mind. Her approach to health is a testament to the power of nature and the human spirit to overcome challenges and find balance in life.

How To Use This Book

Welcome to "The Lost Book of Natural Remedies," a comprehensive guide to the healing power of nature. This book is designed to empower you with knowledge and practical tools to enhance your health and well-being. Here's how you can navigate and make the most of this valuable resource:

Navigating the Book

Explore the Table of Contents: Begin by reviewing the table of contents to familiarize yourself with the structure and range of topics covered. Each part is organized to guide you through different aspects of natural healing, from homemade antibiotics to mindfulness practices.

Read the Introductions to Each Section: Each major section begins with an introduction that provides context and insights into the remedies and practices within. These introductions help you understand the importance and application of each category of remedies.

Use the Index and Glossary: The index at the back of the book allows you to quickly find specific remedies, herbs, or topics. The glossary of common herbs and their uses is a valuable reference to understand the properties and benefits of each herb featured in the book.

Safety Precautions

Start Small: When trying a new remedy or herbal treatment, begin with small dosages to see how your body responds. Gradually increase the dosage as necessary, but always within the recommended limits.

Allergy Check: Before using any new herb or ingredient, especially if applied topically or ingested, conduct a patch test or a small trial to ensure you are not allergic.

Pregnancy and Children: Special caution should be taken when using herbal remedies for pregnant women, nursing mothers, and children. Consult the specific warnings provided in each remedy and seek advice from a healthcare professional.

Proper Dosages

Follow the Guidelines: Each remedy in this book includes dosage recommendations. Adhere to these guidelines to ensure effectiveness and safety.

Adjust for Personal Needs: Understand that individual responses to herbs can vary. Adjust dosages according to your age, health status, and any specific conditions you have, but always within safe limits.

Sourcing High-Quality Ingredients

Choose Organic and Ethical Sources: To ensure the potency and safety of your remedies, use ingredients that are organic and sourced from reputable suppliers. This minimizes exposure to pesticides and ensures a higher quality of the herbal properties.

Grow Your Own: Whenever possible, consider growing your own herbs. This not only ensures freshness and quality but also deepens your connection to the healing process.

Consulting Professionals

Seek Guidance: While this book provides extensive information, it's crucial to consult with healthcare professionals, especially in cases of severe or chronic health issues. This is particularly important for diagnosing conditions and integrating herbal remedies with existing treatments.

Collaborate with Herbalists: For personalized advice and deeper exploration of herbal remedies, consider working with a certified herbalist. They can offer tailored guidance and support for your unique health journey.

By following these guidelines and using "The Lost Book of Natural Remedies" as your guide, you are taking a significant step towards a healthier, more balanced life in harmony with nature. Enjoy this journey into the world of natural healing, and may it bring you health, knowledge, and peace.

PART 01

HOMEMADE
ANTIBIOTICS (1-30)

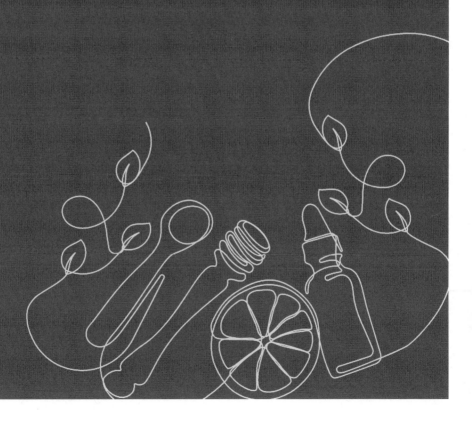

Introduction to Part I: Homemade Antibiotics

In our journey through the world of natural healing, we begin with the powerful, yet often overlooked, realm of homemade antibiotics. Nature has provided us with an array of plants and substances that possess remarkable antibacterial and antiviral properties. These natural agents offer a gentler alternative to synthetic antibiotics, working in harmony with our bodies to foster healing and resist infections.

This section, Part I: Homemade Antibiotics, explores 30 diverse remedies, each crafted from ingredients that you may find in your garden, local health food store, or even your kitchen. From the robust Garlic and Honey Tonic, known for its immune-boosting qualities, to the soothing and protective Propolis Throat Lozenges, each remedy is designed to address common ailments and enhance your body's natural defenses.

As you examine these remedies, you'll encounter familiar ingredients like Oregano Oil and Elderberry Syrup, alongside less common but equally potent options like Usnea Lichen Tincture and Cryptolepis Root Tincture. Each has been chosen for its unique healing properties and ease of preparation.

Before you begin, remember to source high-quality, organic ingredients whenever possible and to heed the dosages and preparation methods outlined. These precautions ensure that you harness the full healing potential of each remedy while respecting the delicate balance of nature and your health.

Embrace these natural antibiotics as part of your journey towards holistic wellness, and discover how simple and effective it can be to integrate the gifts of nature into your everyday health practices.

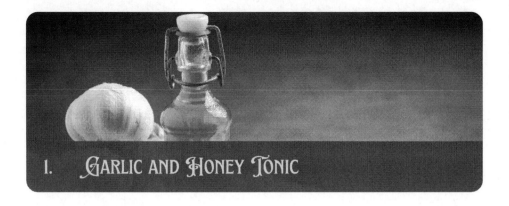

I. GARLIC AND HONEY TONIC

Introduction:

Garlic and Honey Tonic is a time-tested natural remedy known for its pote nt antimicrobial and immune-boosting properties. Garlic, rich in allicin, offers powerful antibacterial and antiviral effects, while honey, especially when raw and organic, serves as a soothing and healing agent. This tonic is ideal for strengthening the immune system, especially during cold and flu season.

Ingredients & Measurements:

- 1 cup of raw, organic honey
- 10 cloves of fresh garlic, peeled and finely minced.

Preparation:

☞ Begin by peeling and finely mincing the garlic cloves. The finer the mince, the more allicin is released, enhancing the tonic's potency.

☞ In a clean jar, combine the minced garlic with 1 cup of raw, organic honey. Stir the mixture thoroughly to ensure the garlic is evenly distributed throughout the honey.

☞ Seal the jar tightly and let it sit at room temperature for 3-5 days. This resting period allows the garlic to infuse into the honey, melding their properties.

☞ After the infusion period, strain the garlic from the honey using a fine sieve or cheesecloth. Press or squeeze the garlic to extract as much of the honey as possible.

☞ Transfer the strained honey to a clean jar and store it in a cool, dark place.

How to Use:

✎ For general immune support, take 1 teaspoon of the Garlic and Honey Tonic each morning on an empty stomach.

✎ If you're feeling the onset of a cold or flu, increase the dosage to 1 teaspoon three times a day until symptoms subside.

✎ This tonic can also be used as a soothing throat remedy. Simply take a teaspoon as needed to relieve soreness or irritation.

Duration:

◎ For preventive care, you can use the Garlic and Honey Tonic daily during the colder months or when you're exposed to illness.

◎ Continue usage for up to two weeks when addressing acute symptoms like a cold or sore throat. If symptoms persist beyond this period, consult a healthcare professional.

◎ This Garlic and Honey Tonic is not only effective but also simple to prepare and use, making it an excellent first line of defense against common respiratory ailments and to boost overall immunity.

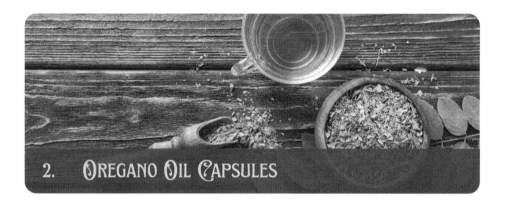

2. OREGANO OIL CAPSULES

Introduction:

Oregano Oil Capsules are a powerful natural antibiotic known for their strong antiviral, antibacterial, and antifungal properties. Oregano oil, derived from the leaves of the oregano plant, contains carvacrol and thymol, compounds that help fight infections and boost the immune system. These capsules are an excellent choice for targeting intestinal parasites, respiratory infections, and even skin conditions.

Ingredients & Measurements:

• Oregano essential oil (high-quality, therapeutic grade)

• Empty gelatin or vegetarian capsules
• A small dropper or pipette

Preparation:

☞ Ensure you have high-quality, therapeutic-grade oregano essential oil. This is crucial for both safety and efficacy.

☞ Take an empty capsule and carefully open it to expose the two halves.

☞ Using a dropper or pipette, fill one half of the capsule with oregano oil. Typically, 2-4 drops are sufficient, but never exceed this amount unless directed by a healthcare professional.

- Once filled, reassemble the two halves of the capsule to seal the oregano oil inside.

- Repeat the process for the desired number of capsules. Store the prepared capsules in a cool, dark place, ideally in an airtight container.

How to Use:

- For general immune support or to address minor infections, take 1 oregano oil capsule once or twice a day with meals.

- In the case of more severe infections or outbreaks, you may increase the dosage to 1 capsule three times a day, but only for short-term use (7-10 days).

- Always take the capsules with a full glass of water to aid absorption and minimize any potential digestive discomfort.

Duration:

- Oregano oil capsules should typically be used for short-term treatment due to their potency. A usual course lasts 7-10 days.

- For preventive measures or milder conditions, limit use to one capsule per day for up to two weeks.

- If symptoms persist or worsen, it is essential to consult a healthcare professional for further guidance.

Oregano Oil Capsules are a convenient and potent way to harness the natural antibiotic properties of oregano. They offer a targeted approach to combatting various infections and boosting overall health without the side effects often associated with synthetic antibiotics.

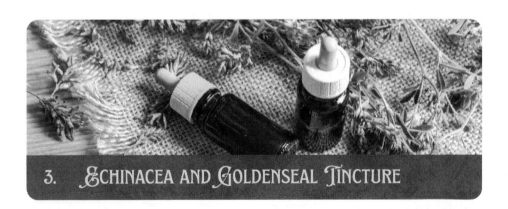

3. ECHINACEA AND GOLDENSEAL TINCTURE

Introduction:

Echinacea and Goldenseal Tincture is a potent herbal combination renowned for its immune-boosting and antimicrobial properties. Echinacea, known for stimulating the immune system, works synergistically with Goldenseal, which contains berberine, a compound effective against bacteria and inflammation. This tincture is ideal for preventing and treating colds, flu, and other infections, especially during times of increased susceptibility.

Ingredients & Measurements:

- Dried Echinacea root or leaves
- Dried Goldenseal root
- Vegetable glycerin (as a non-alcoholic solvent)
- Distilled water
- A clean glass jar with a lid
- A fine strainer or cheesecloth

Preparation:

- Combine equal parts of dried Echinacea and Goldenseal in the glass jar. A typical ratio is 1 part dried herb to 5 parts liquid (vegetable glycerin and water mixture).

- Mix three parts vegetable glycerin with one part distilled water. This mixture will extract the medicinal properties without using alcohol.

- Pour the glycerin and water mixture over the herbs, ensuring they are completely submerged.

- Seal the jar tightly and place it in a cool, dark place. Shake the jar daily to mix the herbs and liquid.

- Allow the mixture to macerate for 4 to 6 weeks.

- After the maceration period, strain the mixture through a fine strainer or cheesecloth into another clean jar. Press or squeeze the herbs to extract as much liquid as possible.

- Store the strained tincture in a dark glass bottle in a cool, dark place to preserve its potency.

How to Use:

- For immune support or to combat an onset of symptoms, take 1 teaspoon of the tincture up to three times a day.

- Dilute the tincture in a small amount of water or juice if the taste is too strong.

- For preventive care, you can take the tincture once daily, especially during seasons when you're more vulnerable to illness.

Duration:

- Use the tincture for up to 7-10 days during acute infections.

- For prevention, it's safe to use the tincture intermittently throughout high-risk periods, such as cold and flu season.

- Consult a healthcare professional if symptoms persist or worsen, or for long-term use guidance.

Echinacea and Goldenseal Tincture offers a natural and effective way to enhance your body's defenses and treat infections without relying on alcohol-based preparations, making it suitable for all ages and various health needs.

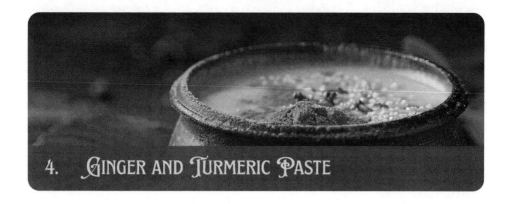

4. GINGER AND TURMERIC PASTE

Introduction:

Ginger and Turmeric Paste is a vibrant, anti-inflammatory blend that harnesses the healing powers of two potent roots. Ginger, with its warming and soothing properties, works alongside turmeric, known for its curcumin content that significantly reduces inflammation. This paste is excellent for relieving pain, improving digestion, and boosting overall health.

Ingredients and Measurements:

- 1/2 cup of fresh ginger root, peeled and finely grated
- 1/2 cup of fresh turmeric root, peeled and finely grated
- 1/4 cup of raw, organic honey or pure maple syrup (for a vegan option)
- 2 tablespoons of virgin coconut oil
- A pinch of black pepper (to enhance turmeric absorption)

Preparation:

☞ Peel and finely grate the ginger and turmeric roots. The finer the grate, the more surface area is exposed for extracting the active compounds.

☞ In a small bowl, combine the grated ginger and turmeric with the honey or maple syrup. Mix thoroughly to create a homogenous blend.

☞ Add the coconut oil and a pinch of black pepper to the mixture. The fat from the coconut oil helps with the absorption of turmeric's curcumin, while the black pepper increases its bioavailability.

☞ Stir all the ingredients until well combined into a smooth paste.

☞ Transfer the paste into a clean glass jar with a tight-fitting lid and store it in the refrigerator.

How to Use:

☞ Take 1 teaspoon of the paste daily, either directly or mixed into warm water or tea, to benefit from its anti-inflammatory and digestive properties.

☞ For pain relief, especially joint or muscle pain, you can increase the intake to 1 teaspoon twice a day.

- Use the paste as a base for curries, soups, or smoothies to add flavor and health benefits to your meals.

Duration:

- The paste can be safely consumed daily for general health benefits.

- For specific conditions like arthritis or acute inflammation, use for at least 2 weeks to notice significant improvements.

- Always consult with a healthcare professional for prolonged use or if you are on medication, as turmeric can interact with certain drugs.

Ginger and Turmeric Paste is not just a remedy but also a versatile addition to your culinary arsenal, making it easy to incorporate these powerful roots into your daily routine for better health and vitality.

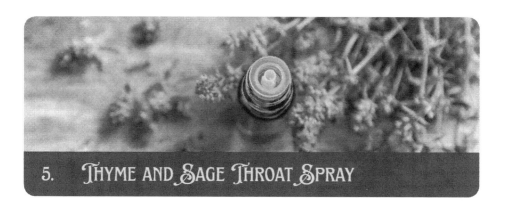

5. THYME AND SAGE THROAT SPRAY

Introduction:

Thyme and Sage Throat Spray is an herbal remedy designed to soothe sore throats and reduce inflammation. Thyme is known for its antibacterial and antiviral properties, while sage offers astringent and antiseptic benefits. This combination makes the spray an effective solution for throat discomfort, coughs, and minor infections.

Ingredients and Measurements:

- 1/4 cup of fresh thyme leaves
- 1/4 cup of fresh sage leaves
- 1 cup of distilled water
- 1 tablespoon of raw, organic honey or vegetable glycerin (for a vegan option)
- A small spray bottle

Preparation:

☞ Rinse the thyme and sage leaves thoroughly to remove any dirt or impurities.

☞ In a small saucepan, bring the distilled water to a boil. Add the thyme and sage leaves, then reduce the heat and let them simmer for 10 minutes. This process extracts the essential oils and medicinal properties of the herbs.

☞ Remove the saucepan from the heat and let the mixture cool to room temperature.

☞ Strain the herbal infusion through a fine mesh sieve or cheesecloth, ensuring all plant material is removed.

☞ Stir in the honey or vegetable glycerin into the cooled herbal liquid. This step not only sweetens the spray but also adds a soothing texture.

☞ Pour the mixture into a clean spray bottle. If needed, use a funnel to avoid spills.

☞ Store the throat spray in the refrigerator to preserve its freshness and potency.

How to Use:

↳ Shake the bottle well before each use.

↳ Spray directly into the throat 2-3 times every few hours or as needed to relieve soreness and discomfort.

↳ For best results, use at the first sign of throat irritation or when exposed to potential irritants like dry air or pollutants.

Duration:

⊘ Use the throat spray for up to 7 days for acute conditions.

⊘ If symptoms persist beyond this period or if you experience worsening pain, consult a healthcare professional.

⊘ The spray should be used within 2 weeks of preparation for optimal effectiveness and then discarded or remade.

Thyme and Sage Throat Spray is a gentle, natural way to manage throat discomfort and support respiratory health. Its herbal blend provides quick relief and can be a comforting addition to your wellness routine during cold and flu season.

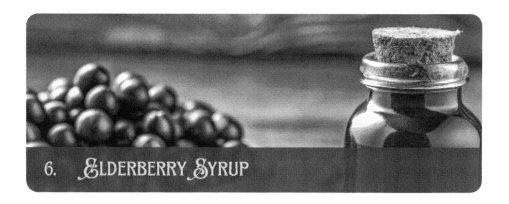

6. ELDERBERRY SYRUP

Introduction:

Elderberry Syrup is a popular natural remedy celebrated for its immune-boosting and antiviral properties. Elderberries are rich in antioxidants and vitamins that help combat colds, flu, and other respiratory infections. This syrup is a family-friendly option that can be taken as a preventive measure or at the first signs of illness to reduce the duration and severity of symptoms.

Ingredients and Measurements:

- 1 cup of dried elderberries
- 4 cups of distilled water
- 1 cup of raw, organic honey or pure maple syrup (for a vegan alternative)
- 2 tablespoons of fresh ginger root, grated
- 1 cinnamon stick
- 1 teaspoon of whole cloves

Preparation:

☞ Combine the dried elderberries, ginger, cinnamon stick, and cloves with the distilled water in a large saucepan.

☞ Bring the mixture to a boil, then reduce the heat and allow it to simmer gently for about 45 minutes to an hour, or until the liquid has reduced by half.

☞ Remove the saucepan from the heat and let the mixture cool to a manageable temperature.

☞ Mash the berries and other ingredients using a spoon or potato masher to release their juices and flavors.

☞ Strain the mixture through a fine mesh sieve or cheesecloth into a large bowl. Press or squeeze to extract as much liquid as possible.

☞ Once the liquid has cooled to lukewarm, stir in the honey or maple syrup. It's important to add the sweetener at this stage to preserve its natural enzymes and benefits.

☞ Transfer the syrup to a clean glass bottle or jar and seal it tightly.

How to Use:

✎ For preventive care during cold and flu season, adults can take 1 tablespoon of elderberry syrup daily, and children over one year old can take 1 teaspoon daily.

ℒ At the first sign of illness, increase the dosage to 1 tablespoon every 3-4 hours for adults and 1 teaspoon every 3-4 hours for children, not exceeding 4 doses per day.

ℒ The syrup can also be mixed into teas, smoothies, or drizzled over yogurt or pancakes for a tasty and healthy treat.

Duration:

⊘ Continue taking elderberry syrup throughout the duration of cold or flu symptoms, typically for 5-7 days.

⊘ As a preventive measure, it can be used throughout the high-risk months of cold and flu season.

⊘ Always consult a healthcare professional if symptoms persist or worsen, or for advice on long-term use.

Elderberry Syrup is not only effective but also a pleasant remedy that both adults and children can enjoy, making it a staple in natural health arsenals for its protective and healing qualities.

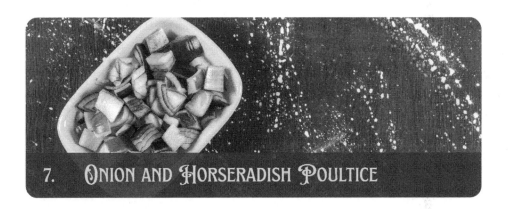

7. ONION AND HORSERADISH POULTICE

Introduction:

Onion and Horseradish Poultice is an effective traditional remedy used to treat congestion and respiratory issues. Onion has natural antibacterial properties and can help break up mucus, while horseradish is known for its ability to clear sinuses and stimulate circulation. This poultice is particularly

beneficial for relieving chest congestion, sinusitis, and cold symptoms.

Ingredients and Measurements:

- 1 large onion, finely grated
- 1/4 cup of fresh horseradish root, finely grated

- 1 tablespoon of olive oil or coconut oil (to help bind and soothe the skin)
- A clean cloth or gauze

Preparation:

Grate the onion and horseradish root as finely as possible to release their active compounds.

Mix the grated onion and horseradish with the olive or coconut oil in a bowl. The oil helps to prevent skin irritation and makes the mixture easier to apply.

Spread the mixture onto a clean cloth or gauze, leaving enough room to fold the cloth over and create a sealed packet.

Warm the poultice slightly by placing it in a microwave for a few seconds or using a double boiler. Ensure it is comfortably warm but not hot to avoid burns.

How to Use:

Place the warm poultice on the chest or back to relieve congestion. If applying near the face for sinus relief, be cautious as the vapors can be very strong.

Cover the poultice with a piece of plastic wrap and then a towel to keep the warmth in.

Leave the poultice in place for up to 20 minutes, checking periodically to ensure comfort and safety.

After removing, gently wipe the skin with a warm, damp cloth to clean off any residue.

Duration:

Use the poultice once a day as needed during acute congestion or sinus issues.

For ongoing issues, it can be used for a few days in a row, but if symptoms persist, seek advice from a healthcare professional.

Onion and Horseradish Poultice is a potent natural remedy that provides quick relief for respiratory discomfort and congestion, helping to restore easier breathing and comfort during cold and flu season.

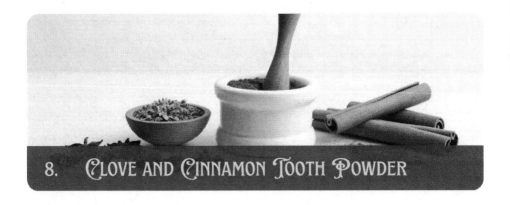

8. CLOVE AND CINNAMON TOOTH POWDER

Introduction:

Clove and Cinnamon Tooth Powder is a natural dental care remedy known for its antibacterial and pain-relieving properties. Clove oil is often used in dentistry for its eugenol content, which numbs pain and reduces inflammation, while cinnamon adds a pleasant flavor and additional antimicrobial benefits. This tooth powder can help maintain oral hygiene, freshen breath, and soothe toothaches and gum discomfort.

Ingredients and Measurements:

- 2 tablespoons of ground cloves
- 2 tablespoons of ground cinnamon
- 1 tablespoon of baking soda (for gentle cleaning and whitening)
- 1 tablespoon of fine sea salt (optional, for extra cleaning power)

Preparation:

🥣 In a small bowl, thoroughly mix the ground cloves and ground cinnamon. These spices are the active ingredients that provide the primary benefits and flavor.

🥣 Add the baking soda to the mixture. Baking soda helps clean teeth by gently scrubbing away surface stains and neutralizing acids in the mouth.

🥣 If using, incorporate the fine sea salt into the mix. The salt acts as an abrasive that can enhance the cleaning effect and support gum health.

🥣 Transfer the combined ingredients into a small jar with a tight-fitting lid to keep the powder dry and fresh.

How to Use:

🪥 Wet your toothbrush and dip it into the tooth powder. Tap off the excess powder.

🪥 Brush your teeth as you would with regular toothpaste, paying special attention to all surfaces and your gums.

🪥 Rinse your mouth thoroughly with water after brushing.

🪥 Use this tooth powder once or twice a day, as part of your regular oral hygiene routine.

Duration:

- The tooth powder can be used daily as a replacement or supplement to your regular toothpaste.

- For those with sensitive teeth or gums, start by using it a few times a week and observe how your mouth responds.

- Consult with your dentist if you have concerns about long-term use, especially if you have pre-existing dental conditions.

Clove and Cinnamon Tooth Powder is not only effective in promoting oral health but also provides a naturally fresh taste, making your daily dental care routine both enjoyable and beneficial.

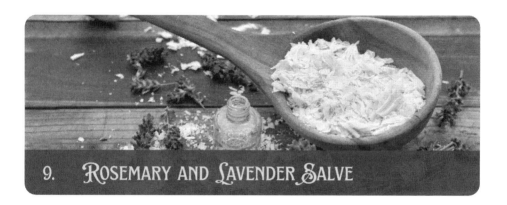

9.   ROSEMARY AND LAVENDER SALVE

Introduction:

Rosemary and Lavender Salve is a soothing and therapeutic balm perfect for nourishing the skin and calming the senses. Rosemary is known for its antioxidant properties and ability to improve circulation, while lavender is celebrated for its relaxing and healing effects on the skin. This salve is ideal for moisturizing dry skin, soothing minor burns or irritations, and providing a gentle aroma that can aid relaxation and sleep.

Ingredients and Measurements:

- 1/2 cup of coconut oil
- 1/4 cup of shea butter
- 2 tablespoons of dried rosemary leaves
- 2 tablespoons of dried lavender flowers
- 1 tablespoon of beeswax pellets (or carnauba wax for a vegan alternative)

Preparation:

- Combine the coconut oil, shea butter, and beeswax in a double boiler or a heat-safe bowl over simmering water. Heat gently until the mixture is fully melted and combined.

- Add the dried rosemary and lavender to the oil mixture. Allow the herbs to infuse in the warm oils for about 30 minutes, ensuring the heat is low enough to prevent burning.

- After infusion, strain the mixture through a fine sieve or cheesecloth to remove the herb particles, pressing to extract as much oil as possible.

- Pour the strained, aromatic oil mixture into clean tins or small glass jars. Allow the salve to cool and solidify at room temperature or hasten the process by placing it in the refrigerator.

How to Use:

- Apply a small amount of the salve to the skin as needed, particularly on dry or irritated areas. The salve spreads easily and absorbs into the skin, providing moisture and a protective barrier.

- Use the salve as part of a nightly routine to benefit from its soothing properties, especially on hands, feet, and areas exposed to the elements.

- For relaxation, massage the salve into temples or wrists before bedtime to enjoy the calming scent of lavender and rosemary.

Duration:

- The salve can be used daily as a moisturizer and skin protector.

- Store the salve in a cool, dry place, and it should remain effective for up to 6 months. If the scent fades or the texture changes, it's time to make a fresh batch.

- As with all topical products, if irritation occurs, discontinue use and consult a healthcare professional.

Rosemary and Lavender Salve is a versatile and delightful addition to any wellness routine, offering both skin care benefits and aromatic therapy that enhances overall well-being.

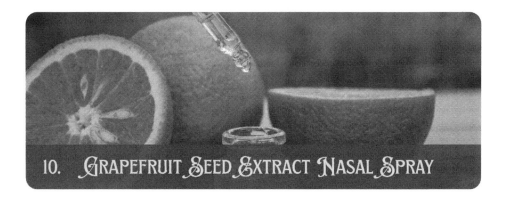

10. GRAPEFRUIT SEED EXTRACT NASAL SPRAY

Introduction:

Grapefruit Seed Extract Nasal Spray is a natural remedy known for its potent antimicrobial and anti-inflammatory properties. Grapefruit seed extract is effective in combating sinus infections, allergies, and other nasal irritations due to its ability to cleanse and soothe inflamed nasal passages. This nasal spray offers a gentle yet effective way to alleviate congestion and promote clear breathing.

Ingredients and Measurements:

- 1 teaspoon of grapefruit seed extract
- 1 cup of distilled water
- 1/4 teaspoon of non-iodized salt (to match the body's natural saline balance)
- A small spray bottle

Preparation:

☞ In a clean bowl, dissolve the non-iodized salt in the distilled water. The salt helps to create a saline solution that is gentle on the nasal passages.

☞ Add the grapefruit seed extract to the saline solution and stir well to ensure it is thoroughly mixed.

☞ Using a funnel, pour the solution into the small spray bottle. Ensure the bottle is clean and dry before filling.

☞ Secure the spray nozzle and shake the bottle gently to mix the contents.

How to Use:

✎ Gently shake the bottle before each use.

✎ Tilt your head slightly forward and insert the nozzle into one nostril.

✎ Press the spray nozzle to release a mist of the solution while gently inhaling to draw the mist into the nasal passages.

✎ Repeat the process for the other nostril.

✎ Use the nasal spray 2-3 times a day or as needed to relieve congestion and nasal discomfort.

Duration:

- Use the nasal spray as needed during periods of nasal congestion or when experiencing allergy symptoms.

- The solution should be fresh for up to one week if stored in the refrigerator. Discard any unused solution after this period and prepare a new batch.

- If symptoms persist or worsen, or if you experience any adverse reactions, consult a healthcare professional.

Grapefruit Seed Extract Nasal Spray is a simple and natural option for maintaining nasal health and relieving discomfort without the harsh chemicals found in many over-the-counter nasal sprays.

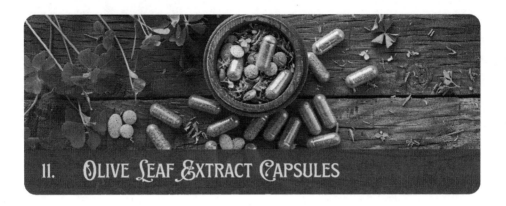

II. OLIVE LEAF EXTRACT CAPSULES

Introduction:

Olive Leaf Extract Capsules are a powerful natural supplement celebrated for their robust antioxidant and immune-boosting properties. Derived from the leaves of the olive tree, this extract contains oleuropein, a compound known for its ability to fight infections, lower blood pressure, and enhance overall cardiovascular health. These capsules are an excellent way to harness the health benefits of olive leaves in a convenient form.

Ingredients and Measurements:

- High-quality olive leaf extract powder
- Empty vegetarian or gelatin capsules

- A small capsule-filling machine or a manual method using a spoon and a steady hand

Preparation:

- Ensure you have a high-quality olive leaf extract powder, standardized to contain a specific percentage of oleuropein for consistency and effectiveness.

- If using a capsule-filling machine, follow the manufacturer's instructions to fill the capsules. Typically, this involves spreading the extract powder over the base of the machine and using the tamper to fill the capsules evenly.

- If manually filling the capsules, carefully open each capsule half. Use a small spoon to fill one half with the olive leaf extract powder. Pack the powder lightly to fit as much as possible without forcing it.

- Carefully reassemble the two halves of each capsule to seal the powder inside.

- Store the filled capsules in a cool, dry place, preferably in an airtight container to preserve their potency.

How to Use:

- Take one capsule daily with a meal, or as directed by your healthcare provider.

- For increased immune support, especially during times of stress or during cold and flu season, you may take one capsule twice daily.

Duration:

- Olive leaf extract capsules can be taken as part of a daily health regimen for ongoing support.

- If using for specific health issues, such as during an infection or for blood pressure management, follow the guidance of a healthcare professional.

- Regularly review your supplement intake with your healthcare provider to adjust dosages as needed based on your health status and response to the supplement.

Olive Leaf Extract Capsules offer a straightforward and effective way to benefit from the natural health-enhancing properties of olive leaves, making them a valuable addition to your wellness routine.

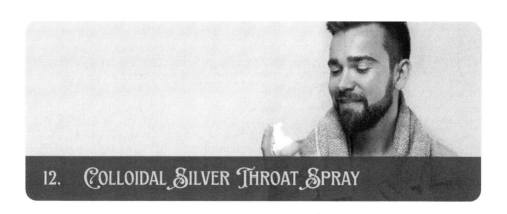

12. COLLOIDAL SILVER THROAT SPRAY

Introduction:

Colloidal Silver Throat Spray is a natural remedy used to alleviate throat discomfort and fight infections. Colloidal silver is known for its antimicrobial properties, effectively targeting bacteria, viruses, and fungi without harming beneficial bacteria. This spray provides quick relief for sore throats, minor infections, and can support overall throat health.

Ingredients and Measurements:

- 1/2 cup of colloidal silver (10-30 ppm strength)
- 1 tablespoon of raw, organic honey or vegetable glycerin (for soothing and taste)
- A few drops of essential oils like peppermint or eucalyptus (optional, for additional relief and freshness)
- A small spray bottle

Preparation:

- Ensure the colloidal silver you use is of a reliable quality, typically within the 10-30 ppm range for safety and effectiveness.

- In a clean bowl, mix the colloidal silver with the honey or vegetable glycerin. Stir until well combined. The honey or glycerin adds a soothing texture and taste, enhancing the spray's effectiveness.

- If using essential oils, add a few drops to the mixture. Essential oils like peppermint or eucalyptus can provide additional antimicrobial benefits and a cooling sensation that further soothes the throat.

- Using a funnel, carefully pour the mixture into the spray bottle. Ensure the bottle is clean and dry to maintain the purity of the spray.

- Close the bottle and shake gently to ensure all ingredients are evenly distributed.

How to Use:

- Shake the bottle well before each use.

- Spray directly into the throat 2-3 times as needed to relieve discomfort and irritation.

- Use the spray every few hours, especially after eating or drinking, to maintain the protective and healing effects.

Duration:

- Use the spray as needed during periods of throat discomfort or at the first signs of infection.

- For acute conditions, continue using the spray for up to a week. If symptoms persist or if there is no improvement, consult a healthcare professional.

- Store the throat spray in a cool, dark place, and use within 1-2 weeks for best results.

Colloidal Silver Throat Spray is a gentle yet potent solution for maintaining throat health and providing quick relief from irritation and infection. Its natural ingredients work synergistically to soothe and protect the throat without the harsh side effects of many over-the-counter options.

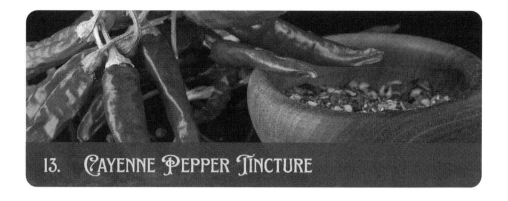

13. CAYENNE PEPPER TINCTURE

Introduction:

Cayenne Pepper Tincture is a powerful natural remedy known for its ability to stimulate circulation and relieve pain. The active compound in cayenne pepper, capsaicin, is celebrated for its pain-relieving properties, particularly in managing joint and muscle pain, as well as its benefits in enhancing digestion and metabolism. This tincture offers a convenient way to use cayenne's potent effects in a controlled and targeted manner.

Ingredients and Measurements:

- 1/4 cup of dried cayenne pepper (ground or crushed)
- 1 cup of vegetable glycerin (as a non-alcoholic solvent)
- A clean glass jar with a tight-fitting lid
- A fine strainer or cheesecloth

Preparation:

🗑 Place the dried cayenne pepper in the glass jar. If using whole dried peppers, crush them slightly to expose more surface area.

🗑 Pour the vegetable glycerin over the cayenne peppers, ensuring they are fully submerged. The glycerin will extract the capsaicin and other beneficial compounds from the peppers without the harshness of alcohol.

🗑 Seal the jar tightly and shake it to mix the contents.

🗑 Store the jar in a cool, dark place, shaking it daily for at least 2-4 weeks to facilitate the extraction process.

🗑 After the infusion period, strain the mixture through a fine strainer or cheesecloth into another clean jar, squeezing or pressing to extract as much liquid as possible.

🗑 Transfer the strained tincture to a dropper bottle for easy use.

How to Use:

🔖 For pain relief, apply a few drops of the tincture to the affected area and gently massage it in. Be cautious with the amount, as cayenne can cause a warming or burning sensation on sensitive skin.

- To aid digestion, add 1-2 drops of the tincture to a glass of water and drink before meals.

- Start with a small dose and increase gradually, observing your body's response to avoid discomfort.

Duration:

- Use the tincture as needed for pain or digestive support.

- For topical application, if irritation or excessive heat occurs, discontinue use and wash the area with cool water.

- The tincture can be stored in a cool, dark place and should remain potent for up to a year.

Cayenne Pepper Tincture is a versatile and effective remedy that leverages the natural heat and healing properties of cayenne pepper to provide relief and support for various health challenges.

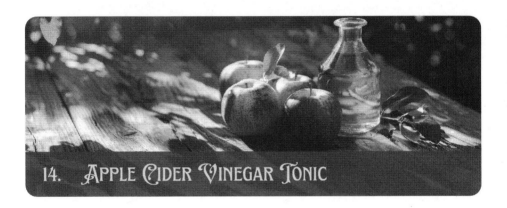

14. APPLE CIDER VINEGAR TONIC

Introduction:

Apple Cider Vinegar Tonic is a popular natural remedy recognized for its numerous health benefits, including aiding digestion, balancing pH levels, and supporting weight management. Rich in acetic acid, this tonic can also help regulate blood sugar levels and improve skin health. Its simplicity and effectiveness make it a staple in many health-conscious households.

Ingredients and Measurements:

- 1 cup of organic apple cider vinegar (with "the mother" for beneficial enzymes)

- 2 cups of filtered water

- 2 tablespoons of raw, organic honey or maple syrup (for sweetness and additional health benefits)

- 1 teaspoon of ground cinnamon (for flavor and its anti-inflammatory properties)

- 1/2 teaspoon of ground ginger (for digestive aid and added spice)

Preparation:

🏺 In a large pitcher or jar, combine the apple cider vinegar and filtered water.

🏺 Add the raw honey or maple syrup to the mixture and stir until fully dissolved. This step not only sweetens the tonic but also enhances its health-promoting qualities.

🏺 Stir in the ground cinnamon and ground ginger, blending thoroughly to ensure even distribution of flavors and health benefits.

🏺 Transfer the tonic to a clean glass bottle or jar with a tight-fitting lid for storage.

How to Use:

🥄 Shake the bottle well before each use to mix the settled ingredients.

🥄 Drink 1-2 tablespoons of the tonic diluted in a glass of water, ideally 15-30 minutes before meals to aid digestion and boost metabolism.

🥄 For a soothing throat remedy, take 1 tablespoon of the undiluted tonic to help relieve irritation and support immune health.

Duration:

🕐 Regular daily use of the tonic can help maintain optimal health and digestive function.

🕐 Store the apple cider vinegar tonic in the refrigerator and consume within 2-3 weeks for best quality and effectiveness.

Apple Cider Vinegar Tonic is an easy-to-make, versatile remedy that offers a range of health benefits, making it an excellent addition to your daily routine for overall wellness.

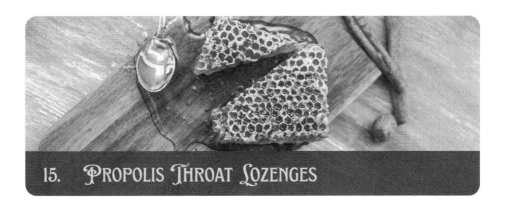

15. PROPOLIS THROAT LOZENGES

Introduction:

Propolis Throat Lozenges are an effective natural remedy designed to soothe sore throats and boost the immune system. Propolis, a resinous substance collected by bees, is known for its potent antimicrobial and anti-inflammatory properties. These lozenges are ideal for relieving throat pain, reducing inflammation, and supporting the body's natural defense mechanisms against infections.

Ingredients and Measurements:

- 1/4 cup of propolis extract
- 1/2 cup of raw, organic honey
- 1 tablespoon of lemon juice (for added vitamin C and flavor)
- 1 teaspoon of ground ginger (for its soothing properties and extra kick)
- Powdered sugar or cornstarch (for dusting, to prevent sticking)

Preparation:

☞ In a small saucepan, combine the propolis extract and honey. Heat gently over low heat, stirring constantly, until the mixture becomes homogeneous and slightly thinner.

☞ Add the lemon juice and ground ginger to the saucepan, continuing to stir to ensure even distribution of all ingredients.

☞ Allow the mixture to simmer gently for about 5-10 minutes until it thickens slightly and reaches the consistency of a syrup.

☞ Remove the saucepan from the heat and let the mixture cool until it's warm but manageable to touch.

☞ Dust a clean surface with powdered sugar or cornstarch to prevent sticking. Pour the mixture onto the dusted surface and allow it to cool further.

☞ Once the mixture is cool enough to handle, shape it into small, lozenge-sized pieces with your hands or use a small candy mold. Dust each lozenge with more powdered sugar or cornstarch to prevent them from sticking together.

☞ Place the lozenges on a parchment-lined tray or container and allow them to harden at room temperature or in the refrigerator.

How to Use:

🥄 Dissolve one lozenge slowly in your mouth as needed to soothe a sore throat, reduce irritation, or support your immune system.

🥄 Do not consume more than 5-6 lozenges per day to avoid excessive intake of propolis.

Duration:

◎ Use the lozenges during periods of throat discomfort or when you feel the onset of a cold or infection.

◎ Store the lozenges in an airtight container in a cool, dry place for up to 2 weeks for optimal freshness and efficacy.

Propolis Throat Lozenges offer a soothing, natural solution for throat discomfort and are a handy remedy to have during cold and flu season or whenever your throat needs extra care.

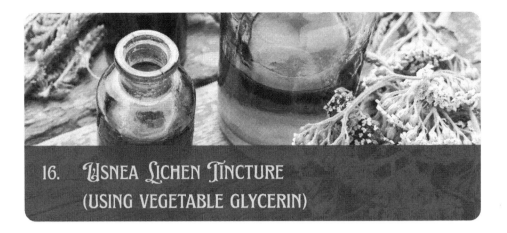

16. USNEA LICHEN TINCTURE (USING VEGETABLE GLYCERIN)

Introduction:

Usnea Lichen Tincture is a natural remedy made from Usnea, a lichen known for its potent antibacterial and antifungal properties. This tincture is particularly effective in supporting respiratory health, treating skin infections, and boosting the immune system. Using vegetable glycerin as the solvent makes this tincture suitable for those who prefer a non-alcoholic option.

Ingredients and Measurements:

- 1 cup of dried Usnea lichen, finely chopped
- 2 cups of vegetable glycerin
- 1 cup of distilled water
- A clean glass jar with a tight-fitting lid
- A fine strainer or cheesecloth

Preparation:

☞ In the glass jar, combine the finely chopped Usnea lichen with the vegetable glycerin and distilled water. The water helps extract water-soluble compounds, while the glycerin is effective for those that are alcohol-soluble.

☞ Seal the jar tightly and shake it to mix the contents thoroughly.

☞ Place the jar in a cool, dark place, shaking it daily for 4-6 weeks to facilitate the extraction process.

☞ After the infusion period, strain the mixture through a fine strainer or cheesecloth into another clean jar, pressing or squeezing to extract as much liquid as possible.

☞ Transfer the strained tincture to a dropper bottle for easy use.

How to Use:

✎ For respiratory health and immune support, take 1-2 dropperfuls (about 30-60 drops) of the tincture up to three times a day, diluted in a small amount of water or juice.

✎ For external use on skin infections, apply the tincture directly to the affected area using a clean cotton ball or pad, up to three times a day.

Duration:

- Use the tincture as needed for respiratory or skin conditions.

- For immune support, it can be used regularly during periods of increased risk, such as cold and flu season.

- Store the tincture in a cool, dark place, and it should remain effective for up to a year.

Usnea Lichen Tincture, made with vegetable glycerin, offers a gentle yet effective way to harness the healing properties of Usnea lichen, providing support for a range of health issues in a non-alcoholic formula.

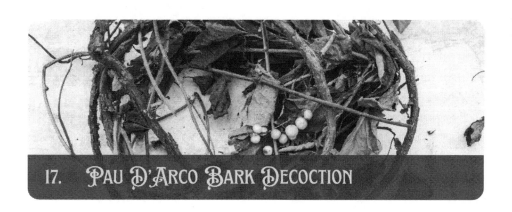

17. PAU D'ARCO BARK DECOCTION

Introduction:

Pau D'Arco Bark Decoction is a traditional herbal remedy known for its potent antifungal, antibacterial, and anti-inflammatory properties. Extracted from the bark of the Pau D'Arco tree, this decoction is especially effective in supporting immune health, combating fungal infections, and reducing inflammation. The preparation involves simmering the bark to release its active compounds into the water, making it an accessible and alcohol-free option for natural healing.

Ingredients and Measurements:

- 1/4 cup of dried Pau D'Arco bark
- 4 cups of distilled water
- A large pot for simmering
- A fine strainer or cheesecloth

Preparation:

- Place the dried Pau D'Arco bark into the large pot and cover it with the distilled water.

- Bring the mixture to a boil over high heat, then reduce the heat and let it simmer gently for at least 20-30 minutes. This process allows the water to extract the healing compounds from the bark effectively.

☞ After simmering, remove the pot from the heat and let the decoction cool to room temperature.

☞ Strain the liquid through a fine strainer or cheesecloth to remove the bark pieces, ensuring a clear liquid remains.

☞ Transfer the strained decoction into a clean glass bottle or jar for storage.

How to Use:

🥄 Drink 1/2 to 1 cup of the decoction up to three times a day to support immune health, fight infections, or reduce inflammation.

🥄 For topical use on skin infections or irritations, apply the decoction directly to the affected area using a clean cloth or cotton pad.

Duration:

🕐 Use the decoction as needed for health concerns or as part of a regular wellness routine for up to 2-3 weeks.

🕐 If symptoms persist or if there are concerns about long-term use, consult a healthcare professional for guidance.

🕐 Store the decoction in the refrigerator and use within 1 week for best quality and effectiveness.

Pau D'Arco Bark Decoction offers a straightforward and effective way to harness the medicinal benefits of Pau D'Arco bark in a natural, alcohol-free format, suitable for various therapeutic needs.

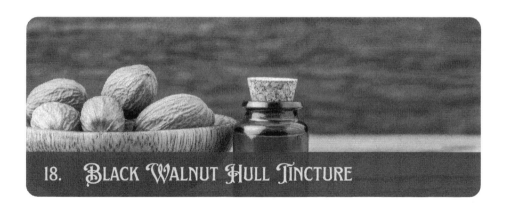

18. BLACK WALNUT HULL TINCTURE

Introduction:

Black Walnut Hull Tincture is a powerful herbal remedy known for its antiparasitic, antifungal, and antibacterial properties.

Made from the green outer hulls of black walnuts, this tincture is particularly effective in treating intestinal parasites, skin infections, and supporting overall digestive health. Using vegetable glycerin as a solvent makes this tincture alcohol-free and suitable for a wider range of users.

Ingredients and Measurements:

- 1 cup of fresh or dried black walnut hulls, finely chopped
- 2 cups of vegetable glycerin
- 1 cup of distilled water
- A clean glass jar with a tight-fitting lid
- A fine strainer or cheesecloth

Preparation:

Place the finely chopped black walnut hulls in the glass jar.

Combine the vegetable glycerin and distilled water in a separate container, mixing them thoroughly.

Pour the glycerin and water mixture over the black walnut hulls in the jar, ensuring the hulls are completely submerged.

Seal the jar tightly and shake it to mix the contents well.

Store the jar in a cool, dark place, shaking it daily for 4-6 weeks to facilitate the extraction of the medicinal compounds from the hulls.

After the infusion period, strain the mixture through a fine strainer or cheesecloth into another clean jar, pressing or squeezing to extract as much liquid as possible.

Transfer the strained tincture to a dropper bottle for easy use.

How to Use:

For internal use, especially for parasitic infections, take 1-2 dropperfuls (about 30-60 drops) of the tincture up to three times a day, diluted in water or juice.

For skin issues, apply the tincture directly to the affected area using a clean cotton ball or pad, up to three times a day.

Duration:

Use the tincture as needed for specific health concerns, such as during a parasitic infection or to treat a skin condition.

Consult a healthcare professional for guidance on duration, especially for internal use, to ensure safe and effective treatment.

Store the tincture in a cool, dark place, and it should remain effective for up to a year.

Black Walnut Hull Tincture, prepared with vegetable glycerin, offers a natural and effective way to benefit from the potent properties of black walnut hulls, providing a non-alcoholic solution for various health challenges.

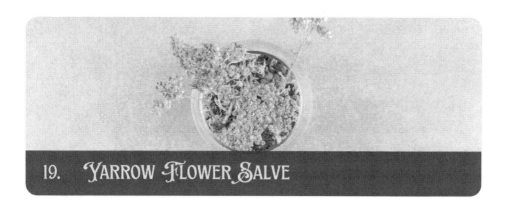

19. Yarrow Flower Salve

Introduction:

Yarrow Flower Salve is a natural remedy celebrated for its healing properties, particularly in treating wounds, reducing inflammation, and soothing skin irritations. Yarrow, known for its astringent and antimicrobial qualities, is effective in speeding up the healing process of cuts, bruises, and rashes. This salve combines the benefits of yarrow with other soothing ingredients to create a gentle yet potent topical treatment.

Ingredients and Measurements:

- 1/2 cup of dried yarrow flowers
- 1 cup of coconut oil
- 1/4 cup of beeswax pellets (or carnauba wax for a vegan option)
- 1 tablespoon of shea butter or cocoa butter (for extra moisturization)
- A few drops of lavender essential oil (for additional healing and a pleasant scent)
- A clean glass jar or metal tin for storage
- A double boiler
- A fine strainer or cheesecloth

Preparation:

☞ Combine the coconut oil and dried yarrow flowers in the top of a double boiler. Heat the mixture over low heat, allowing the yarrow flowers to infuse the oil for 1-2 hours. Keep the heat gentle to preserve the medicinal properties.

☞ After infusion, strain the oil through a fine strainer or cheesecloth into a clean bowl, pressing the flowers to extract as much oil as possible. Discard the used flowers.

☞ Return the infused oil to the double boiler and add the beeswax pellets and shea or cocoa butter. Stir continuously until the beeswax and butter are completely melted and the mixture is well combined.

☞ Remove the mixture from the heat and allow it to cool slightly before adding a few drops of lavender essential oil. Stir well to ensure the essential oil is evenly distributed.

☞ Pour the finished salve into the clean glass jar or metal tin and allow it to cool and solidify at room temperature.

How to Use:

⤷ Apply a small amount of the yarrow flower salve to the affected area 2-3 times a day or as needed to soothe and heal the skin.

⤷ Massage gently into the skin until fully absorbed, especially on wounds, bruises, or irritated areas.

Duration:

⊘ Use the salve as needed for skin issues. If no improvement is seen within a few days or if the condition worsens, consult a healthcare professional.

⊘ Store the salve in a cool, dry place, and it should remain effective for up to 6 months. If the scent changes or the texture breaks down, it's time to make a fresh batch.

Yarrow Flower Salve is an effective and gentle option for natural skin care, providing relief and promoting healing with the combined powers of yarrow and other soothing ingredients.

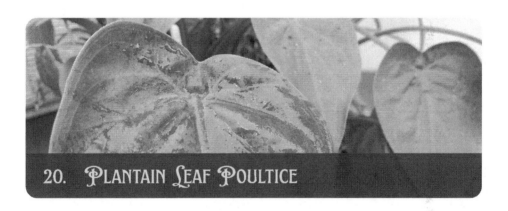

20. PLANTAIN LEAF POULTICE

Introduction:

Plantain Leaf Poultice is a traditional remedy renowned for its ability to soothe skin irritations, heal wounds, and reduce inflammation. The plantain leaf, common in many backyards, is packed with natural anti-inflammatory and antimicrobial properties. This poultice is especially effective for insect bites, cuts, rashes, and minor burns, providing quick and soothing relief.

Ingredients and Measurements:

• Fresh plantain leaves, thoroughly washed

• A small amount of water (if needed to help form the paste)

• A clean cloth or gauze

Preparation:

🫕 Crush the fresh plantain leaves using a mortar and pestle until a paste-like consistency is achieved. If the leaves are tough or dry, add a small amount of water to assist in forming a smooth paste.

🫕 If a mortar and pestile are not available, you can also chop the leaves finely and then mash them with the back of a spoon or in a blender with a little water.

🫕 Spread the plantain leaf paste evenly onto a clean cloth or gauze.

How to Use:

🩹 Apply the cloth or gauze with the plantain paste directly to the affected area of the skin.

🩹 Secure the poultice in place with a bandage or medical tape if necessary.

🩹 Leave the poultice on for up to an hour, or longer if treating a severe irritation or wound.

🩹 Remove the poultice and gently wash the area with cool water. Reapply a fresh poultice if needed.

Duration:

🕐 Use the poultice as needed for immediate relief of skin issues. For ongoing problems, you can apply a new poultice several times a day.

🕐 Consult a healthcare professional if there is no improvement or if the condition worsens after a few days of treatment.

Plantain Leaf Poultice is a simple yet powerful way to harness the healing properties of nature directly on the skin, offering relief and promoting healing without the need for complex preparations or synthetic ingredients.

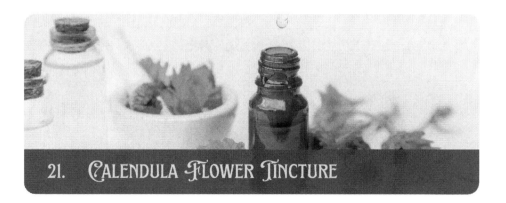

21. CALENDULA FLOWER TINCTURE

Introduction:

Calendula Flower Tincture is a gentle yet effective herbal remedy known for its healing, anti-inflammatory, and antimicrobial properties. Calendula, often used in skin care, is particularly beneficial for soothing and repairing the skin, treating minor wounds, and reducing inflammation. This tincture, made with vegetable glycerin, provides a non-alcoholic method to extract and utilize the healing properties of calendula flowers, making it suitable for all ages and sensitive individuals.

Ingredients and Measurements:

- 1 cup of dried calendula flowers
- 2 cups of vegetable glycerin
- 1 cup of distilled water
- A clean glass jar with a tight-fitting lid
- A fine strainer or cheesecloth

Preparation:

- Place the dried calendula flowers in the glass jar.
- Mix the vegetable glycerin and distilled water in a separate bowl to create a diluted glycerin solution. This combination helps extract both water-soluble and glycerin-soluble compounds from the flowers.
- Pour the glycerin and water mixture over the calendula flowers, ensuring they are fully submerged.
- Seal the jar tightly and shake it to mix the contents thoroughly.
- Store the jar in a cool, dark place, shaking it daily for 4-6 weeks to facilitate the extraction process.
- After the infusion period, strain the mixture through a fine strainer or cheesecloth into another clean jar, pressing the flowers to extract as much liquid as possible.

- Transfer the strained tincture to a dropper bottle for easy use.

How to Use:

- For skin issues like cuts, scrapes, or rashes, apply a few drops of the calendula tincture directly to the affected area up to three times a day.
- To soothe and heal inflamed skin or for general skincare, mix a few drops of the tincture with a carrier oil or lotion and apply as needed.
- Internally, to support immune function and reduce inflammation, take 1-2 dropperfuls (about 30-60 drops) diluted in water or tea, up to three times a day.

Duration:

- Use the tincture as needed for skin conditions or general health support.
- If using for an acute condition, continue for a week or until symptoms improve. Consult a healthcare professional for longer-term use or if the condition persists or worsens.
- Store the tincture in a cool, dark place, and it should remain effective for up to a year.

Calendula Flower Tincture made with vegetable glycerin is an excellent choice for those seeking the soothing and restorative benefits of calendula in a gentle, alcohol-free form, suitable for a variety of health and skincare needs.

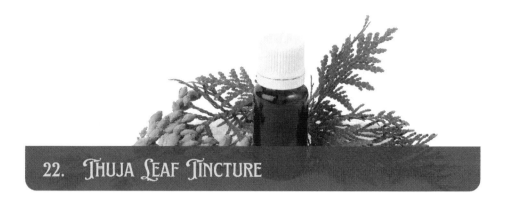

22. THUJA LEAF TINCTURE

Introduction:

Thuja Leaf Tincture is a valued herbal remedy derived from the leaves of the Thuja tree, known for its antiviral and immune-stimulating properties. Thuja is commonly used to treat skin conditions such as warts and molluscum contagiosum, as well as to support respiratory health. Using vegetable glycerin to extract its beneficial compounds, this tincture offers a non-alcoholic option suitable for various users, including those sensitive to alcohol.

Ingredients and Measurements:

- 1 cup of fresh or dried Thuja leaves
- 2 cups of vegetable glycerin
- 1 cup of distilled water
- A clean glass jar with a tight-fitting lid
- A fine strainer or cheesecloth

Preparation:

- Place the fresh or dried Thuja leaves into the glass jar.
- Combine the vegetable glycerin and distilled water in a separate container, ensuring a thorough mix. This solution helps to efficiently extract both water-soluble and glycerin-soluble compounds from the leaves.
- Pour the glycerin-water mixture over the Thuja leaves, making sure they are completely submerged.
- Seal the jar tightly and shake it well to mix the contents.
- Store the jar in a cool, dark place, shaking it daily for 4-6 weeks to facilitate the extraction process.
- After the infusion period, strain the mixture through a fine strainer or cheesecloth into another clean jar, pressing the leaves to extract as much liquid as possible.
- Transfer the strained tincture to a dropper bottle for convenient dosing and use.

How to Use:

🖎 For skin conditions such as warts, apply a few drops of the tincture directly to the affected area up to three times a day. Be cautious and consult a healthcare professional, as Thuja can be potent and may irritate sensitive skin.

🖎 To support respiratory health, take 1-2 dropperfuls (about 30-60 drops) of the tincture diluted in water or tea, up to three times a day.

Duration:

🕐 Use the tincture as needed for specific health concerns. For skin conditions, continue until improvement is observed or as directed by a healthcare professional.

🕐 Consult a healthcare professional for advice on duration and dosage, especially for internal use or if using for extended periods.

🕐 Store the tincture in a cool, dark place, and it should remain effective for up to a year.

Thuja Leaf Tincture made with vegetable glycerin is an effective and gentle alternative to alcohol-based tinctures, providing targeted support for skin and respiratory health with the therapeutic benefits of Thuja leaves.

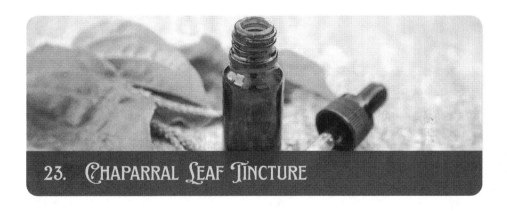

23. CHAPARRAL LEAF TINCTURE

Introduction:

Chaparral Leaf Tincture is an herbal remedy known for its strong antioxidant and anti-inflammatory properties. Extracted from the leaves of the chaparral plant, this tincture is particularly effective in supporting liver health, addressing skin conditions, and providing antimicrobial benefits. Using vegetable glycerin as the solvent allows for a non-alcoholic and gentler extraction, making it suitable for a wide range of users.

Ingredients and Measurements:

- 1 cup of dried chaparral leaves
- 2 cups of vegetable glycerin
- 1 cup of distilled water
- A clean glass jar with a tight-fitting lid
- A fine strainer or cheesecloth

Preparation:

- Place the dried chaparral leaves into the glass jar.

- Mix the vegetable glycerin and distilled water in a separate bowl to create a blended solvent. This mixture ensures efficient extraction of both water-soluble and glycerin-soluble compounds from the chaparral leaves.

- Pour the glycerin and water mixture over the chaparral leaves, ensuring they are completely submerged.

- Seal the jar tightly and shake it well to integrate the contents.

- Store the jar in a cool, dark place, shaking it daily for 4-6 weeks to promote thorough extraction of the chaparral's medicinal properties.

- After the infusion period, strain the mixture through a fine strainer or cheesecloth into another clean jar, pressing the leaves to maximize the extraction of liquid.

- Transfer the strained tincture to a dropper bottle for easy application and dosage control.

How to Use:

- For skin issues such as eczema or psoriasis, apply a few drops of the tincture directly to the affected area up to three times a day, being mindful of chaparral's potency and potential skin sensitivity.

- To support liver health and overall detoxification, take 1-2 dropperfuls (about 30-60 drops) of the tincture diluted in water or juice, up to three times a day. Consult a healthcare professional before starting this regimen, especially for internal use.

Duration:

- Use the tincture as needed for specific health issues. For ongoing conditions, consult with a healthcare professional for guidance on duration and appropriate use.

- Store the tincture in a cool, dark place. It should remain effective for up to a year if properly stored.

Chaparral Leaf Tincture made with vegetable glycerin is an effective herbal solution that leverages the potent properties of chaparral for health and wellness, offering a non-alcoholic option for users seeking natural remedies.

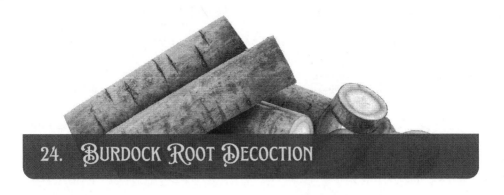

24. Burdock Root Decoction

Introduction:

Burdock Root Decoction is a traditional herbal remedy valued for its ability to purify the blood, support liver health, and improve skin conditions. Burdock root is rich in antioxidants and has natural diuretic properties, making it effective in detoxifying the body and promoting overall health. This decoction is a straightforward method to extract the beneficial compounds from burdock root, offering a potent and healing drink.

Ingredients and Measurements:

- 1/2 cup of dried burdock root, chopped or sliced
- 4 cups of water
- A large pot
- A fine strainer or cheesecloth

Preparation:

- Place the dried burdock root into the large pot.
- Add the water to the pot and bring the mixture to a boil over high heat.

- Once boiling, reduce the heat and allow the mixture to simmer gently for 30-40 minutes. This slow simmering helps to release the active compounds from the burdock root into the water.
- After simmering, remove the pot from the heat and let the decoction cool slightly.
- Strain the liquid through a fine strainer or cheesecloth to remove the root pieces, ensuring a clear liquid remains.
- Transfer the strained decoction into a clean glass container for storage and use.

How to Use:

- Drink 1/2 to 1 cup of the burdock root decoction up to three times a day to support detoxification, improve skin health, or aid digestion.
- The decoction can also be used externally as a rinse for skin issues or scalp conditions, thanks to its soothing and healing properties.

Duration:

- Use the decoction as part of a short-term health regimen, typically for 2-3 weeks, to observe benefits and ensure compatibility with your body.

- If using for an ongoing condition, consult a healthcare professional for guidance on safe and effective long-term use.

- Store the decoction in the refrigerator and consume within 5-7 days for optimal freshness and efficacy.

Burdock Root Decoction is a simple yet powerful way to utilize the natural healing properties of burdock root, providing a versatile remedy for internal and external health challenges.

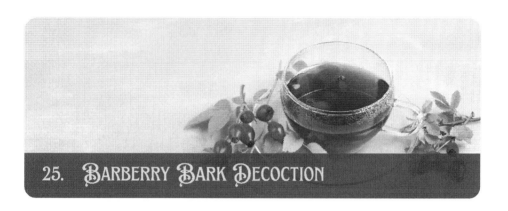

25. BARBERRY BARK DECOCTION

Introduction:

Barberry Bark Decoction is a potent herbal remedy known for its antibacterial, antifungal, and liver-supportive properties. Barberry bark contains berberine, a compound that helps regulate blood sugar levels, improve digestion, and combat infections. This decoction is an effective way to harness the medicinal benefits of barberry bark for health and wellness.

Ingredients and Measurements:

- 1/4 cup of dried barberry bark
- 4 cups of water

- A large pot
- A fine strainer or cheesecloth

Preparation:

- Place the dried barberry bark in the large pot.

- Add the water and bring the mixture to a boil over high heat.

- Once boiling, reduce the heat to a simmer and allow the bark to steep in the water for about 30-40 minutes. The slow simmer helps to extract the active compounds from the bark effectively.

- After the allotted time, remove the pot from the heat and let the decoction cool slightly.

- Strain the liquid through a fine strainer or cheesecloth, ensuring all the bark pieces are removed, and a clear liquid remains.

- Transfer the strained decoction into a clean glass container for storage and use.

How to Use:

- Drink 1/2 to 1 cup of the barberry bark decoction up to three times a day to benefit from its blood sugar regulation, digestive support, and infection-fighting properties.

- Consult a healthcare professional before using the decoction, especially for children or if you have a pre-existing medical condition, as barberry can interact with certain medications.

Duration:

- Typically, use the decoction as part of a short-term health regimen, usually for a few weeks, to observe the benefits and ensure it is well-tolerated.

- For long-term use or chronic conditions, seek guidance from a healthcare provider to determine the appropriate duration and dosage.

- Store the decoction in the refrigerator and consume within 5-7 days for the best quality and effectiveness.

Barberry Bark Decoction offers a natural approach to health, utilizing the powerful properties of barberry bark to support various bodily functions and promote overall wellness.

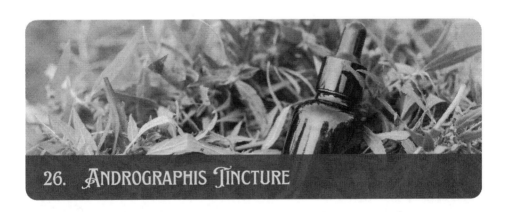

26. ANDROGRAPHIS TINCTURE

Introduction:

Andrographis Tincture, made with vegetable glycerin, is a powerful herbal remedy known for its immune-boosting, anti-inflammatory, and antiviral properties. Andrographis is often called the "King of Bitters" due to its potent flavor and is frequently used to prevent and treat colds, flu, and other infections. This glycerin-based tincture provides a non-alcoholic alternative for extracting the active compounds of Andrographis, making it suitable for a broader range of users including those who prefer alcohol-free options.

Ingredients and Measurements:

- 1 cup of dried Andrographis leaves, finely chopped or powdered

- 2 cups of vegetable glycerin

- 1 cup of distilled water

- A clean glass jar with a tight-fitting lid

- A fine strainer or cheesecloth

Preparation:

- Place the dried Andrographis leaves into the glass jar.

- Mix the vegetable glycerin and distilled water in a separate bowl, ensuring they are well combined. This mixture will serve as the solvent to extract the beneficial compounds from the Andrographis leaves effectively.

- Pour the glycerin and water mixture over the Andrographis leaves, making sure they are fully submerged.

- Seal the jar tightly and shake it to thoroughly mix the contents.

- Store the jar in a cool, dark place, shaking it daily for 4-6 weeks to facilitate the extraction process.

- After the infusion period, strain the mixture through a fine strainer or cheesecloth into another clean jar, pressing the leaves to extract as much liquid as possible.

- Transfer the strained tincture to a dropper bottle for convenient dosing and use.

How to Use:

- To support immune function and combat infections, take 1-2 dropperfuls (about 30-60 drops) of the tincture diluted in water or juice, up to three times a day, especially during times of increased risk like cold and flu season.

- For preventative care, particularly during peak illness times, a lower dose of 1 dropperful once or twice a day may be used.

Duration:

- Use the tincture as needed during illness or as a preventive measure during vulnerable periods.

- Consult a healthcare professional for advice on duration and dosage, particularly for long-term use or in combination with other medications.

- Store the tincture in a cool, dark place, and it should remain effective for up to a year.

Andrographis Tincture made with vegetable glycerin is an effective and accessible way to benefit from the therapeutic properties of Andrographis, providing a natural boost to the immune system and helping to fight off infections without the use of alcohol.

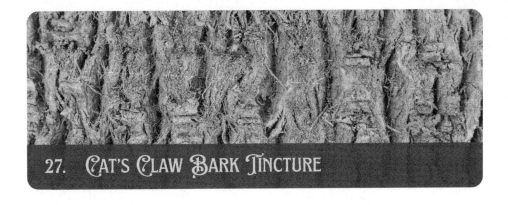

27. CAT'S CLAW BARK TINCTURE

Introduction:

Cat's Claw Bark Tincture is a renowned herbal remedy known for its powerful anti-inflammatory, immune-boosting, and antiviral properties. Derived from the bark of the Cat's Claw vine, this tincture is effective in supporting joint health, enhancing immune response, and promoting overall wellness. Using vegetable glycerin as the extraction solvent creates an alcohol-free tincture suitable for a variety of users, including those who prefer or require non-alcoholic options.

Ingredients and Measurements:

- 1 cup of dried Cat's Claw bark, finely chopped or powdered
- 2 cups of vegetable glycerin
- 1 cup of distilled water
- A clean glass jar with a tight-fitting lid
- A fine strainer or cheesecloth

Preparation:

- Place the dried Cat's Claw bark into the glass jar.

- In a separate container, mix the vegetable glycerin and distilled water thoroughly. This mixture will help extract both water-soluble and glycerin-soluble compounds from the bark.

- Pour the glycerin-water solution over the Cat's Claw bark, ensuring it is completely submerged.

- Seal the jar tightly and shake it well to integrate all the components.

- Store the jar in a cool, dark place, shaking it daily for 4-6 weeks to facilitate the extraction process.

- After the infusion period, strain the mixture through a fine strainer or cheesecloth into another clean jar, pressing the bark to maximize the extraction of the liquid.

- Transfer the strained tincture to a dropper bottle for easy application and dosage.

How to Use:

🥄 To support immune function and reduce inflammation, particularly in cases of arthritis or similar conditions, take 1-2 dropperfuls (about 30-60 drops) of the tincture diluted in water or juice, up to three times a day.

🥄 For general wellness and preventive care, especially during periods of increased health risks, a lower dose of 1 dropperful once or twice a day can be beneficial.

Duration:

☺ Use the tincture as needed for specific health concerns or as part of a routine wellness regimen.

☺ Consult a healthcare professional for guidance on long-term use and to ensure the tincture's compatibility with any existing treatments or conditions.

☺ Store the tincture in a cool, dark place, and it should remain potent for up to a year.

Cat's Claw Bark Tincture made with vegetable glycerin offers a potent and natural way to harness the healing properties of Cat's Claw bark, providing a valuable addition to health routines without the need for alcohol.

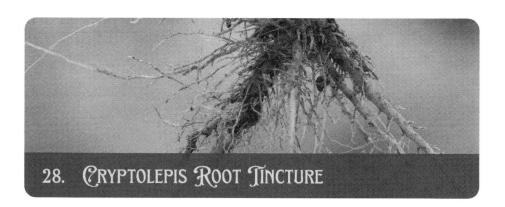

28. CRYPTOLEPIS ROOT TINCTURE

Introduction:

Cryptolepis Root Tincture is a potent herbal remedy recognized for its broad-spectrum antimicrobial, antimalarial, and immune-boosting properties. Derived from the root of the Cryptolepis sanguinolenta plant, this tincture is particularly effective in treating various infections, including respiratory and urinary tract infections. Using vegetable glycerin as the solvent allows for an alcohol-free extraction, making it suitable for all users, including those who avoid alcohol.

Ingredients and Measurements:

- 1 cup of dried Cryptolepis root, finely chopped or powdered
- 2 cups of vegetable glycerin
- 1 cup of distilled water
- A clean glass jar with a tight-fitting lid
- A fine strainer or cheesecloth

Preparation:

- Place the dried Cryptolepis root into the glass jar.
- Mix the vegetable glycerin and distilled water in a separate bowl to ensure a thorough blend. This mixture will effectively extract the beneficial compounds from the Cryptolepis root.
- Pour the glycerin-water solution over the Cryptolepis root, making sure the root is fully submerged.
- Seal the jar tightly and shake it to mix the contents thoroughly.
- Store the jar in a cool, dark place, shaking it daily for 4-6 weeks to facilitate the extraction process.
- After the infusion period, strain the mixture through a fine strainer or cheesecloth into another clean jar, pressing the root to extract as much liquid as possible.
- Transfer the strained tincture to a dropper bottle for convenient use.

How to Use:

- For treating infections or supporting the immune system, take 1-2 dropperfuls (about 30-60 drops) of the tincture diluted in water or juice, up to three times a day.
- Begin with the lower dose and increase as needed, monitoring your body's response to the tincture.

Duration:

- Use the tincture as needed during illness or as a preventive measure during high-risk times for infections.
- Consult a healthcare professional for advice on duration and dosage, especially for long-term use or when treating severe infections.
- Store the tincture in a cool, dark place, and it should remain effective for up to a year.

Cryptolepis Root Tincture made with vegetable glycerin is an effective, natural way to harness the healing properties of Cryptolepis root, providing a non-alcoholic solution for combating infections and boosting overall health.

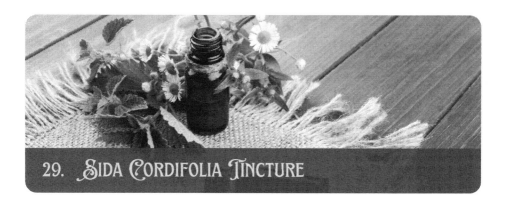

29. Sida Cordifolia Tincture

Introduction:

Sida Cordifolia Tincture is an herbal remedy known for its stimulating and anti-inflammatory properties. Extracted from the Sida Cordifolia plant, often referred to as "country mallow," this tincture is effective in enhancing energy levels, supporting respiratory health, and providing relief from pain and inflammation. Utilizing vegetable glycerin as a solvent ensures an alcohol-free tincture, making it accessible to those who avoid alcohol for health or personal reasons.

Ingredients and Measurements:

- 1 cup of dried Sida Cordifolia leaves or roots, finely chopped or powdered

- 2 cups of vegetable glycerin

- 1 cup of distilled water

- A clean glass jar with a tight-fitting lid

- A fine strainer or cheesecloth

Preparation:

☞ Place the dried Sida Cordifolia leaves or roots into the glass jar.

☞ In a separate container, mix the vegetable glycerin and distilled water, creating a balanced solvent to extract the plant's active compounds effectively.

☞ Pour the glycerin-water mixture over the Sida Cordifolia, ensuring all plant material is submerged.

☞ Seal the jar tightly and shake well to integrate the contents.

☞ Store the jar in a cool, dark place, shaking it daily for 4-6 weeks to promote optimal extraction of the medicinal properties.

☞ After the infusion period, strain the mixture through a fine strainer or cheesecloth into another clean jar, pressing the plant material to extract as much liquid as possible.

☞ Transfer the strained tincture to a dropper bottle for ease of use.

How to Use:

✎ To boost energy and support respiratory health, take 1-2 dropperfuls (about 30-60 drops) of the tincture diluted in water or juice, up to three times a day.

For pain and inflammation relief, the same dosage can be used, adjusting based on response and need.

Duration:

- Use the tincture as necessary for specific health needs or as part of a wellness routine.

- Consult a healthcare professional for guidance on long-term use, particularly if using for chronic conditions or alongside other treatments.

- Store the tincture in a cool, dark place, and it should remain effective for up to a year.

Sida Cordifolia Tincture made with vegetable glycerin is a versatile and effective way to utilize the beneficial properties of the Sida Cordifolia plant, providing a natural, non-alcoholic option for enhancing health and well-being.

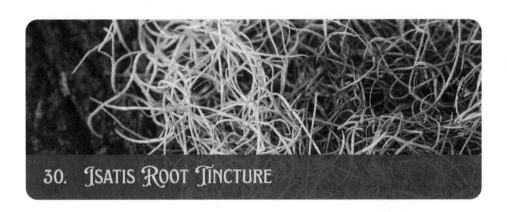

30. ISATIS ROOT TINCTURE

Introduction:

Isatis Root Tincture is a potent herbal remedy known for its antiviral, antibacterial, and anti-inflammatory properties. Extracted from the root of the Isatis plant, this tincture is especially effective in treating viral infections, reducing inflammation, and boosting immune health. Using vegetable glycerin as a solvent creates an alcohol-free tincture, suitable for a wide range of users, including those who avoid alcohol for health or personal reasons.

Ingredients and Measurements:

- 1 cup of dried Isatis root, finely chopped or powdered

- 2 cups of vegetable glycerin

- 1 cup of distilled water

- A clean glass jar with a tight-fitting lid

- A fine strainer or cheesecloth

Preparation:

Place the dried Isatis root into the glass jar.

- Mix the vegetable glycerin and distilled water in a separate bowl to create a diluted glycerin solution. This mixture ensures a thorough extraction of the beneficial compounds from the Isatis root.

- Pour the glycerin-water mixture over the Isatis root, ensuring the root is fully submerged.

- Seal the jar tightly and shake it well to combine the contents.

- Store the jar in a cool, dark place, shaking it daily for 4-6 weeks to facilitate the extraction process.

- After the infusion period, strain the mixture through a fine strainer or cheesecloth into another clean jar, pressing the root to extract as much liquid as possible.

- Transfer the strained tincture to a dropper bottle for ease of use.

How to Use:

- To combat viral infections and support immune health, take 1-2 dropperfuls (about 30-60 drops) of the tincture diluted in water or juice, up to three times a day.

- For reducing inflammation and enhancing general health, use the same dosage, adjusting based on your response and specific needs.

Duration:

- Use the tincture as needed for addressing acute health issues or as part of a preventive health regimen.

- Consult a healthcare professional for guidance on duration and dosage, especially for long-term use or when treating severe conditions.

- Store the tincture in a cool, dark place, and it should remain effective for up to a year.

Isatis Root Tincture made with vegetable glycerin is an effective way to harness the healing properties of Isatis root, offering a natural, non-alcoholic solution for improving health and combating infections.

PART 02

HERBAL
REMEDIES (31-70)

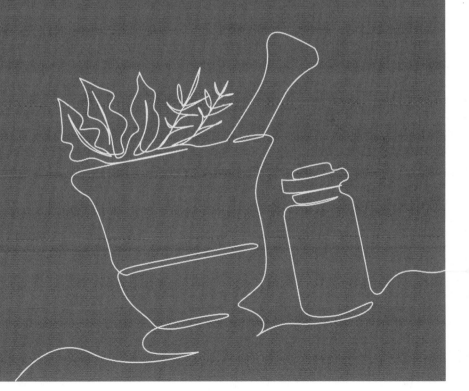

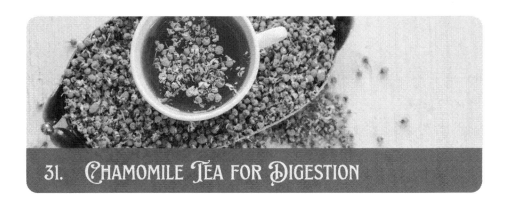

31. CHAMOMILE TEA FOR DIGESTION

Introduction:

Chamomile Tea is renowned for its soothing effects on the digestive system. This gentle herbal tea is perfect for easing stomach discomfort, reducing bloating, and promoting a healthy digestive process. Its calming properties also help alleviate stress and anxiety, which can contribute to digestive issues.

Ingredients & Measurements:

- 2 teaspoons of dried chamomile flowers
- 1 cup of boiling water
- Optional: Honey or lemon to enhance flavor and add extra benefits

Preparation:

🍵 Place the dried chamomile flowers in a teapot or a heat-resistant cup.

🍵 Pour boiling water over the flowers, ensuring they are fully submerged.

🍵 Cover the teapot or cup to keep the essential oils intact and let the tea steep for 5-10 minutes, depending on your preference for strength.

🍵 Strain the tea to remove the flowers and pour the clear tea into a cup.

How to Use:

🍵 Enjoy a cup of chamomile tea after meals to aid digestion or when you feel stomach discomfort.

🍵 Sweeten with honey or add a twist of lemon for flavor and additional digestive support.

Duration:

🕐 Chamomile tea can be consumed regularly, up to 2-3 times daily, especially after meals or before bedtime to maximize its digestive and calming benefits.

🕐 Continue using as part of your daily routine for ongoing digestive health. Consult a healthcare provider if digestive issues persist or for personalized advice.

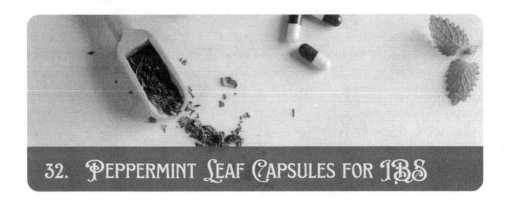

32. Peppermint Leaf Capsules for IBS

Introduction:

Peppermint Leaf Capsules are a natural and effective treatment for Irritable Bowel Syndrome (IBS). Peppermint is known for its antispasmodic properties, which help relax the muscles of the digestive tract, reducing the symptoms of bloating, gas, and abdominal pain associated with IBS. These capsules provide a convenient way to deliver the benefits of peppermint directly to the digestive system, helping to manage and alleviate IBS symptoms.

Ingredients & Measurements:

- High-quality peppermint leaf powder
- Empty vegetarian or gelatin capsules
- A small capsule-filling machine or a manual method using a spoon and a steady hand

Preparation:

☞ Ensure you have high-quality peppermint leaf powder, which retains the essential oils and active compounds of peppermint.

☞ If using a capsule-filling machine, follow the manufacturer's instructions to fill the capsules. Typically, this involves spreading the peppermint powder over the base of the machine and using the tamper to fill the capsules evenly.

☞ If manually filling the capsules, carefully open each capsule half. Use a small spoon to fill one half with the peppermint leaf powder. Pack the powder lightly to fit as much as possible without forcing it.

☞ Carefully reassemble the two halves of each capsule to seal the powder inside.

☞ Store the filled capsules in a cool, dry place, preferably in an airtight container to preserve their potency.

How to Use:

↳ Take one peppermint leaf capsule 1-2 times a day, ideally 30 minutes before meals, to help prevent or reduce IBS symptoms.

↳ Start with the lower dosage and increase if necessary, observing how your body responds to the treatment.

Duration:

- Peppermint leaf capsules can be used as part of a daily routine to manage IBS symptoms.

- If symptoms persist or worsen, consult a healthcare professional for further evaluation and advice.

- Regularly review your supplement intake with your healthcare provider to adjust dosages as needed based on your health status and response to the supplement.

Peppermint Leaf Capsules are a practical and efficient way to use the natural soothing and antispasmodic benefits of peppermint for managing IBS, providing targeted relief and improving digestive health.

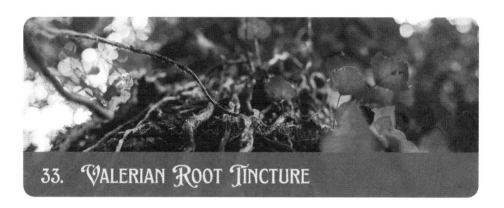

33. VALERIAN ROOT TINCTURE

Introduction:

Valerian Root Tincture is a renowned herbal remedy known for its ability to promote relaxation and improve sleep quality. Valerian root has natural sedative and anxiolytic properties, making it effective in treating insomnia, reducing anxiety, and calming nervous tension. Using vegetable glycerin as the extraction medium creates an alcohol-free tincture, suitable for a wide range of users, including those who prefer or need to avoid alcohol.

Ingredients & Measurements:

- 1 cup of dried valerian root, finely chopped or powdered

- 2 cups of vegetable glycerin

- 1 cup of distilled water

- A clean glass jar with a tight-fitting lid

- A fine strainer or cheesecloth

Preparation:

- Place the dried valerian root into the glass jar.

- In a separate container, mix the vegetable glycerin and distilled water to create a diluted glycerin solution. This solution will help extract the active compounds from the valerian root effectively.

- Pour the glycerin-water mixture over the valerian root, ensuring the root is fully submerged.

- Seal the jar tightly and shake it well to integrate all the ingredients.

- Store the jar in a cool, dark place, shaking it daily for 4-6 weeks to facilitate the extraction process.

- After the infusion period, strain the mixture through a fine strainer or cheesecloth into another clean jar, pressing the root to extract as much liquid as possible.

- Transfer the strained tincture to a dropper bottle for ease of use.

How to Use:

- To aid relaxation and promote better sleep, take 1-2 dropperfuls (about 30-60 drops) of the tincture diluted in water or a beverage of your choice, 30 minutes to an hour before bedtime.

- For anxiety or stress, the same dosage can be taken during the day, up to three times if needed.

Duration:

- Use the tincture as needed for relaxation or sleep improvement. For chronic conditions or regular use, consult a healthcare professional for guidance on duration and dosage.

- Store the tincture in a cool, dark place, and it should remain effective for up to a year.

Valerian Root Tincture made with vegetable glycerin is an effective and gentle way to utilize the calming properties of valerian root, offering a natural solution to enhance sleep and reduce anxiety without the use of alcohol.

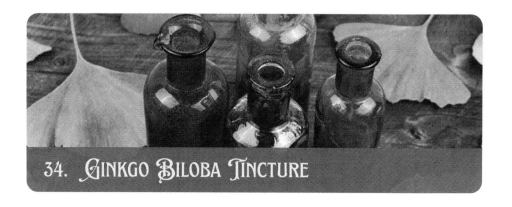

34. Ginkgo Biloba Tincture

Introduction:

Ginkgo Biloba Tincture is a powerful herbal supplement known for its ability to enhance cognitive function, improve circulation, and support overall brain health. Ginkgo biloba, one of the oldest living tree species, contains potent antioxidants that protect against cellular damage and improve blood flow. Using vegetable glycerin as the solvent, this tincture offers an alcohol-free option that is suitable for a broad audience, including those who avoid alcohol for health or personal reasons.

Ingredients and Measurements:

- 1 cup of dried ginkgo biloba leaves, finely chopped or powdered
- 2 cups of vegetable glycerin
- 1 cup of distilled water
- A clean glass jar with a tight-fitting lid
- A fine strainer or cheesecloth

Preparation:

- Place the dried ginkgo biloba leaves into the glass jar.

- Mix the vegetable glycerin and distilled water in a separate container to create a consistent solution. This blend ensures an efficient extraction of both water-soluble and glycerin-soluble compounds from the ginkgo leaves.

- Pour the glycerin-water mixture over the ginkgo biloba leaves, making sure they are fully submerged.

- Seal the jar tightly and shake it to mix the contents thoroughly.

- Store the jar in a cool, dark place, shaking it daily for 4-6 weeks to promote the extraction process.

- After the infusion period, strain the mixture through a fine strainer or cheesecloth into another clean jar, pressing the leaves to extract as much liquid as possible.

- Transfer the strained tincture to a dropper bottle for easy application and dosage.

How to Use:

- To support cognitive function and enhance circulation, take 1-2 dropperfuls (about 30-60 drops) of the tincture diluted in water or juice, up to three times a day.

- Begin with a lower dose to observe how your body responds, and adjust as needed based on your health goals and response to the supplement.

Duration:

- Use the tincture as part of a regular health regimen for cognitive and circulatory support.

- Consult a healthcare professional for guidance on long-term use, especially if you are taking other medications or have underlying health conditions.

- Store the tincture in a cool, dark place, and it should remain potent for up to a year.

Ginkgo Biloba Tincture made with vegetable glycerin is an effective way to harness the cognitive-enhancing and circulatory benefits of ginkgo biloba, providing a natural and alcohol-free option for improving mental performance and overall well-being.

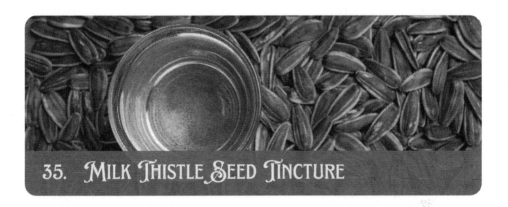

35. MILK THISTLE SEED TINCTURE

Introduction:

Milk Thistle Seed Tincture is a revered herbal remedy celebrated for its liver-protective and detoxifying properties. Milk thistle, with its active ingredient silymarin, is known to support liver function, promote the regeneration of liver cells, and protect against toxins and pollutants. Using vegetable glycerin as a solvent for this tincture ensures an alcohol-free preparation, making it suitable for individuals of all ages and those who prefer to avoid alcohol.

Ingredients and Measurements:

- 1 cup of dried milk thistle seeds, finely ground

- 2 cups of vegetable glycerin

- 1 cup of distilled water

- A clean glass jar with a tight-fitting lid
- A fine strainer or cheesecloth

Preparation:

☞ Place the finely ground milk thistle seeds into the glass jar.

☞ Combine the vegetable glycerin and distilled water in a separate bowl to create a diluted glycerin solution. This mixture facilitates an effective extraction of silymarin and other beneficial compounds from the seeds.

☞ Pour the glycerin-water mixture over the milk thistle seeds, ensuring they are completely submerged.

☞ Seal the jar tightly and shake it to mix the contents thoroughly.

☞ Store the jar in a cool, dark place, shaking it daily for 4-6 weeks to promote the extraction process.

☞ After the infusion period, strain the mixture through a fine strainer or cheesecloth into another clean jar, pressing the seeds to extract as much liquid as possible.

☞ Transfer the strained tincture to a dropper bottle for ease of use.

How to Use:

✎ To support liver health and detoxification, take 1-2 dropperfuls (about 30-60 drops) of the tincture diluted in water or juice, up to three times a day.

✎ Start with a lower dose to observe how your body responds and adjust as necessary based on your health goals and response.

Duration:

◷ Use the tincture regularly as part of a health regimen focused on liver support and detoxification.

◷ Consult a healthcare professional for guidance on long-term use, especially if you have existing liver conditions or are taking medications that affect liver function.

◷ Store the tincture in a cool, dark place, and it should remain effective for up to a year.

Milk Thistle Seed Tincture made with vegetable glycerin is a safe and effective way to utilize the liver-protective benefits of milk thistle, offering a natural and alcohol-free option for enhancing liver health and overall well-being.

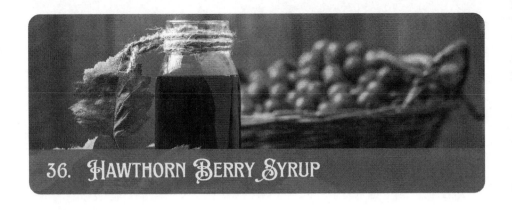

36. Hawthorn Berry Syrup

Introduction:

Hawthorn Berry Syrup is a traditional herbal remedy known for its ability to support heart health and improve circulation. Hawthorn berries are rich in antioxidants and bioflavonoids, which help to strengthen heart function, regulate blood pressure, and enhance overall cardiovascular health. This syrup offers a pleasant and effective way to incorporate the benefits of hawthorn berries into your daily routine.

Ingredients and Measurements:

- 1 cup of dried hawthorn berries
- 4 cups of water
- 1 cup of raw, organic honey or pure maple syrup (for a vegan alternative)
- A large pot
- A fine strainer or cheesecloth

Preparation:

- Place the dried hawthorn berries in the large pot and add the water.
- Bring the mixture to a boil over high heat, then reduce the heat and let it simmer for 30-40 minutes, or until the liquid has reduced by about half. This slow simmering helps to extract the therapeutic compounds from the berries.
- Remove the pot from the heat and allow the mixture to cool slightly.
- Strain the liquid through a fine strainer or cheesecloth to remove the berry solids, pressing the berries to extract as much liquid as possible.
- Return the strained liquid to the pot, add the honey or maple syrup, and heat gently, stirring until fully dissolved.
- Once the syrup has cooled, pour it into a clean glass bottle or jar for storage.

How to Use:

- Take 1-2 tablespoons of Hawthorn Berry Syrup daily, either directly or mixed into a beverage of your choice, to support cardiovascular health.
- The syrup can also be used as a natural sweetener in teas, smoothies, or yogurt.

Duration:

- Hawthorn Berry Syrup can be part of a daily health regimen, especially for those focusing on heart health and circulation.

- If symptoms persist or you have a specific heart condition, consult a healthcare professional for advice on long-term use and appropriate dosages.

- Store the syrup in the refrigerator and consume within 4-6 weeks for optimal freshness and potency.

Hawthorn Berry Syrup is a delicious and beneficial way to support heart health and improve circulation, leveraging the natural therapeutic properties of hawthorn berries in a convenient and enjoyable form.

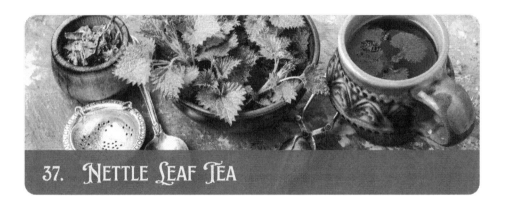

37. NETTLE LEAF TEA

Introduction:

Nettle Leaf Tea is a nutrient-rich herbal beverage celebrated for its wide array of health benefits. Nettle leaves are loaded with vitamins, minerals, and antioxidants that support overall health, including reducing inflammation, alleviating allergy symptoms, and enhancing urinary function. This tea is an excellent way to enjoy the therapeutic qualities of nettles in a soothing and easily digestible form.

Ingredients and Measurements:

- 2 tablespoons of dried nettle leaves

- 2 cups of boiling water

- Optional: honey or lemon for flavor

Preparation:

- Place the dried nettle leaves in a teapot or a heat-resistant infuser.

- Pour the boiling water over the nettles and cover to prevent the steam and essential oils from escaping.

- Allow the tea to steep for 10-15 minutes. Steeping for a longer period helps to extract more of the beneficial compounds from the nettles.

- Strain the tea into a cup to remove the nettle leaves.

How to Use:

- Drink a cup of nettle leaf tea up to three times a day to benefit from its anti-inflammatory, diuretic, and antihistamine properties.

- For added flavor and health benefits, sweeten the tea with a teaspoon of honey or a squeeze of lemon.

Duration:

- Nettle leaf tea can be consumed daily as part of a healthy routine to maintain optimal health and wellness.

- If using nettle tea to address specific health issues like allergies or inflammation, observe how your body responds and adjust your consumption accordingly.

- Consult a healthcare professional if you have ongoing health concerns or are taking medications, as nettle can interact with certain drugs.

Nettle Leaf Tea is an easy and effective way to incorporate the health-enhancing properties of nettles into your daily routine, offering a natural solution to support a variety of health needs.

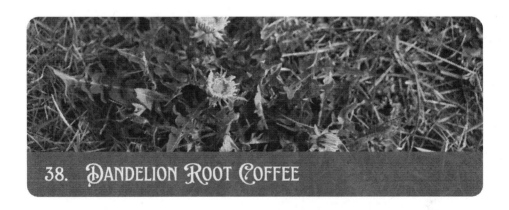

38. DANDELION ROOT COFFEE

Introduction:

Dandelion Root Coffee is a healthful alternative to traditional coffee, celebrated for its detoxifying properties and ability to support liver function. Made from roasted dandelion roots, this beverage is rich in vitamins, minerals, and antioxidants. It offers a coffee-like flavor without the caffeine, making it ideal for those looking to reduce their caffeine intake while still enjoying a warm, comforting drink.

Ingredients and Measurements:

- 1 cup of dried and roasted dandelion roots

- 4 cups of water

- Optional: milk, honey, or sweetener of choice for flavor

Preparation:

- Grind the roasted dandelion roots into a coarse powder, similar to coffee grounds.

- Bring the water to a boil in a large pot.

- Add the ground dandelion root to the boiling water and reduce the heat. Let it simmer for 10-15 minutes. The longer it simmers, the stronger and more flavorful the "coffee" will be.

- Remove from heat and allow it to steep for a few minutes.

- Strain the mixture through a fine strainer or coffee filter into a cup or pot, removing the dandelion root grounds.

How to Use:

- Serve the dandelion root coffee hot, as you would regular coffee.

- Enhance the flavor by adding milk, honey, or your preferred sweetener.

- Enjoy this beverage in the morning or throughout the day as a caffeine-free alternative to coffee.

Duration:

- Dandelion root coffee can be consumed daily as part of a balanced diet to support detoxification and liver health.

- If you have specific health conditions or are on medication, consult with a healthcare professional before making it a regular part of your routine, especially if using it for therapeutic purposes.

Dandelion Root Coffee is a delightful and beneficial way to enjoy the robust flavors and health benefits of dandelion root, offering a natural, caffeine-free alternative that supports overall wellness.

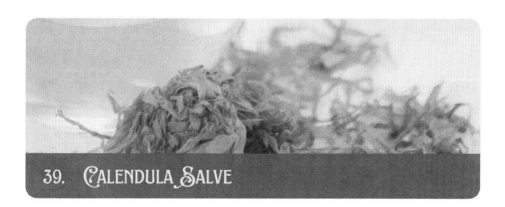

39. CALENDULA SALVE

Introduction:

Calendula Salve is a soothing and healing ointment renowned for its ability to repair skin, alleviate irritations, and reduce inflammation. Made from calendula flowers, which are rich in anti-inflammatory and antimicrobial compounds, this salve is excellent for treating cuts, scrapes, burns, rashes, and dry skin. Its gentle formulation makes it suitable for all skin types, including sensitive skin.

Ingredients and Measurements:

- 1/2 cup of dried calendula petals
- 1 cup of coconut oil or olive oil
- 1/4 cup of beeswax pellets (or carnauba wax for a vegan alternative)
- Optional: a few drops of lavender essential oil for added healing properties and fragrance
- A clean glass jar or tin for storage
- A double boiler
- A fine strainer or cheesecloth

Preparation:

- Infuse the calendula petals in the coconut or olive oil. Place both in a double boiler, heat gently, and allow the petals to simmer in the oil for 1-2 hours to extract the active compounds.

- Strain the oil through a fine strainer or cheesecloth into a clean bowl, removing the calendula petals.

- Return the infused oil to the double boiler, add the beeswax pellets, and stir continuously until the beeswax is fully melted and combined with the oil.

- If using, add a few drops of lavender essential oil to the mixture after removing it from the heat. Stir well to ensure the essential oil is evenly distributed.

- Pour the finished salve into the clean glass jar or tin and allow it to cool and solidify at room temperature.

How to Use:

- Apply a small amount of calendula salve to the affected area 2-3 times a day or as needed to soothe and heal the skin.

- Gently massage the salve into the skin until it is fully absorbed, particularly focusing on areas with cuts, burns, rashes, or dryness.

Duration:

- Use the salve as needed for skin issues. If there is no improvement within a few days or if the condition worsens, consult a healthcare professional.

- Store the salve in a cool, dry place, and it should remain effective for up to 6 months. If the scent changes or the texture breaks down, it's time to make a fresh batch.

Calendula Salve is an effective and gentle option for natural skin care, providing relief and promoting healing with the combined powers of calendula and other soothing ingredients.

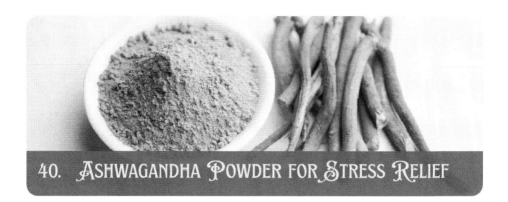

Introduction:

Ashwagandha Powder is a highly revered adaptogenic herb known for its ability to reduce stress, improve mood, and enhance overall vitality. This ancient remedy, used extensively in Ayurvedic medicine, helps balance the body's response to physical and emotional stress by regulating hormones and improving nervous system function. Ashwagandha is particularly beneficial for those looking to naturally manage anxiety, improve sleep, and boost energy levels.

Ingredients and Measurements:

- 1 teaspoon of ashwagandha powder
- 1 cup of warm milk or a milk alternative
- Optional: honey or a sweetener of choice to enhance flavor

Preparation:

- Measure out 1 teaspoon of ashwagandha powder.
- Mix the ashwagandha powder into a cup of warm milk or a suitable milk alternative. Stir thoroughly to ensure the powder is fully dissolved and the mixture is smooth.
- If desired, add honey or another sweetener to taste for improved flavor.

How to Use:

- Drink this ashwagandha-infused beverage once a day, preferably in the evening, to help calm the mind and prepare for a restful night's sleep.
- Consistent use can help reduce stress levels and improve overall well-being.

Duration:

- Ashwagandha can be taken daily as part of a routine to manage stress and support overall health.
- If you are new to ashwagandha, start with a lower dose and gradually increase as needed to monitor your body's response.
- Consult a healthcare professional if you have any health conditions or are taking medications, as ashwagandha can interact with certain drugs.

Ashwagandha Powder is an effective and natural way to combat stress, enhance mood, and promote a balanced lifestyle, making it an invaluable addition to any wellness regimen.

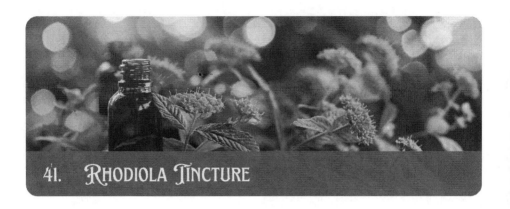

41. RHODIOLA TINCTURE

Introduction:

Rhodiola Tincture is a powerful adaptogenic remedy known for its ability to enhance mental clarity, increase physical endurance, and improve stress resilience. Rhodiola, often referred to as "golden root," is celebrated for its potent effects on reducing fatigue and boosting mood. By using vegetable glycerin as the extraction medium, this tincture provides a non-alcoholic method to harness the therapeutic benefits of Rhodiola, making it accessible to a broader range of users.

Ingredients and Measurements:

- 1 cup of dried Rhodiola root, finely chopped or powdered
- 2 cups of vegetable glycerin
- 1 cup of distilled water
- A clean glass jar with a tight-fitting lid
- A fine strainer or cheesecloth

Preparation:

- Place the dried Rhodiola root into the glass jar.

- Mix the vegetable glycerin and distilled water in a separate bowl to create a diluted glycerin solution. This solution ensures an effective extraction of the active compounds from Rhodiola.

- Pour the glycerin-water mixture over the Rhodiola root, ensuring the root is completely submerged.

- Seal the jar tightly and shake it to mix the contents well.

- Store the jar in a cool, dark place, shaking it daily for 4-6 weeks to facilitate the extraction process.

- After the infusion period, strain the mixture through a fine strainer or cheesecloth into another clean jar, pressing the root to extract as much liquid as possible.

Transfer the strained tincture to a dropper bottle for easy use.

How to Use:

- To combat mental fatigue and enhance physical energy, take 1-2 dropperfuls (about 30-60 drops) of the tincture diluted in water or juice, up to three times a day.

- For stress relief and mood enhancement, the same dosage can be taken, adjusting based on your body's response and needs.

Duration:

- Use the tincture as part of a regular health regimen for cognitive and physical support.

- Consult a healthcare professional for advice on long-term use and to ensure the tincture's compatibility with any existing treatments or conditions.

- Store the tincture in a cool, dark place, and it should remain effective for up to a year.

Rhodiola Tincture made with vegetable glycerin is an effective way to leverage the adaptogenic and health-boosting properties of Rhodiola, offering a natural solution to improve mental performance and manage stress without alcohol.

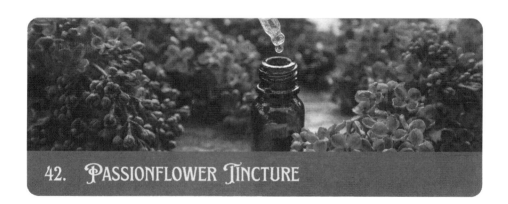

42. PASSIONFLOWER TINCTURE

Introduction:

Passionflower Tincture is a natural remedy known for its calming and sedative properties, making it an excellent choice for alleviating anxiety, insomnia, and nervous tension. Passionflower works by increasing levels of gamma-aminobutyric acid (GABA) in the brain, which helps to promote relaxation and improve sleep quality. Utilizing vegetable glycerin for this tincture ensures an alcohol-free option that is gentle and suitable for a wide range of users.

Ingredients and Measurements:

- 1 cup of dried passionflower leaves and flowers, finely chopped or powdered
- 2 cups of vegetable glycerin
- 1 cup of distilled water
- A clean glass jar with a tight-fitting lid
- A fine strainer or cheesecloth

Preparation:

- Place the dried passionflower into the glass jar.

- In a separate container, mix the vegetable glycerin and distilled water to create a consistent solution. This blend facilitates an efficient extraction of the active compounds from the passionflower.

- Pour the glycerin-water mixture over the passionflower, ensuring all plant material is submerged.

- Seal the jar tightly and shake it to thoroughly mix the contents.

- Store the jar in a cool, dark place, shaking it daily for 4-6 weeks to promote the extraction process.

- After the infusion period, strain the mixture through a fine strainer or cheesecloth into another clean jar, pressing the plant material to extract as much liquid as possible.

- Transfer the strained tincture to a dropper bottle for ease of use.

How to Use:

- To help relieve anxiety and promote relaxation, take 1-2 dropperfuls (about 30-60 drops) of the tincture diluted in water or juice, up to three times a day, especially during stressful periods or before bedtime.

- For aiding sleep, take the tincture 30 minutes to an hour before going to bed to help unwind and encourage a restful night.

Duration:

- Use the tincture as needed to manage symptoms of anxiety or sleep disturbances.

- Consult a healthcare professional for guidance on long-term use, particularly if you have existing health conditions or are taking other medications.

- Store the tincture in a cool, dark place, and it should remain effective for up to a year.

Passionflower Tincture made with vegetable glycerin offers a natural and effective way to harness the soothing properties of passionflower, providing a gentle solution to improve relaxation and sleep without the use of alcohol.

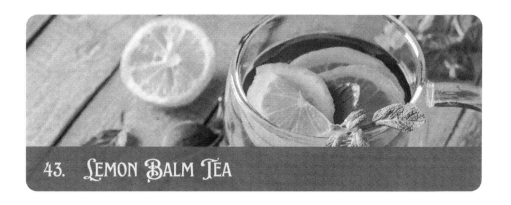

43. LEMON BALM TEA

Introduction:

Lemon Balm Tea is a delightful and therapeutic herbal beverage known for its calming effects on the mind and body. Lemon balm, a member of the mint family, has a mild lemon scent and flavor, and is used to reduce stress, ease anxiety, and improve sleep quality. Rich in antioxidants and anti-inflammatory compounds, this tea is also beneficial for digestive health and boosting the immune system.

Ingredients and Measurements:

- 2 tablespoons of fresh or 1 tablespoon of dried lemon balm leaves
- 1 cup of boiling water
- Optional: honey or a slice of lemon to enhance flavor

Preparation:

☕ If using fresh lemon balm, gently bruise the leaves with your fingers to release the essential oils.

☕ Place the lemon balm leaves in a teapot or a heat-resistant infuser.

☕ Pour the boiling water over the leaves and cover the teapot or cup to keep the steam and aromatic oils contained.

☕ Let the tea steep for 5-10 minutes, depending on your preferred strength and flavor intensity.

☕ Strain the tea into a cup to remove the leaves.

How to Use:

☕ Enjoy a cup of lemon balm tea in the evening to wind down before bed, or throughout the day to reduce stress and anxiety.

☕ Enhance the flavor and health benefits by adding a teaspoon of honey or a slice of lemon, if desired.

Duration:

☕ Lemon balm tea can be consumed daily as part of a healthy routine to maintain calm and support overall wellness.

☕ If you are using lemon balm tea to address specific health issues like insomnia or severe anxiety, monitor your response and consult a healthcare professional if symptoms persist or for guidance on long-term use.

Lemon Balm Tea is an easy and enjoyable way to incorporate the soothing properties of lemon balm into your daily life, offering a natural and effective remedy to promote relaxation and enhance well-being.

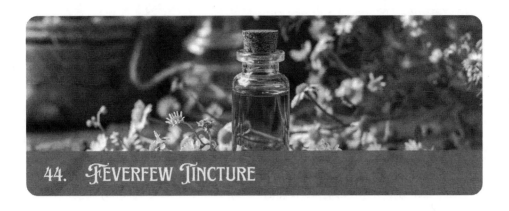

44. FEVERFEW TINCTURE

Introduction:

Feverfew Tincture is a well-known herbal remedy primarily used for its effectiveness in preventing and reducing the frequency of migraines and headaches. Feverfew, a plant with potent anti-inflammatory properties, also helps alleviate arthritis pain and reduce fever. Using vegetable glycerin as the solvent, this tincture provides an alcohol-free option that is gentle and suitable for various users, including those who prefer to avoid alcohol.

Ingredients and Measurements:

- 1 cup of dried feverfew leaves and flowers, finely chopped or powdered
- 2 cups of vegetable glycerin
- 1 cup of distilled water
- A clean glass jar with a tight-fitting lid
- A fine strainer or cheesecloth

Preparation:

- Place the dried feverfew into the glass jar.
- Mix the vegetable glycerin and distilled water in a separate bowl to create a consistent solution. This blend ensures an efficient extraction of the active compounds from feverfew.
- Pour the glycerin-water mixture over the feverfew, making sure all plant material is submerged.
- Seal the jar tightly and shake it to thoroughly mix the contents.
- Store the jar in a cool, dark place, shaking it daily for 4-6 weeks to promote the extraction process.
- After the infusion period, strain the mixture through a fine strainer or cheesecloth into another clean jar, pressing the plant material to extract as much liquid as possible.
- Transfer the strained tincture to a dropper bottle for ease of use.

How to Use:

- To prevent migraines and reduce headache severity, take 1-2 dropperfuls (about 30-60 drops) of the tincture diluted in water or juice, up to three times a day.

- For reducing inflammation and pain related to arthritis, the same dosage can be taken, adjusting based on your body's response and needs.

Duration:

- Use the tincture regularly as part of a preventive regimen for migraines or as needed for pain relief.

- Consult a healthcare professional for guidance on long-term use, particularly if you have existing health conditions or are taking other medications.

- Store the tincture in a cool, dark place, and it should remain effective for up to a year.

Feverfew Tincture made with vegetable glycerin is a natural and effective way to leverage the medicinal properties of feverfew, providing a non-alcoholic solution for managing migraines, headaches, and inflammation.

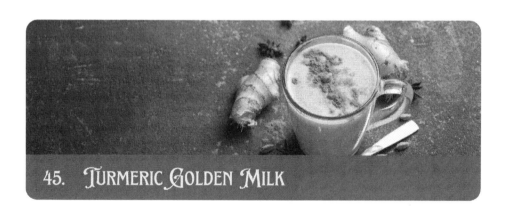

45. TURMERIC GOLDEN MILK

Introduction:

Turmeric Golden Milk is a warming and healthful beverage renowned for its anti-inflammatory and antioxidant properties. The key ingredient, turmeric, contains curcumin, which is responsible for its vibrant color and numerous health benefits, including reducing inflammation, boosting immunity, and supporting digestion. This drink is often enhanced with other spices like ginger and cinnamon, making it not only delicious but also highly beneficial for overall wellness.

Ingredients and Measurements:

- 1 teaspoon of turmeric powder
- 1/2 teaspoon of ground ginger
- 1/4 teaspoon of ground cinnamon

- A pinch of black pepper (to enhance curcumin absorption)
- 1 cup of milk or a milk alternative (like almond, coconut, or oat milk)
- 1 teaspoon of honey or maple syrup (optional, for sweetness)

Preparation:

- In a small saucepan, combine the turmeric powder, ground ginger, ground cinnamon, and black pepper.

- Add the milk or milk alternative and stir well to blend the spices evenly.

- Heat the mixture over medium heat, stirring constantly, until it is hot but not boiling. This gentle heating allows the spices to infuse the milk without losing their beneficial properties.

- Once heated, remove the saucepan from the heat. If desired, sweeten with honey or maple syrup to taste.

How to Use:

- Drink a cup of Turmeric Golden Milk daily, preferably in the evening, to help relax and benefit from its anti-inflammatory and antioxidant effects.

- This beverage can also be enjoyed in the morning or after meals to aid digestion and boost overall vitality.

Duration:

- Turmeric Golden Milk can be a regular part of your daily routine to support health and well-being.

- If you are using it to address specific health issues, observe your body's response and adjust your intake accordingly.

- Consult a healthcare professional if you have any health conditions or are taking medications, as turmeric can interact with certain drugs.

Turmeric Golden Milk is a delightful and beneficial way to enjoy the therapeutic properties of turmeric and other spices, providing a comforting and health-promoting drink suitable for any time of day.

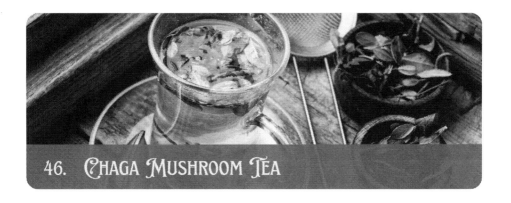

46. Chaga Mushroom Tea

Introduction:

Chaga Mushroom Tea is a nutrient-dense beverage celebrated for its powerful antioxidant and immune-boosting properties. Derived from the Chaga mushroom, which grows on birch trees in colder climates, this tea is rich in betulinic acid, melanin, and other compounds that support overall health, enhance the immune system, and provide anti-aging benefits. Chaga tea offers a unique, earthy flavor and is a natural way to bolster wellness.

Ingredients and Measurements:

- 1-2 tablespoons of dried Chaga mushroom chunks or powder
- 4 cups of water
- Optional: honey or maple syrup for sweetness

Preparation:

☞ Place the dried Chaga mushroom chunks or powder in a pot.

☞ Add the water and bring the mixture to a boil.

☞ Once boiling, reduce the heat and let the tea simmer for at least 30 minutes to an hour. The longer you simmer, the more concentrated and potent the tea will become.

☞ After simmering, strain the tea to remove the Chaga chunks or sediment if using powder.

☞ Pour the tea into a cup or a teapot.

How to Use:

✎ Drink a cup of Chaga Mushroom Tea daily to benefit from its immune-boosting and antioxidant properties.

✎ If desired, enhance the flavor with a bit of honey or maple syrup.

Duration:

☺ Chaga Mushroom Tea can be a part of your daily routine, especially during seasons when immune support is crucial, such as the colder months or periods of high stress.

☺ Monitor your body's response to the tea, and adjust your intake as necessary.

Consult a healthcare professional if you have any underlying health conditions or are taking medications, as Chaga can interact with certain drugs.

Chaga Mushroom Tea is an excellent way to incorporate the health benefits of Chaga mushrooms into your diet, offering a simple, natural approach to enhancing immunity and overall well-being.

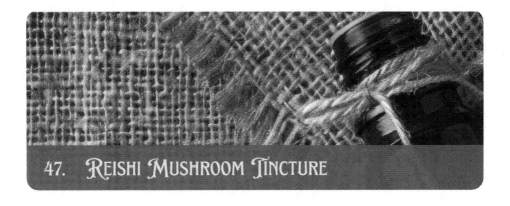

47. REISHI MUSHROOM TINCTURE

Introduction:

Reishi Mushroom Tincture is an esteemed herbal supplement recognized for its adaptogenic properties, which help the body manage stress, enhance immune function, and support overall wellness. Reishi mushrooms, often referred to as the "mushroom of immortality," contain a range of bioactive compounds including polysaccharides and triterpenoids that provide anti-inflammatory, antioxidant, and immune-modulating effects. Using vegetable glycerin as the extraction medium makes this tincture an alcohol-free option suitable for various users, including those who prefer to avoid alcohol.

Ingredients and Measurements:

- 1 cup of dried Reishi mushroom slices or powder

- 2 cups of vegetable glycerin
- 1 cup of distilled water
- A clean glass jar with a tight-fitting lid
- A fine strainer or cheesecloth

Preparation:

▭ Place the dried Reishi mushroom slices or powder into the glass jar.

▭ Mix the vegetable glycerin and distilled water in a separate container to create a diluted glycerin solution. This solution ensures efficient extraction of the medicinal compounds from the Reishi mushrooms.

▭ Pour the glycerin-water mixture over the Reishi mushrooms, making sure they are fully submerged.

▭ Seal the jar tightly and shake it to mix the contents thoroughly.

- Store the jar in a cool, dark place, shaking it daily for 4-6 weeks to facilitate the extraction process.

- After the infusion period, strain the mixture through a fine strainer or cheesecloth into another clean jar, pressing the mushrooms to extract as much liquid as possible.

- Transfer the strained tincture to a dropper bottle for easy use.

How to Use:

- To support immune function and reduce stress, take 1-2 dropperfuls (about 30-60 drops) of the tincture diluted in water or juice, up to three times a day.

- Start with a lower dose to observe how your body responds, and adjust as necessary based on your health goals and reaction to the supplement.

Duration:

- Use the tincture regularly as part of a health regimen for immune support and stress management.

- Consult a healthcare professional for advice on long-term use and to ensure the tincture's compatibility with any existing treatments or conditions.

- Store the tincture in a cool, dark place, and it should remain effective for up to a year.

Reishi Mushroom Tincture made with vegetable glycerin is an effective way to leverage the adaptogenic and health-boosting properties of Reishi mushrooms, offering a natural solution to improve wellness without the use of alcohol.

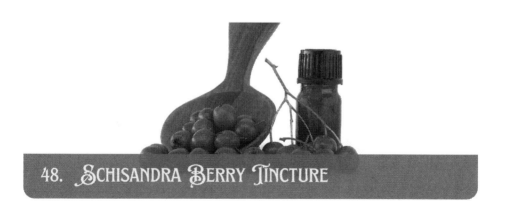

48. SCHISANDRA BERRY TINCTURE

Introduction:

Schisandra Berry Tincture is a powerful adaptogenic supplement renowned for enhancing mental clarity, boosting liver function, and increasing energy levels. Schisandra berries, known for their unique five-flavor profile (sweet, sour, salty, bitter, and pungent), contain a range of beneficial compounds, including lignans, which contribute to their antioxidant, anti-inflammatory, and stress-reducing properties. Using vegetable glycerin as a solvent creates an alcohol-free tincture, suitable for individuals who prefer or need to avoid alcohol.

Ingredients and Measurements:

- 1 cup of dried Schisandra berries, finely chopped or powdered
- 2 cups of vegetable glycerin
- 1 cup of distilled water
- A clean glass jar with a tight-fitting lid
- A fine strainer or cheesecloth

Preparation:

- Place the dried Schisandra berries into the glass jar.
- In a separate container, mix the vegetable glycerin and distilled water to create a consistent solution. This blend ensures an efficient extraction of the active compounds from the Schisandra berries.
- Pour the glycerin-water mixture over the Schisandra berries, ensuring they are fully submerged.
- Seal the jar tightly and shake it well to mix the contents.
- Store the jar in a cool, dark place, shaking it daily for 4-6 weeks to facilitate the extraction process.

- After the infusion period, strain the mixture through a fine strainer or cheesecloth into another clean jar, pressing the berries to extract as much liquid as possible.
- Transfer the strained tincture to a dropper bottle for easy use.

How to Use:

- To enhance mental clarity and boost energy, take 1-2 dropperfuls (about 30-60 drops) of the tincture diluted in water or juice, up to three times a day.
- For liver support and overall wellness, the same dosage can be used, adjusting based on your body's response and needs.

Duration:

- Use the tincture regularly as part of a health regimen for cognitive and physical enhancement.
- Consult a healthcare professional for guidance on long-term use, particularly if you have existing health conditions or are taking other medications.
- Store the tincture in a cool, dark place, and it should remain effective for up to a year.
- Schisandra Berry Tincture made with vegetable glycerin is an effective way to leverage the adaptogenic and health-boosting properties of Schisandra berries, offering a natural solution to improve mental and physical performance without alcohol.

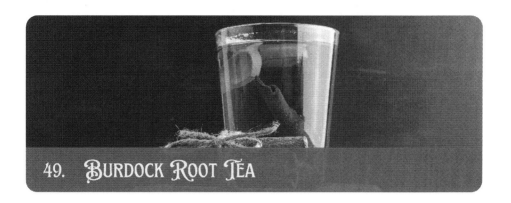

49. BURDOCK ROOT TEA

Introduction:

Burdock Root Tea is a nourishing herbal beverage known for its blood-purifying and detoxifying properties. Rich in antioxidants, vitamins, and minerals, burdock root supports liver function, promotes healthy skin, and aids in digestion. This tea has a mildly sweet, earthy flavor and serves as a gentle way to cleanse the body and boost overall health.

Ingredients and Measurements:

- 1 tablespoon of dried burdock root
- 2 cups of water
- Optional: honey or lemon to taste

Preparation:

☞ Place the dried burdock root in a pot.

☞ Add the water and bring the mixture to a boil.

☞ Once boiling, reduce the heat and allow the tea to simmer for 15-20 minutes. This slow simmer helps to extract the beneficial compounds from the burdock root effectively.

☞ Remove the pot from the heat and let the tea steep for an additional 10 minutes.

☞ Strain the tea into a cup or teapot, removing the burdock root.

How to Use:

☟ Enjoy a cup of Burdock Root Tea daily, especially in the morning or before meals, to aid in detoxification and improve digestion.

☟ Enhance the flavor and health benefits by adding a teaspoon of honey or a squeeze of lemon, if desired.

Duration:

⊘ Burdock Root Tea can be consumed regularly as part of a healthy routine to maintain detoxification and support liver health.

⊘ If using burdock root tea to address specific health issues, observe how your body responds and consult a healthcare professional if symptoms persist or for guidance on long-term use.

Burdock Root Tea is a simple and effective way to incorporate the health benefits of burdock root into your diet, offering a natural approach to enhancing detoxification and promoting overall wellness.

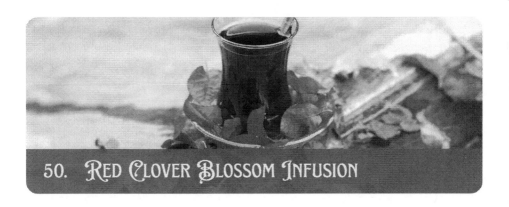

50. Red Clover Blossom Infusion

Introduction:

Red Clover Blossom Infusion is a herbal tea celebrated for its numerous health benefits, including supporting hormonal balance, improving cardiovascular health, and providing essential nutrients. Rich in isoflavones, a type of phytoestrogen, red clover blossoms help alleviate menopausal symptoms, reduce inflammation, and enhance skin health. This infusion has a mild, sweet flavor and is an excellent way to harness the therapeutic properties of red clover in a gentle, soothing form.

Ingredients and Measurements:

- 2 tablespoons of dried red clover blossoms
- 2 cups of boiling water
- Optional: honey or lemon to enhance flavor

Preparation:

- Place the dried red clover blossoms in a teapot or heat-resistant infuser.
- Pour the boiling water over the blossoms and cover to keep the essential oils and flavors intact.
- Allow the infusion to steep for 10-15 minutes, depending on your preferred strength and flavor intensity.
- Strain the infusion into a cup or teapot to remove the blossoms.

How to Use:

- Drink a cup of Red Clover Blossom Infusion once or twice daily to benefit from its hormonal balancing and cardiovascular health properties.
- If desired, sweeten the infusion with a teaspoon of honey or add a slice of lemon for extra flavor and additional health benefits.

Duration:

◉ Red Clover Blossom Infusion can be a part of your daily routine, particularly for those seeking natural support for hormonal balance and cardiovascular health.

◉ Monitor your body's response to the infusion, especially if using it for specific health concerns. Consult a healthcare professional if you have any conditions or are taking medications, as red clover can interact with certain drugs.

Red Clover Blossom Infusion offers a natural and enjoyable way to enjoy the health benefits of red clover, providing a nurturing and beneficial addition to a wellness-focused lifestyle.

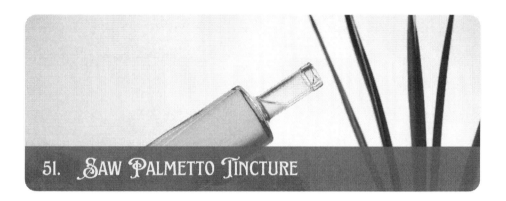

51. SAW PALMETTO TINCTURE

Introduction:

Saw Palmetto Tincture is a well-regarded herbal remedy primarily used for its benefits in supporting prostate health and balancing hormone levels. Extracted from the berries of the saw palmetto plant, this tincture is known for its ability to improve urinary function and reduce symptoms associated with benign prostatic hyperplasia (BPH). Using vegetable glycerin as the solvent makes this tincture an alcohol-free option suitable for various users, including those who prefer or need to avoid alcohol.

Ingredients and Measurements:

• 1 cup of dried saw palmetto berries, finely chopped or powdered

• 2 cups of vegetable glycerin

• 1 cup of distilled water

• A clean glass jar with a tight-fitting lid

• A fine strainer or cheesecloth

Preparation:

🖮 Place the dried saw palmetto berries into the glass jar.

🖮 In a separate container, mix the vegetable glycerin and distilled water to create a consistent solution.

This mixture ensures an effective extraction of the active compounds from the saw palmetto berries.

- Pour the glycerin-water mixture over the saw palmetto berries, ensuring they are fully submerged.
- Seal the jar tightly and shake it well to mix the contents.
- Store the jar in a cool, dark place, shaking it daily for 4-6 weeks to facilitate the extraction process.
- After the infusion period, strain the mixture through a fine strainer or cheesecloth into another clean jar, pressing the berries to extract as much liquid as possible.
- Transfer the strained tincture to a dropper bottle for ease of use.

How to Use:

- To support prostate health and improve urinary function, take 1-2 dropperfuls (about 30-60 drops) of the tincture diluted in water or juice, up to three times a day.

- Begin with a lower dose to observe how your body responds, and adjust as needed based on your health goals and response to the supplement.

Duration:

- Use the tincture regularly as part of a health regimen focused on maintaining prostate health and hormonal balance.
- Consult a healthcare professional for guidance on long-term use and to ensure the tincture's compatibility with any existing treatments or conditions.
- Store the tincture in a cool, dark place, and it should remain effective for up to a year.

Saw Palmetto Tincture made with vegetable glycerin is an effective way to harness the beneficial properties of saw palmetto, offering a natural solution to support prostate health and improve urinary function without the use of alcohol.

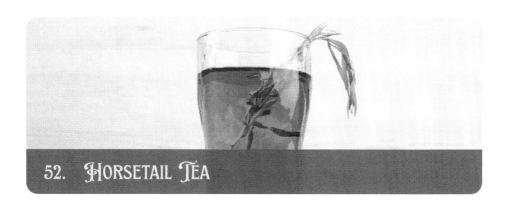

52. HORSETAIL TEA

Introduction:

Horsetail Tea is an herbal beverage known for its high silica content, which supports strong hair, nails, and bones. Horsetail, a plant with a long history of medicinal use, also has diuretic properties that aid in detoxification and reduce inflammation, particularly in the joints and urinary tract. This tea has a mild, slightly grassy flavor and is a simple way to incorporate the benefits of horsetail into your daily wellness routine.

Ingredients and Measurements:

- 1-2 teaspoons of dried horsetail
- 2 cups of boiling water
- Optional: honey or lemon to taste

Preparation:

⚗ Place the dried horsetail in a teapot or heat-resistant infuser.

⚗ Pour the boiling water over the horsetail and cover to preserve the essential nutrients and flavors.

⚗ Let the tea steep for 10-15 minutes, depending on how strong you prefer the flavor.

⚗ Strain the tea into a cup to remove the horsetail.

How to Use:

🌿 Enjoy a cup of Horsetail Tea once or twice a day to benefit from its supportive properties for hair, nails, and bones, as well as its detoxifying effects.

🌿 Enhance the flavor and additional health benefits by adding a teaspoon of honey or a slice of lemon, if desired.

Duration:

⊘ Horsetail Tea can be consumed regularly as part of a healthy routine to maintain and support overall wellness.

⊘ If using horsetail tea to address specific health concerns, such as joint inflammation or urinary tract issues, observe your body's response and consult a healthcare professional if symptoms persist or for guidance on long-term use.

Horsetail Tea is an effective and enjoyable way to enjoy the natural benefits of horsetail, offering a straightforward approach to enhancing health and wellness.

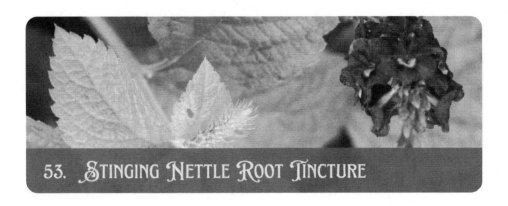

53. STINGING NETTLE ROOT TINCTURE

Introduction:

Stinging Nettle Root Tincture is a potent herbal extract known for its anti-inflammatory and diuretic properties. This tincture is particularly effective in supporting prostate health, alleviating symptoms of benign prostatic hyperplasia (BPH), and enhancing urinary function. Nettle root also contains compounds that can help balance hormones and reduce inflammation throughout the body. Using vegetable glycerin as the extraction medium ensures an alcohol-free tincture, making it suitable for a wide range of users, including those who avoid alcohol.

Ingredients and Measurements:

- 1 cup of dried stinging nettle root, finely chopped or powdered
- 2 cups of vegetable glycerin
- 1 cup of distilled water
- A clean glass jar with a tight-fitting lid
- A fine strainer or cheesecloth

Preparation:

☞ Place the dried stinging nettle root into the glass jar.

☞ Mix the vegetable glycerin and distilled water in a separate container to create a consistent solution. This mixture ensures efficient extraction of the active compounds from the nettle root.

☞ Pour the glycerin-water mixture over the nettle root, making sure the root is fully submerged.

☞ Seal the jar tightly and shake it well to combine the contents.

☞ Store the jar in a cool, dark place, shaking it daily for 4-6 weeks to facilitate the extraction process.

After the infusion period, strain the mixture through a fine strainer or cheesecloth into another clean jar, pressing the root to extract as much liquid as possible.

Transfer the strained tincture to a dropper bottle for easy use.

How to Use:

To support prostate health and improve urinary function, take 1-2 dropperfuls (about 30-60 drops) of the tincture diluted in water or juice, up to three times a day.

For reducing inflammation and balancing hormones, the same dosage can be used, adjusting based on your body's response and needs.

Duration:

Use the tincture regularly as part of a health regimen focused on maintaining prostate health and hormonal balance.

Consult a healthcare professional for guidance on long-term use and to ensure the tincture's compatibility with any existing treatments or conditions.

Store the tincture in a cool, dark place, and it should remain effective for up to a year.

Stinging Nettle Root Tincture made with vegetable glycerin is an effective way to harness the beneficial properties of stinging nettle root, offering a natural solution to support prostate health, urinary function, and overall wellness without the use of alcohol.

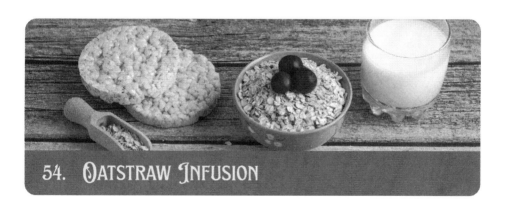

54. OATSTRAW INFUSION

Introduction:

Oatstraw Infusion is a nourishing herbal drink known for its soothing and restorative properties. Made from the green stems and leaves of the oat plant, this infusion is rich in vitamins, minerals, and antioxidants. It supports nervous system health, aids in stress reduction, and improves bone density. Oatstraw has a mild, slightly sweet taste and is a gentle way to enhance overall vitality and wellness.

Ingredients and Measurements:

- 1/4 cup of dried oatstraw
- 4 cups of boiling water
- Optional: honey or lemon to taste

Preparation:

- Place the dried oatstraw in a large heat-resistant jar or teapot.

- Pour the boiling water over the oatstraw and cover to keep the essential nutrients intact.

- Allow the infusion to steep for 4-8 hours or overnight for a stronger and more nutrient-rich drink.

- Strain the infusion into a cup or pitcher, removing the oatstraw.

How to Use:

- Drink 1-2 cups of Oatstraw Infusion daily to benefit from its supportive properties for the nervous system, bone health, and overall vitality.

- If desired, enhance the flavor with a teaspoon of honey or a slice of lemon.

Duration:

- Oatstraw Infusion can be consumed regularly as part of a balanced diet to maintain health and wellness.

- Monitor your body's response to the infusion, especially if using it for specific health concerns, and adjust your intake accordingly. Consult a healthcare professional if you have any conditions or are taking medications, as oatstraw can interact with certain drugs.

Oatstraw Infusion is a simple and effective way to incorporate the health benefits of oatstraw into your daily routine, providing a natural and nurturing approach to supporting health and wellness.

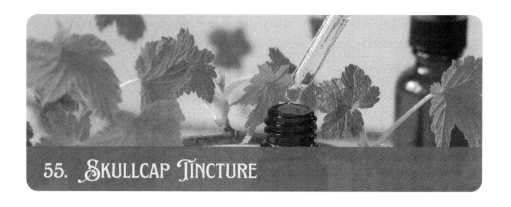

55. SKULLCAP TINCTURE

Introduction:

Skullcap Tincture is a valuable herbal extract known for its calming and neuroprotective properties. Skullcap, particularly the American variety (Scutellaria lateriflora), is used to alleviate anxiety, improve sleep, and support overall nervous system health. Its active compounds, including flavonoids and glycosides, help reduce stress and promote a balanced mood. Using vegetable glycerin as the solvent ensures this tincture is alcohol-free, making it suitable for a variety of users.

Ingredients and Measurements:

- 1 cup of dried skullcap leaves and flowers, finely chopped or powdered
- 2 cups of vegetable glycerin
- 1 cup of distilled water
- A clean glass jar with a tight-fitting lid
- A fine strainer or cheesecloth

Preparation:

☞ Place the dried skullcap into the glass jar.

☞ In a separate container, mix the vegetable glycerin and distilled water to create a consistent solution. This mixture will effectively extract the beneficial compounds from the skullcap.

☞ Pour the glycerin-water mixture over the skullcap, ensuring the plant material is fully submerged.

☞ Seal the jar tightly and shake it to mix the contents thoroughly.

☞ Store the jar in a cool, dark place, shaking it daily for 4-6 weeks to facilitate the extraction process.

☞ After the infusion period, strain the mixture through a fine strainer or cheesecloth into another clean jar, pressing the plant material to extract as much liquid as possible.

☞ Transfer the strained tincture to a dropper bottle for ease of use.

How to Use:

⟴ To help reduce anxiety and support relaxation, take 1-2 dropperfuls (about 30-60 drops) of the tincture diluted in water or juice, up to three times a day.

For improving sleep, take the tincture 30 minutes to an hour before bedtime.

Duration:

- Use the tincture regularly as part of a health regimen for managing stress and enhancing nervous system health.
- Consult a healthcare professional for guidance on long-term use, especially if you have existing health conditions or are taking other medications.

Store the tincture in a cool, dark place, and it should remain effective for up to a year.

Skullcap Tincture made with vegetable glycerin is an effective way to leverage the soothing and neuroprotective properties of skullcap, offering a natural solution to improve mental well-being and support a balanced lifestyle without the use of alcohol.

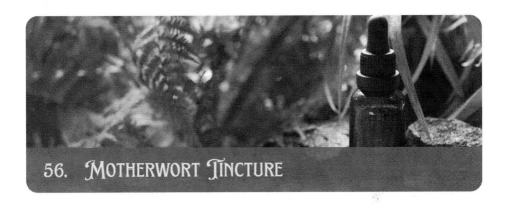

56. MOTHERWORT TINCTURE

Introduction:

Motherwort Tincture is an esteemed herbal remedy known for its ability to soothe the heart and calm the nerves. Motherwort, scientifically known as Leonurus cardiaca, is particularly beneficial for managing heart palpitations, reducing anxiety, and easing symptoms of menopause. Its active compounds, including leonurine and stachydrine, promote relaxation and support cardiovascular health. Using vegetable glylycerin as the extraction medium creates an alcohol-free tincture, suitable for various users, especially those who avoid alcohol.

Ingredients and Measurements:

- 1 cup of dried motherwort herb, finely chopped or powdered
- 2 cups of vegetable glycerin
- 1 cup of distilled water

- A clean glass jar with a tight-fitting lid
- A fine strainer or cheesecloth

Preparation:

☞ Place the dried motherwort into the glass jar.

☞ Mix the vegetable glycerin and distilled water in a separate container to ensure a homogeneous solution. This blend effectively extracts the beneficial compounds from the motherwort.

☞ Pour the glycerin-water mixture over the motherwort, ensuring the herb is fully submerged.

☞ Seal the jar tightly and shake it well to combine the ingredients.

☞ Store the jar in a cool, dark place, shaking it daily for 4-6 weeks to promote the extraction process.

☞ After the infusion period, strain the mixture through a fine strainer or cheesecloth into another clean jar, pressing the herb to extract as much liquid as possible.

☞ Transfer the strained tincture to a dropper bottle for ease of use.

How to Use:

↳ To alleviate heart palpitations and reduce anxiety, take 1-2 dropperfuls (about 30-60 drops) of the tincture diluted in water or juice, up to three times a day.

↳ For easing menopausal symptoms, particularly hot flashes and mood swings, the same dosage can be taken.

Duration:

◎ Use the tincture regularly as part of a health regimen for cardiovascular and nervous system support.

◎ Consult a healthcare professional for guidance on long-term use, especially if you have existing health conditions or are taking other medications.

◎ Store the tincture in a cool, dark place, and it should remain effective for up to a year.

Motherwort Tincture made with vegetable glycerin is an effective way to harness the soothing and heart-supportive properties of motherwort, offering a natural solution to improve emotional balance and heart health without alcohol.

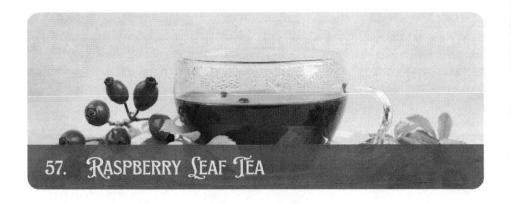

57. RASPBERRY LEAF TEA

Introduction:

Raspberry Leaf Tea is a traditional herbal beverage renowned for its benefits to women's reproductive health, particularly during pregnancy. Raspberry leaves are rich in vitamins and minerals like magnesium, potassium, iron, and B vitamins. These nutrients contribute to toning the uterine muscles, easing menstrual cramps, and supporting overall reproductive health. This tea has a subtle, pleasant taste similar to black tea but without the caffeine.

Ingredients and Measurements:

- 1-2 tablespoons of dried raspberry leaves
- 2 cups of boiling water
- Optional: honey or lemon to taste

Preparation:

🫖 Place the dried raspberry leaves in a teapot or a heat-resistant infuser.

🫖 Pour the boiling water over the leaves and cover to preserve the essential nutrients and flavors.

🫖 Let the tea steep for 10-15 minutes, depending on your preferred strength and flavor intensity.

🫖 Strain the tea into a cup to remove the leaves.

How to Use:

🥄 Drink 1-2 cups of Raspberry Leaf Tea daily, especially beneficial for women during the second and third trimesters of pregnancy, to help prepare the uterus for labor.

🥄 Enjoy the tea regularly to alleviate menstrual cramps and support reproductive health.

🥄 Enhance the flavor and additional health benefits by adding a teaspoon of honey or a slice of lemon, if desired.

Duration:

⊘ Raspberry Leaf Tea can be consumed regularly as part of a healthy routine to maintain reproductive health and ease menstrual discomfort.

Pregnant women should consult a healthcare professional before starting or continuing raspberry leaf tea, especially in the first trimester, to ensure it's appropriate for their specific health situation.

Raspberry Leaf Tea is a simple and effective way to incorporate the health benefits of raspberry leaves into your daily life, offering a natural approach to enhancing reproductive health and well-being.

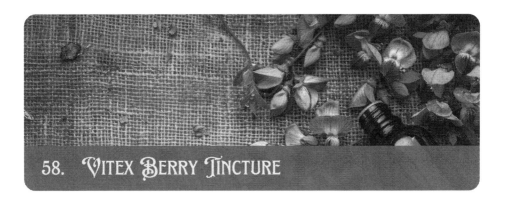

58. VITEX BERRY TINCTURE

Introduction:

Vitex Berry Tincture is an acclaimed herbal remedy known for its effectiveness in balancing hormones and supporting reproductive health in women. Vitex, also known as chaste tree or chasteberry, helps regulate menstrual cycles, alleviate symptoms of premenstrual syndrome (PMS), and improve fertility. Using vegetable glycerin as the solvent for this tincture ensures an alcohol-free product, making it suitable for a wide range of users, including those who prefer or need to avoid alcohol.

Ingredients and Measurements:

- 1 cup of dried Vitex berries, finely chopped or powdered

- 2 cups of vegetable glycerin

- 1 cup of distilled water

- A clean glass jar with a tight-fitting lid

- A fine strainer or cheesecloth

Preparation:

☞ Place the dried Vitex berries into the glass jar.

☞ In a separate container, mix the vegetable glycerin and distilled water to create a consistent solution. This mixture ensures an efficient extraction of the active compounds from the Vitex berries.

☞ Pour the glycerin-water mixture over the Vitex berries, ensuring they are fully submerged.

☞ Seal the jar tightly and shake it to mix the contents well.

- Store the jar in a cool, dark place, shaking it daily for 4-6 weeks to promote the extraction process.
- After the infusion period, strain the mixture through a fine strainer or cheesecloth into another clean jar, pressing the berries to extract as much liquid as possible.
- Transfer the strained tincture to a dropper bottle for ease of use.

How to Use:

- To help balance hormones and alleviate PMS or menopausal symptoms, take 1-2 dropperfuls (about 30-60 drops) of the tincture diluted in water or juice, once or twice a day.
- For fertility support, the same dosage can be taken, adjusting based on your body's response and specific health goals.

Duration:

- Use the tincture regularly as part of a health regimen for hormonal balance and reproductive health.
- Consult a healthcare professional for guidance on long-term use, especially if you have existing health conditions or are taking other medications.
- Store the tincture in a cool, dark place, and it should remain effective for up to a year.

Vitex Berry Tincture made with vegetable glycerin is an effective way to harness the hormone-balancing and reproductive health-supporting properties of Vitex, offering a natural solution to improve well-being without the use of alcohol.

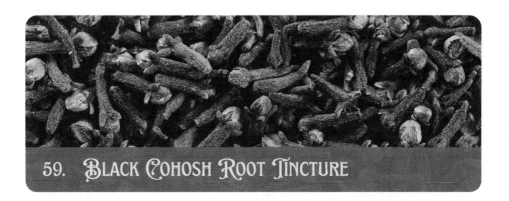

59. BLACK COHOSH ROOT TINCTURE

Introduction:

Black Cohosh Root Tincture is a respected herbal remedy commonly used to manage menopausal symptoms such as hot flashes, mood swings, and sleep disturbances. Black cohosh, a plant native to North America, contains compounds that mimic estrogenic activity, helping to balance hormone levels and provide relief during menopause. Using vegetable glycerin as the solvent creates an alcohol-free tincture, making it suitable for a variety of users, especially those who prefer or need to avoid alcohol.

Ingredients and Measurements:

- 1 cup of dried black cohosh root, finely chopped or powdered
- 2 cups of vegetable glycerin
- 1 cup of distilled water
- A clean glass jar with a tight-fitting lid
- A fine strainer or cheesecloth

Preparation:

- Place the dried black cohosh root into the glass jar.
- Mix the vegetable glycerin and distilled water in a separate container to ensure a uniform solution. This mixture effectively extracts the active compounds from the black cohosh root.
- Pour the glycerin-water mixture over the black cohosh root, ensuring it is completely submerged.
- Seal the jar tightly and shake it well to mix the contents thoroughly.
- Store the jar in a cool, dark place, shaking it daily for 4-6 weeks to facilitate the extraction process.
- After the infusion period, strain the mixture through a fine strainer or cheesecloth into another clean jar, pressing the root to extract as much liquid as possible.
- Transfer the strained tincture to a dropper bottle for ease of use.

How to Use:

- To alleviate menopausal symptoms such as hot flashes and mood swings, take 1-2 dropperfuls (about 30-60 drops) of the tincture diluted in water or juice, once or twice a day.
- Start with a lower dose to observe how your body responds, and adjust as necessary based on your health goals and reaction to the supplement.

Duration:

- Use the tincture regularly as part of a health regimen for managing menopausal symptoms.
- Consult a healthcare professional for guidance on long-term use, especially if you have existing health conditions or are taking other medications.
- Store the tincture in a cool, dark place, and it should remain effective for up to a year.

Black Cohosh Root Tincture made with vegetable glycerin is an effective way to leverage the hormone-balancing and menopausal symptom-relieving properties of black cohosh, offering a natural solution to improve well-being without the use of alcohol.

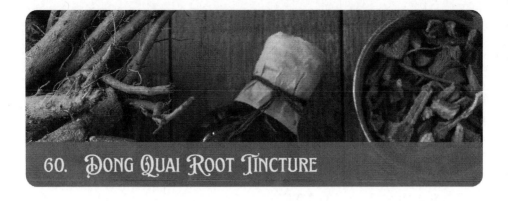

60. Dong Quai Root Tincture

Introduction:

Dong Quai Root Tincture is a powerful herbal supplement renowned for its ability to support women's reproductive health. Often referred to as "female ginseng," Dong Quai is used to balance hormones, alleviate menstrual cramps, and improve blood circulation. Its active compounds, including phytoestrogens, make it particularly beneficial for managing PMS and menopausal symptoms. Using vegetable glycerin as the solvent ensures this tincture is alcohol-free, suitable for individuals who prefer or need to avoid alcohol.

Ingredients and Measurements:

- 1 cup of dried Dong Quai root, finely chopped or powdered
- 2 cups of vegetable glycerin
- 1 cup of distilled water
- A clean glass jar with a tight-fitting lid
- A fine strainer or cheesecloth

Preparation:

🝑 Place the dried Dong Quai root into the glass jar.

🝑 In a separate container, mix the vegetable glycerin and distilled water to create a consistent solution. This blend ensures an effective extraction of the active compounds from Dong Quai.

🝑 Pour the glycerin-water mixture over the Dong Quai root, ensuring the root is fully submerged.

🝑 Seal the jar tightly and shake it well to combine the ingredients.

🝑 Store the jar in a cool, dark place, shaking it daily for 4-6 weeks to promote the extraction process.

🝑 After the infusion period, strain the mixture through a fine strainer or cheesecloth into another clean jar, pressing the root to extract as much liquid as possible.

🝑 Transfer the strained tincture to a dropper bottle for ease of use.

How to Use:

🝑 To support hormonal balance and alleviate menstrual cramps, take 1-2 dropperfuls (about 30-60 drops) of the tincture diluted in water or juice, once or twice a day, especially during the menstrual cycle or when experiencing symptoms.

- ↳ For menopausal support, the same dosage can be taken, adjusting based on your body's response and specific health goals.

Duration:

- ⊘ Use the tincture regularly as part of a health regimen for reproductive health and hormonal balance.

- ⊘ Consult a healthcare professional for guidance on long-term use, particularly if you have existing health conditions or are taking other medications.

- ⊘ Store the tincture in a cool, dark place, and it should remain effective for up to a year.

Dong Quai Root Tincture made with vegetable glycerin is an effective way to harness the reproductive health-supporting and hormone-balancing properties of Dong Quai, offering a natural solution to improve well-being without the use of alcohol.

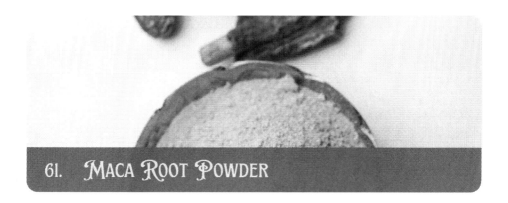

61. MACA ROOT POWDER

Introduction:

Maca Root Powder is a highly nutritious supplement derived from the maca plant, traditionally grown in the Andes Mountains of Peru. Renowned for its energy-boosting, hormone-balancing, and libido-enhancing properties, maca is rich in essential vitamins, minerals, and amino acids. Its adaptogenic qualities help the body manage stress and improve overall vitality, making it a popular choice for enhancing physical and mental performance.

Ingredients and Measurements:

- • Pure maca root powder (no additional ingredients required for preparation)

Preparation:

⬚ Maca root powder is ready to use and does not require preparation. It can be directly incorporated into various foods and beverages.

How to Use:

✎ Add 1-2 teaspoons of maca root powder to smoothies, juices, yogurt, or hot cereals to boost nutritional content and energy levels.

✎ Incorporate maca powder into baking recipes or energy bars for an added health benefit.

✎ For a simple beverage, mix maca powder with warm milk or a milk alternative, and sweeten with honey or maple syrup if desired.

Duration:

⊘ Maca root powder can be consumed daily as part of a balanced diet to support energy, hormonal balance, and overall wellness.

⊘ Start with a lower dose to see how your body reacts, and adjust the amount based on your health goals and response to the supplement.

⊘ Consult a healthcare professional if you have any health conditions or are taking medications, as maca can interact with certain drugs.

Maca Root Powder is an effective and versatile way to enhance your diet and improve health, offering a natural approach to increasing energy, balancing hormones, and boosting libido.

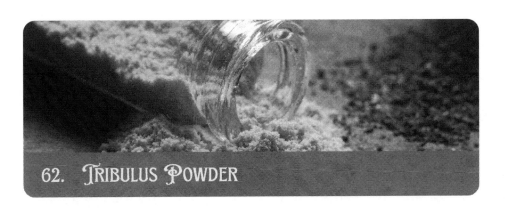

62. TRIBULUS POWDER

Introduction:

Tribulus Powder is derived from the Tribulus terrestris plant, known for its potential to enhance athletic performance, increase libido, and support overall vitality. This herbal supplement is popular among athletes and those seeking natural ways to improve sexual health and hormone balance. Tribulus contains active compounds like saponins, which are believed to boost testosterone levels and improve muscle strength and recovery.

Ingredients and Measurements:

- Pure Tribulus terrestris powder (ready to use without further preparation)

Preparation:

☞ Tribulus Powder is conveniently ready for immediate use and does not require additional preparation steps.

How to Use:

✎ Mix 1-2 teaspoons of Tribulus powder into smoothies, shakes, or juice to integrate it seamlessly into your diet.

✎ Sprinkle the powder over meals or incorporate it into energy bars or other snacks for an extra health boost.

✎ For a direct approach, you can mix the powder with water or your preferred beverage and consume it once or twice daily.

Duration:

⊘ Tribulus Powder can be part of your daily regimen to enhance athletic performance, support sexual health, and maintain hormone balance.

⊘ Monitor your body's response to the supplement, starting with a smaller dose and adjusting based on your specific health goals and reactions.

⊘ Consult a healthcare professional before starting Tribulus, especially if you have underlying health issues or are taking medications, to avoid potential interactions and ensure safe usage.

Tribulus Powder offers a natural and straightforward way to harness the benefits of Tribulus terrestris, providing support for increased energy, improved sexual health, and enhanced athletic performance.

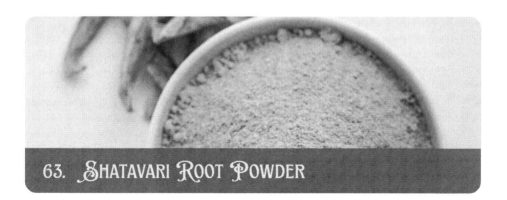

63. SHATAVARI ROOT POWDER

Introduction:

Shatavari Root Powder is a revered herbal supplement in Ayurvedic medicine, known for its potent benefits in supporting women's reproductive health. Shatavari, which means "a woman with a hundred husbands," is often used to enhance fertility, regulate menstrual cycles, and alleviate symptoms of menopause. It is also beneficial for digestive health and immune system support due to its adaptogenic properties.

Ingredients and Measurements:

- Pure Shatavari root powder (ready for use without further preparation)

Preparation:

⛩ Shatavari Root Powder is ready touse and requires no additional steps for preparation.

How to Use:

↳ Mix 1-2 teaspoons of Shatavari root powder into warm milk or a milk alternative to create a nourishing drink. You can sweeten this with honey if desired.

↳ Add the powder to smoothies, juices, or yogurts for an easy way to incorporate it into your daily diet.

↳ For direct intake, the powder can be mixed into a glass of water and consumed once or twice daily.

Duration:

⊘ Shatavari Root Powder can be taken daily as part of a healthy routine to support reproductive health, digestive wellness, and overall vitality.

⊘ Start with a lower dose to observe how your body responds, and adjust the amount based on your health needs and reaction to the supplement..

⊘ Consult a healthcare professional, especially if you are pregnant, breastfeeding, or have any existing health conditions, to ensure the supplement is appropriate for your specific situation.

Shatavari Root Powder is an effective and versatile supplement that offers a natural approach to improving reproductive health, enhancing digestive function, and boosting overall vitality.

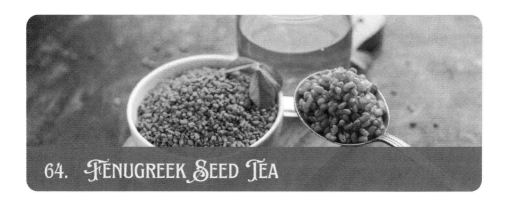

64. FENUGREEK SEED TEA

Introduction:

Fenugreek Seed Tea is a healthful beverage known for its distinct aromatic and slightly sweet flavor, offering a range of benefits from enhancing lactation in nursing mothers to improving glucose metabolism. Rich in fiber, minerals, and phytonutrients, fenugreek seeds help regulate blood sugar levels, reduce inflammation, and support digestive health.

Ingredients and Measurements:

- 1-2 teaspoons of fenugreek seeds
- 2 cups of water
- Optional: honey or lemon to taste

Preparation:

⛶ Lightly crush the fenugreek seeds to release their flavor and active compounds.

⛶ Boil the water in a pot and add the crushed fenugreek seeds.

⛶ Reduce the heat and let the seeds simmer for about 5-10 minutes. The longer you simmer, the stronger the tea will be.

⛶ Remove from heat and let the tea steep for an additional 5-10 minutes.

⛶ Strain the tea into a cup, removing the fenugreek seeds.

How to Use:

↳ Drink a cup of Fenugreek Seed Tea once or twice a day to benefit from its health properties, particularly for blood sugar regulation and digestive support.

↳ If desired, enhance the flavor with a teaspoon of honey or a squeeze of lemon.

Duration:

⊘ Fenugreek Seed Tea can be consumed regularly as part of a healthy lifestyle to maintain blood sugar levels, support digestion, and for nursing mothers, to aid lactation.

⊘ Monitor your body's response to the tea, particularly if using it for specific health issues. Consult a healthcare professional if you have any underlying conditions or are taking medications, as fenugreek can interact with certain drugs.

Fenugreek Seed Tea is an easy and effective way to enjoy the nutritional benefits of fenugreek, offering a natural solution to improve health and well-being.

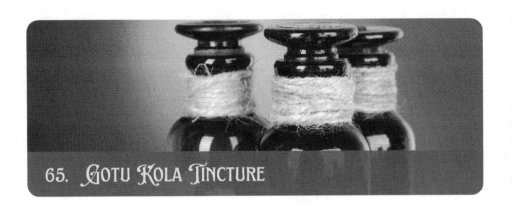

65. GOTU KOLA TINCTURE

Introduction:

Gotu Kola Tincture is a revered herbal extract known for its impressive benefits in enhancing cognitive function, supporting skin health, and promoting wound healing. Gotu Kola, a staple in traditional Asian medicine, is celebrated for its ability to improve circulation, reduce anxiety, and support overall brain health. By utilizing vegetable glycerin as the extraction medium, this tincture provides an alcohol-free alternative suitable for various users, including those who avoid alcohol.

Ingredients and Measurements:

- 1 cup of dried Gotu Kola leaves, finely chopped or powdered
- 2 cups of vegetable glycerin
- 1 cup of distilled water
- A clean glass jar with a tight-fitting lid
- A fine strainer or cheesecloth

Preparation:

- Place the dried Gotu Kola leaves into the glass jar.

- Mix the vegetable glycerin and distilled water in a separate container to create a consistent solution. This mixture ensures an effective extraction of the active compounds from Gotu Kola.

- Pour the glycerin-water mixture over the Gotu Kola leaves, ensuring they are fully submerged.

- Seal the jar tightly and shake it well to combine the ingredients.

- Store the jar in a cool, dark place, shaking it daily for 4-6 weeks to facilitate the extraction process.

- After the infusion period, strain the mixture through a fine strainer or cheesecloth into another clean jar, pressing the leaves to extract as much liquid as possible.

Transfer the strained tincture to a dropper bottle for ease of use.

How to Use:

To enhance cognitive function and reduce anxiety, take 1-2 dropperfuls (about 30-60 drops) of the tincture diluted in water or juice, up to three times a day.

For supporting skin health and promoting wound healing, the same dosage can be applied, adjusting based on your body's response and needs.

Duration:

Use the tincture regularly as part of a health regimen for cognitive enhancement, anxiety reduction, and skin health support.

Consult a healthcare professional for guidance on long-term use, especially if you have existing health conditions or are taking other medications.

Store the tincture in a cool, dark place, and it should remain effective for up to a year.

Gotu Kola Tincture made with vegetable glycerin is an effective way to leverage the healing and cognitive-enhancing properties of Gotu Kola, offering a natural solution to improve mental and physical well-being without the use of alcohol.

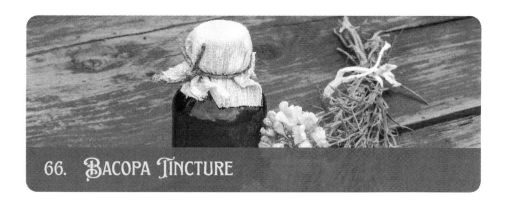

66. BACOPA TINCTURE

Introduction:

Bacopa Tincture is a potent herbal extract derived from Bacopa monnieri, a plant celebrated for its cognitive-enhancing properties. Often used in Ayurvedic medicine, Bacopa is known for improving memory, increasing focus, and reducing stress. This tincture, made with vegetable glycerin, provides an alcohol-free way to harness the benefits of Bacopa, making it suitable for a wide range of users including those who prefer to avoid alcohol.

Ingredients and Measurements:

- 1 cup of dried Bacopa monnieri leaves, finely chopped or powdered
- 2 cups of vegetable glycerin
- 1 cup of distilled water
- A clean glass jar with a tight-fitting lid
- A fine strainer or cheesecloth

Preparation:

🝨 Place the dried Bacopa leaves into the glass jar.

🝨 Mix the vegetable glycerin and distilled water in a separate container to create a consistent solution. This blend ensures efficient extraction of the active compounds from Bacopa.

🝨 Pour the glycerin-water mixture over the Bacopa leaves, ensuring they are fully submerged.

🝨 Seal the jar tightly and shake it well to combine the ingredients.

🝨 Store the jar in a cool, dark place, shaking it daily for 4-6 weeks to promote the extraction process.

🝨 After the infusion period, strain the mixture through a fine strainer or cheesecloth into another clean jar, pressing the leaves to extract as much liquid as possible.

🝨 Transfer the strained tincture to a dropper bottle for ease of use.

How to Use:

🝨 To enhance cognitive function and reduce mental fatigue, take 1-2 dropperfuls (about 30-60 drops) of the tincture diluted in water or juice, up to three times a day.

🝨 Begin with a lower dose to observe how your body responds, and adjust as necessary based on your health goals and reaction to the supplement.

Duration:

⊘ Use the tincture regularly as part of a health regimen for cognitive enhancement and stress reduction.

⊘ Consult a healthcare professional for guidance on long-term use, especially if you have existing health conditions or are taking other medications.

⊘ Store the tincture in a cool, dark place, and it should remain effective for up to a year.

Bacopa Tincture made with vegetable glycerin is an effective way to leverage the cognitive-enhancing properties of Bacopa monnieri, offering a natural solution to improve mental performance and well-being without the use of alcohol.

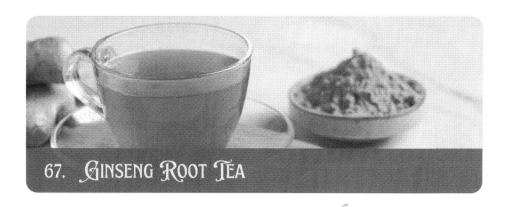

67. GINSENG ROOT TEA

Introduction:

Ginseng Root Tea is a revered herbal drink known for its energy-boosting and immune-enhancing properties. Ginseng, particularly Asian (Panax) ginseng, is celebrated for its adaptogenic effects, helping the body resist stress, improve mental performance, and support overall vitality. This tea has a distinctive, slightly bitter flavor and offers a natural way to increase stamina and reduce fatigue.

Ingredients and Measurements:

- 1-2 teaspoons of dried ginseng root, sliced or chopped
- 2 cups of water
- Optional: honey or lemon to taste

Preparation:

☕ Place the dried ginseng root slices in a pot.

☕ Add the water and bring the mixture to a boil.

☕ Once boiling, reduce the heat and allow the tea to simmer for 15-20 minutes. The longer you simmer, the stronger the tea will be and the more beneficial compounds will be extracted.

☕ Remove from heat and let the tea steep for an additional 5-10 minutes.

☕ Strain the tea into a cup, removing the ginseng root.

How to Use:

🥄 Enjoy a cup of Ginseng Root Tea daily, preferably in the morning or early afternoon, to benefit from its energizing and health-boosting effects.

🥄 If desired, enhance the flavor with a teaspoon of honey or a slice of lemon.

Duration:

⊘ Ginseng Root Tea can be consumed regularly as part of a healthy lifestyle to maintain energy levels, support immune function, and improve mental clarity.

⊘ Monitor your body's response to the tea, especially if using it for specific health benefits. Consult a healthcare professional if you have any underlying conditions or are taking medications, as ginseng can interact with certain drugs.

Ginseng Root Tea is an effective and enjoyable way to incorporate the health benefits of ginseng into your daily routine, offering a natural approach to boosting energy, enhancing immunity, and supporting overall well-being.

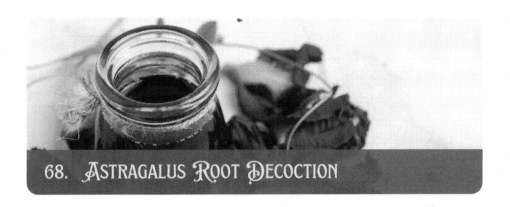

68. ASTRAGALUS ROOT DECOCTION

Introduction:

Astragalus Root Decoction is a powerful herbal brew known for its immune-boosting and adaptogenic properties. Originating from traditional Chinese medicine, Astragalus root helps enhance the body's resistance to stress, supports cardiovascular health, and promotes overall vitality. This decoction has a mild, sweet taste and is effective in fortifying the immune system, especially during times of seasonal change or increased stress.

Ingredients and Measurements:

- 1-2 tablespoons of dried Astragalus root slices
- 4 cups of water
- Optional: honey or lemon to taste

Preparation:

- Place the dried Astragalus root slices in a pot.
- Add the water and bring the mixture to a boil.
- Once boiling, reduce the heat and allow the decoction to simmer for 30-60 minutes. The longer you simmer, the more concentrated and potent the brew will be, extracting more of the beneficial compounds.
- Remove from heat and let the decoction steep for an additional 10-15 minutes.
- Strain the decoction into a cup or pitcher, removing the Astragalus root.

How to Use:

🥄 Drink 1 cup of Astragalus Root Decoction 1-2 times daily to boost the immune system and support overall health.

🥄 Enhance the flavor and add health benefits by sweetening with a teaspoon of honey or a squeeze of lemon, if desired.

Duration:

🕑 Astragalus Root Decoction can be consumed regularly as part of a health-focused routine to maintain immunity, particularly during seasons when you are more susceptible to illness.

🕑 Monitor your body's response to the decoction, especially if using it for specific health issues, and adjust your intake accordingly. Consult a healthcare professional if you have any underlying conditions or are taking medications, as Astragalus can interact with certain drugs.

Astragalus Root Decoction is a simple and effective way to enjoy the health benefits of Astragalus root, providing a natural approach to enhancing immunity and improving overall vitality.

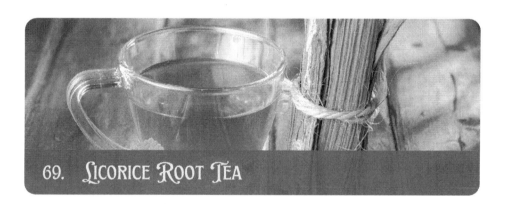

69. Licorice Root Tea

Introduction:

Licorice Root Tea is a sweet and soothing herbal beverage renowned for its beneficial effects on digestive health, respiratory function, and stress relief. Licorice root contains glycyrrhizin, which helps soothe gastrointestinal issues, acts as an expectorant for respiratory ailments, and supports adrenal function to manage stress. Its naturally sweet flavor makes it a popular choice for a comforting tea.

Ingredients and Measurements:

- 1-2 teaspoons of dried licorice root
- 2 cups of water

- Optional: honey or lemon to enhance flavor

Preparation:

☞ Place the dried licorice root in a pot.

☞ Add the water and bring the mixture to a boil.

☞ Once boiling, reduce the heat and let the tea simmer for 10-15 minutes. This allows for a thorough extraction of the licorice root's beneficial compounds.

☞ Remove from heat and let the tea steep for an additional 5-10 minutes.

☞ Strain the tea into a cup, removing the licorice root.

How to Use:

✍ Drink a cup of Licorice Root Tea 1-2 times a day to benefit from its digestive and respiratory support.

✍ If desired, adjust the flavor with a teaspoon of honey or a slice of lemon.

Duration:

🕐 Licorice Root Tea can be part of your daily routine, especially beneficial for soothing digestive discomfort and easing respiratory symptoms.

🕐 Monitor your body's response to the tea, particularly if using it for specific health benefits. Consult a healthcare professional if you have high blood pressure, kidney problems, or are on medication, as licorice can interact with certain drugs and cause side effects due to glycyrrhizin.

Licorice Root Tea is an enjoyable and effective way to incorporate the health benefits of licorice root into your diet, offering a natural solution to improve digestion, respiratory function, and stress management.

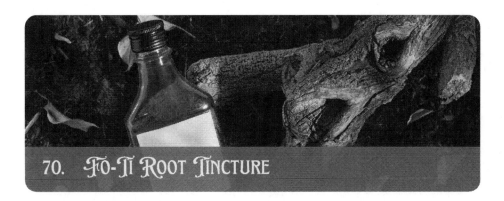

70. FO-TI ROOT TINCTURE

Introduction:

Fo-Ti Root Tincture is a valuable herbal extract derived from a plant also known as He Shou Wu, celebrated in traditional Chinese medicine for its rejuvenating and anti-aging properties. Fo-Ti is believed to enhance longevity, improve hair and skin health, and support liver and kidney function. Utilizing vegetable glycerin as the extraction medium, this tincture provides an alcohol-free option, making it suitable for individuals who prefer or need to avoid alcohol.

Ingredients and Measurements:

- 1 cup of dried Fo-Ti root, finely chopped or powdered
- 2 cups of vegetable glycerin
- 1 cup of distilled water
- A clean glass jar with a tight-fitting lid
- A fine strainer or cheesecloth

Preparation:

☞ Place the dried Fo-Ti root into the glass jar.

☞ In a separate container, mix the vegetable glycerin and distilled water to create a homogeneous solution. This mixture ensures efficient extraction of the active compounds from Fo-Ti.

☞ Pour the glycerin-water mixture over the Fo-Ti root, making sure the root is fully submerged.

☞ Seal the jar tightly and shake it to mix the contents well.

☞ Store the jar in a cool, dark place, shaking it daily for 4-6 weeks to facilitate the extraction process.

☞ After the infusion period, strain the mixture through a fine strainer or cheesecloth into another clean jar, pressing the root to extract as much liquid as possible.

☞ Transfer the strained tincture to a dropper bottle for ease of use.

How to Use:

✎ To support anti-aging, hair and skin health, and overall vitality, take 1-2 dropperfuls (about 30-60 drops) of the tincture diluted in water or juice, up to three times a day.

✎ Begin with a lower dose to observe how your body responds, and adjust as necessary based on your health goals and reaction to the supplement.

Duration:

⊘ Use the tincture regularly as part of a health regimen for longevity and vitality.

⊘ Consult a healthcare professional for guidance on long-term use, especially if you have existing health conditions or are taking other medications.

⊘ Store the tincture in a cool, dark place, and it should remain effective for up to a year.

Fo-Ti Root Tincture made with vegetable glycerin is an effective way to leverage the rejuvenating and health-boosting properties of Fo-Ti, offering a natural solution to enhance well-being without the use of alcohol.

PART 03

RESPIRATORY REMEDIES

(71-85)

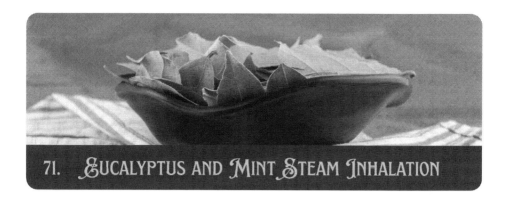

71. Eucalyptus and Mint Steam Inhalation

Introduction:

Eucalyptus and Mint Steam Inhalation is a therapeutic practice used to alleviate respiratory discomfort, clear nasal passages, and reduce inflammation. Eucalyptus oil contains cineole, a compound known for its decongestant and antimicrobial properties, while mint provides a cooling sensation that helps soothe irritated airways. This combination is effective for treating symptoms of colds, sinusitis, and bronchitis.

Ingredients and Measurements:

- 3-5 drops of eucalyptus essential oil
- 3-5 drops of peppermint essential oil
- A large bowl of boiling water

Preparation:

☞ Boil water and pour it into a large, heat-resistant bowl.

☞ Carefully add 3-5 drops each of eucalyptus and peppermint essential oils to the hot water.

How to Use:

↳ Lean over the bowl, keeping a safe distance to avoid burns.

↳ Drape a towel over your head and the bowl to create a tent that traps the steam.

↳ Inhale the steam deeply for 5-10 minutes, allowing the therapeutic vapors to penetrate the respiratory tract.

↳ Breathe normally and take breaks if needed, especially if the steam feels too intense.

Duration:

⊘ Use this steam inhalation method once or twice a day when experiencing respiratory discomfort or congestion.

⊘ If symptoms persist for more than a few days or worsen, consult a healthcare professional.

Eucalyptus and Mint Steam Inhalation is an easy and natural way to relieve respiratory symptoms, providing immediate comfort and promoting clearer breathing.

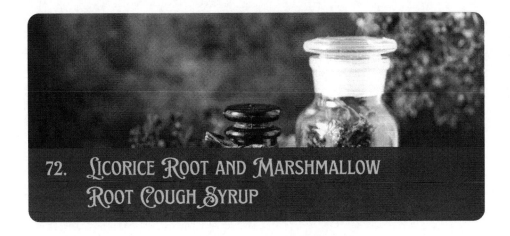

72. Licorice Root and Marshmallow Root Cough Syrup

Introduction:

Licorice Root and Marshmallow Root Cough Syrup is a natural remedy designed to soothe and relieve coughs and sore throats. Licorice root has anti-inflammatory and expectorant properties that help loosen mucus and ease congestion, while marshmallow root provides a protective, soothing coating for irritated mucous membranes. This combination is effective for treating dry, persistent coughs and providing relief for respiratory discomfort.

Ingredients and Measurements:

- 2 tablespoons of dried licorice root
- 2 tablespoons of dried marshmallow root
- 4 cups of water
- 1 cup of honey (or a suitable vegan alternative like maple syrup)

Preparation:

- Combine the licorice and marshmallow roots with the water in a pot.
- Bring the mixture to a boil, then reduce the heat and allow it to simmer until the liquid is reduced by half, about 30-45 minutes.
- Strain the herbs from the liquid using a fine strainer or cheesecloth, ensuring all the herbal essence is extracted.
- While the liquid is still warm (not hot), stir in the honey or maple syrup until it is completely dissolved.
- Pour the finished syrup into a clean glass bottle or jar for storage.

How to Use:

- Take 1-2 teaspoons of the cough syrup every 3-4 hours as needed to relieve coughs and soothe the throat.
- Keep the syrup refrigerated, and gently warm it before use for extra soothing effects.

Duration:

- Use the cough syrup as needed during bouts of cough and throat irritation.

- The syrup can be stored in the refrigerator for up to 2-3 weeks. If you notice any changes in color, smell, or texture, discard the syrup and prepare a fresh batch.

Licorice Root and Marshmallow Root Cough Syrup is an effective and comforting remedy for respiratory ailments, providing a gentle and natural approach to relieving coughs and soothing sore throats.

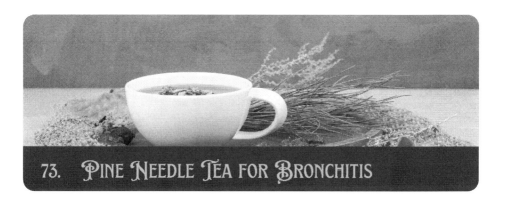

73. PINE NEEDLE TEA FOR BRONCHITIS

Introduction:

Pine Needle Tea is a traditional remedy known for its ability to alleviate respiratory symptoms associated with bronchitis, such as coughing and congestion. Rich in vitamin C and antioxidants, pine needles can help boost the immune system while providing anti-inflammatory benefits that soothe irritated airways. This tea has a distinct, refreshing flavor and acts as a natural expectorant to help clear mucus from the lungs.

Ingredients and Measurements:

- 1-2 tablespoons of fresh or dried pine needles (ensure they are from a non-toxic species like white pine)

- 2 cups of water

- Optional: honey or lemon to taste

Preparation:

- Rinse the pine needles thoroughly to remove any dirt or debris.

- Chop the needles finely to maximize the surface area for extraction.

- Boil the water, then add the chopped pine needles.

- Reduce the heat and simmer for 10-15 minutes to allow the essential oils and nutrients to infuse into the water.
- Strain the tea into a cup, removing the pine needles.

How to Use:

- Drink a cup of Pine Needle Tea 1-2 times daily when experiencing bronchitis symptoms to help reduce inflammation and clear mucus from the respiratory tract.
- Enhance the flavor and health benefits by adding a teaspoon of honey or a slice of lemon, if desired.

Duration:

- Use Pine Needle Tea as needed during periods of respiratory discomfort due to bronchitis or similar conditions.
- If symptoms persist for more than a week or worsen, consult a healthcare professional.

Pine Needle Tea offers a natural and soothing way to relieve symptoms of bronchitis, supporting respiratory health and enhancing overall well-being with its rich nutrient profile and aromatic flavor.

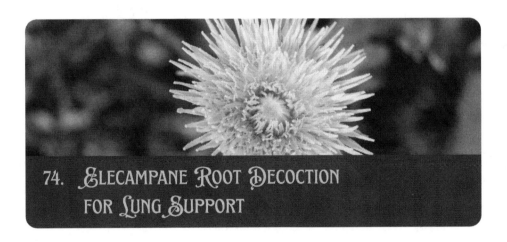

74. ELECAMPANE ROOT DECOCTION FOR LUNG SUPPORT

Introduction:

Elecampane Root Decoction is a robust herbal remedy known for its beneficial impact on lung health and respiratory function. Elecampane, with its high content of inulin and mucilage, acts as an expectorant to help clear excess mucus and soothe irritated airways. It is particularly effective in treating conditions like bronchitis, asthma, and other respiratory ailments due to its antibacterial and antitussive properties.

Ingredients and Measurements:

- 1 tablespoon of dried elecampane root
- 4 cups of water
- Optional: honey or lemon to taste

Preparation:

- Place the dried elecampane root into a pot.

- Add the water and bring the mixture to a boil.

- Once boiling, reduce the heat and allow the decoction to simmer for about 30 minutes until the liquid is reduced by half. This slow simmer helps to extract the medicinal compounds from the elecampane root effectively.

- Strain the decoction into a cup, removing the elecampane root.

How to Use:

- Drink 1 cup of Elecampane Root Decoction up to two times daily to support lung health and ease respiratory symptoms.

- If desired, enhance the flavor and additional health benefits by adding a teaspoon of honey or a squeeze of lemon.

Duration:

- Use Elecampane Root Decoction as needed during periods of respiratory discomfort or as part of a regular routine to maintain respiratory health.

- If respiratory symptoms persist or worsen, it's important to consult a healthcare professional for further evaluation and treatment.

Elecampane Root Decoction is a simple yet effective way to support respiratory health, offering natural relief for those dealing with lung and airway conditions.

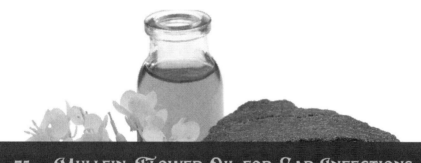

75. MULLEIN FLOWER OIL FOR EAR INFECTIONS

Introduction:

Mullein Flower Oil is a gentle and effective remedy commonly used to treat ear infections and reduce ear pain. Mullein flowers are known for their anti-inflammatory and antibacterial properties, making them ideal for soothing irritated tissues and combating infection. This oil is particularly useful for children and adults alike, providing a natural way to alleviate discomfort and promote healing.

Ingredients and Measurements:

- 1/4 cup of dried mullein flowers
- 1 cup of olive oil or almond oil
- A clean glass jar with a tight-fitting lid
- A fine strainer or cheesecloth

Preparation:

- Place the dried mullein flowers in the glass jar.
- Warm the olive oil or almond oil gently in a saucepan, being careful not to overheat or boil the oil.
- Pour the warm oil over the mullein flowers, ensuring they are fully submerged.
- Seal the jar tightly and place it in a warm, sunny spot for 2-3 weeks, shaking it daily to facilitate the infusion process.
- After the infusion period, strain the oil through a fine strainer or cheesecloth into another clean jar to remove the mullein flowers.
- Store the strained mullein flower oil in a dark, cool place or in the refrigerator to preserve its potency.

How to Use:

- To treat an ear infection or alleviate ear pain, slightly warm a small amount of mullein flower oil (ensure it's comfortably warm, not hot).
- Use a clean dropper to apply 2-3 drops of the oil into the affected ear, gently massaging the area around the outer ear to help the oil penetrate.
- Repeat this treatment 2-3 times a day as needed for relief.

Duration:

- Use mullein flower oil as needed during episodes of ear discomfort or infection until symptoms improve.
- If there is no improvement or if symptoms worsen after a few days, consult a healthcare professional, especially for severe or persistent ear infections.

Mullein Flower Oil provides a soothing and natural treatment for ear infections, helping to reduce pain and inflammation while promoting recovery in a gentle manner.

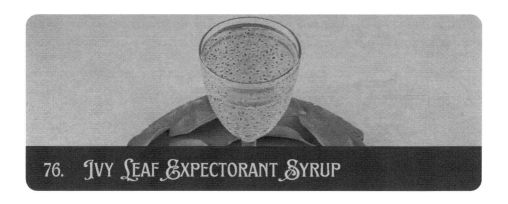

76. IVY LEAF EXPECTORANT SYRUP

Introduction:

Ivy Leaf Expectorant Syrup is a natural remedy designed to alleviate coughs and improve respiratory function by helping to clear mucus from the lungs and airways. Ivy leaf, known for its saponins and antioxidant properties, effectively thins and loosens mucus, making it easier to expel. This makes the syrup particularly useful for treating bronchial conditions like chronic bronchitis and asthma.

Ingredients and Measurements:

- 2 tablespoons of dried ivy leaf
- 2 cups of water
- 1 cup of honey (or a suitable vegan alternative like agave syrup)

Preparation:

☞ Place the dried ivy leaf in a pot and add the water.

☞ Bring the mixture to a boil, then reduce the heat and allow it to simmer until the liquid is reduced by half, about 30-45 minutes.

☞ Strain the liquid through a fine strainer or cheesecloth to remove the ivy leaves.

☞ While the liquid is still warm (not hot), mix in the honey or agave syrup until it is completely dissolved.

☞ Pour the finished syrup into a clean glass bottle or jar for storage.

How to Use:

✎ Take 1-2 teaspoons of Ivy Leaf Expectorant Syrup every 3-4 hours as needed to relieve cough and facilitate mucus expulsion.

✎ Keep the syrup refrigerated, and gently warm it before use for extra soothing effects.

Duration:

⊘ Use the syrup as needed during bouts of cough and respiratory discomfort.

⊘ The syrup can be stored in the refrigerator for up to 2-3 weeks. If you notice any changes in color, smell, or texture, discard the syrup and prepare a fresh batch.

Ivy Leaf Expectorant Syrup is an effective and comforting remedy for respiratory ailments, providing a gentle and natural approach to relieving coughs and facilitating clearer breathing.

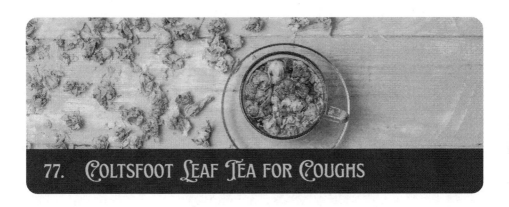

77. COLTSFOOT LEAF TEA FOR COUGHS

Introduction:

Coltsfoot Leaf Tea is an age-old herbal remedy favored for its ability to soothe persistent coughs and relieve respiratory ailments. Coltsfoot, with its mucilaginous and anti-inflammatory properties, acts as an expectorant to help clear mucus from the airways, making it ideal for treating coughs, bronchitis, and asthma. This herbal tea has a mild, slightly sweet taste and offers gentle relief for respiratory discomfort.

Ingredients and Measurements:

- 1-2 teaspoons of dried coltsfoot leaves
- 2 cups of boiling water
- Optional: honey or lemon to enhance flavor

Preparation:

☞ Place the dried coltsfoot leaves in a teapot or a heat-resistant infuser.

☞ Pour the boiling water over the leaves and cover to keep the essential oils and medicinal properties intact.

☞ Allow the tea to steep for 10-15 minutes, depending on your preferred strength and flavor intensity.

☞ Strain the tea into a cup to remove the coltsfoot leaves.

How to Use:

↳ Drink a cup of Coltsfoot Leaf Tea 1-2 times daily to benefit from its soothing properties for coughs and respiratory health.

↳ If desired, sweeten the tea with a teaspoon of honey or add a slice of lemon for extra flavor and health benefits.

Duration:

- Coltsfoot Leaf Tea can be consumed as needed during periods of respiratory discomfort or as part of a regular routine to support lung health.

- If symptoms persist or worsen, it is important to consult a healthcare professional for further evaluation and treatment.

Coltsfoot Leaf Tea is an easy and effective way to incorporate the healing properties of coltsfoot into your daily life, offering a natural approach to soothing coughs and enhancing respiratory health.

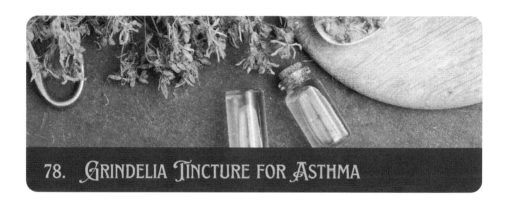

78. GRINDELIA TINCTURE FOR ASTHMA

Introduction:

Grindelia Tincture is a beneficial herbal extract used to manage asthma symptoms and improve respiratory function. Grindelia, known for its potent anti-inflammatory and expectorant properties, helps relax the airways, reduce bronchial spasms, and clear mucus from the lungs. Utilizing vegetable glycerin as the extraction medium provides an alcohol-free alternative, making this tincture suitable for various users, including those who avoid alcohol.

Ingredients and Measurements:

- 1 cup of dried Grindelia flowers and leaves, finely chopped or powdered

- 2 cups of vegetable glycerin

- 1 cup of distilled water

- A clean glass jar with a tight-fitting lid

- A fine strainer or cheesecloth

Preparation:

- Place the dried Grindelia into the glass jar.

- Mix the vegetable glycerin and distilled water in a separate container to create a consistent solution. This mixture ensures an effective extraction of the active compounds from Grindelia.

- Pour the glycerin-water mixture over the Grindelia, ensuring the plant material is fully submerged.

- Seal the jar tightly and shake it well to combine the ingredients.

- Store the jar in a cool, dark place, shaking it daily for 4-6 weeks to promote the extraction process.

- After the infusion period, strain the mixture through a fine strainer or cheesecloth into another clean jar, pressing the plant material to extract as much liquid as possible.

- Transfer the strained tincture to a dropper bottle for ease of use.

How to Use:

- To help manage asthma symptoms and improve respiratory function, take 1-2 dropperfuls (about 30-60 drops) of the tincture diluted in water or juice, up to three times a day.

- Begin with a lower dose to observe how your body responds, and adjust as necessary based on your health goals and reaction to the supplement.

Duration:

- Use the tincture regularly as part of a health regimen for asthma and respiratory support.

- Consult a healthcare professional for guidance on long-term use, especially if you have existing health conditions or are taking other medications.

- Store the tincture in a cool, dark place, and it should remain effective for up to a year.

Grindelia Tincture made with vegetable glycerin is an effective way to leverage the respiratory-supporting and anti-inflammatory properties of Grindelia, offering a natural solution to manage asthma and enhance lung health without the use of alcohol.

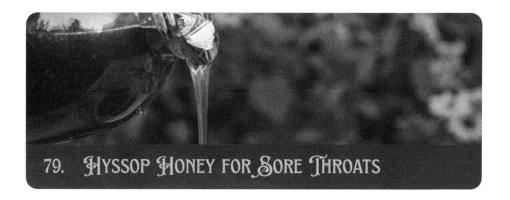

79. Hyssop Honey for Sore Throats

Introduction:

Hyssop Honey is a soothing and therapeutic remedy designed to alleviate sore throats and reduce inflammation. Hyssop, an herb with antiseptic and antimicrobial properties, is combined with honey, known for its healing and soothing effects. This blend is particularly effective for treating sore throats, calming coughs, and boosting the immune system.

Ingredients and Measurements:

- 2 tablespoons of dried hyssop leaves
- 1 cup of honey (preferably raw and organic)
- A clean glass jar with a tight-fitting lid

Preparation:

- Place the dried hyssop leaves in the glass jar.
- Gently warm the honey in a saucepan over low heat, just until it becomes more fluid. Avoid overheating to preserve the honey's natural enzymes and nutrients.
- Pour the warm honey over the hyssop leaves in the jar, ensuring the leaves are fully submerged.
- Seal the jar tightly and let it sit in a warm, dark place for 1-2 weeks, shaking it daily to help the hyssop infuse into the honey.
- After the infusion period, strain the honey through a fine strainer or cheesecloth into another clean jar to remove the hyssop leaves.

How to Use:

- Take 1-2 teaspoons of Hyssop Honey directly or dissolve it in warm water or tea as needed to soothe a sore throat and relieve cough symptoms.
- The honey can also be used as a preventive measure during cold and flu season by taking a small amount daily.

Duration:

- Hyssop Honey can be stored in a cool, dark place and used as needed for sore throat relief and immune support.

- It typically remains potent and effective for up to a year if stored properly.

- If there is no improvement in symptoms after a few days of use or if symptoms worsen, consult a healthcare professional.

Hyssop Honey is an effective and comforting remedy for sore throats, providing a natural and gentle approach to relieving discomfort and enhancing overall well-being.

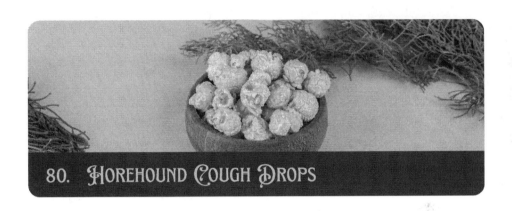

80. Horehound Cough Drops

Introduction:

Horehound Cough Drops are a traditional herbal remedy designed to soothe coughs and sore throats. Horehound, a member of the mint family, is known for its bitter taste and potent expectorant properties, which help to loosen mucus and ease respiratory discomfort. These cough drops combine the benefits of horehound with soothing ingredients like honey to create a natural and effective treatment for coughs and throat irritation.

Ingredients and Measurements:

- 1/2 cup of dried horehound leaves
- 2 cups of water
- 1 cup of honey
- 1 tablespoon of lemon juice
- Powdered sugar or cornstarch, for dusting

Preparation:

- Place the dried horehound leaves in a pot and add the water. Bring the mixture to a boil, then reduce the heat and simmer until the liquid is reduced by half, about 30 minutes.

- Strain the liquid through a fine sieve or cheesecloth, pressing the leaves to extract as much of the infusion as possible. Discard the leaves.

- Return the strained liquid to the pot, add the honey and lemon juice, and stir well.

Heat the mixture over medium heat, stirring constantly, until it reaches the "hard crack" stage (300°F on a candy thermometer).

Remove from heat and allow the mixture to cool slightly until it thickens but is still pourable.

Drop small spoonfuls of the mixture onto a tray lined with parchment paper or a silicone mat dusted with powdered sugar or cornstarch.

Allow the drops to cool and harden completely. Dust with additional powdered sugar or cornstarch to prevent sticking.

How to Use:

Suck on a Horehound Cough Drop as needed to soothe coughs and sore throats.

Do not consume more than 5-6 drops in a 24-hour period to avoid excessive intake of horehound.

Duration:

Store Horehound Cough Drops in an airtight container in a cool, dry place for up to 2 months.

If symptoms persist or worsen, consult a healthcare professional.

Horehound Cough Drops provide a natural and effective way to relieve coughs and sore throats, combining the therapeutic properties of horehound with the soothing effects of honey and lemon.

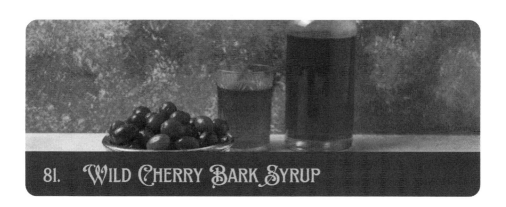

81. WILD CHERRY BARK SYRUP

Introduction:

Wild Cherry Bark Syrup is a natural remedy renowned for its ability to soothe persistent coughs and ease respiratory discomfort. Wild cherry bark contains compounds that help relax the airways, reduce inflammation, and suppress coughing. This syrup combines the healing properties of wild cherry bark with honey to enhance its soothing effects and improve taste.

Ingredients and Measurements:

- 1/4 cup of dried wild cherry bark
- 4 cups of water
- 1 cup of honey
- Optional: lemon juice or ginger for additional flavor and health benefits

Preparation:

- Place the dried wild cherry bark in a pot and add the water.
- Bring the mixture to a boil, then reduce the heat and let it simmer until the liquid is reduced by half, about 30-40 minutes.
- Strain the liquid through a fine sieve or cheesecloth, pressing the bark to extract as much of the infusion as possible. Discard the bark.
- Return the strained liquid to the pot, add the honey, and stir until fully dissolved. If using, add a tablespoon of lemon juice or a few slices of fresh ginger for extra flavor and benefits.
- Continue to simmer the mixture for an additional 10 minutes to ensure a syrupy consistency.
- Remove from heat and let the syrup cool before transferring it to a clean glass bottle or jar.

How to Use:

- Take 1-2 teaspoons of Wild Cherry Bark Syrup every 4 hours as needed to relieve cough and soothe the throat.
- Not suitable for very young children due to the honey content; consult a healthcare provider before giving to children.

Duration:

- Store the syrup in the refrigerator for up to 3 weeks.
- If there is no improvement in symptoms after several days of use or if symptoms worsen, seek medical advice from a healthcare professional.

Wild Cherry Bark Syrup is an effective and comforting remedy for treating coughs and respiratory ailments, providing a soothing and natural approach to improving respiratory health.

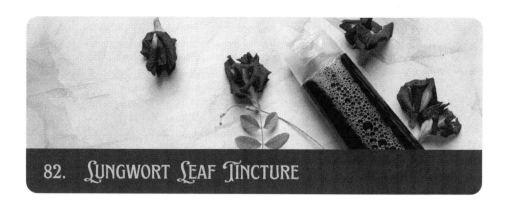

82. Lungwort Leaf Tincture

Introduction:

Lungwort Leaf Tincture is a therapeutic herbal extract known for its beneficial effects on respiratory health. Lungwort, with its high mucilage content, acts as a soothing agent for irritated respiratory tracts and is effective in managing conditions like bronchitis and asthma. Its antioxidant properties also help protect lung tissue. Using vegetable glycerin as the extraction medium makes this tincture alcohol-free, suitable for various users, including those who prefer or need to avoid alcohol.

Ingredients and Measurements:

- 1 cup of dried lungwort leaves, finely chopped or powdered
- 2 cups of vegetable glycerin
- 1 cup of distilled water
- A clean glass jar with a tight-fitting lid
- A fine strainer or cheesecloth

Preparation:

- Place the dried lungwort leaves into the glass jar.

- Mix the vegetable glycerin and distilled water in a separate container to create a consistent solution. This mixture ensures efficient extraction of the active compounds from lungwort.

- Pour the glycerin-water mixture over the lungwort leaves, ensuring they are fully submerged.

- Seal the jar tightly and shake it well to combine the ingredients.

- Store the jar in a cool, dark place, shaking it daily for 4-6 weeks to facilitate the extraction process.

- After the infusion period, strain the mixture through a fine strainer or cheesecloth into another clean jar, pressing the leaves to extract as much liquid as possible.

- Transfer the strained tincture to a dropper bottle for ease of use.

How to Use:

- To support respiratory health and soothe irritated airways, take 1-2 dropperfuls (about 30-60 drops) of the tincture diluted in water or juice, up to three times a day.

Begin with a lower dose to observe how your body responds, and adjust as necessary based on your health goals and reaction to the supplement.

Duration:

- Use the tincture regularly as part of a health regimen for respiratory support.

- Consult a healthcare professional for guidance on long-term use, especially if you have existing health conditions or are taking other medications.

Store the tincture in a cool, dark place, and it should remain effective for up to a year.

Lungwort Leaf Tincture made with vegetable glycerin is an effective way to leverage the respiratory-supporting properties of lungwort, offering a natural solution to improve lung health and ease breathing without the use of alcohol.

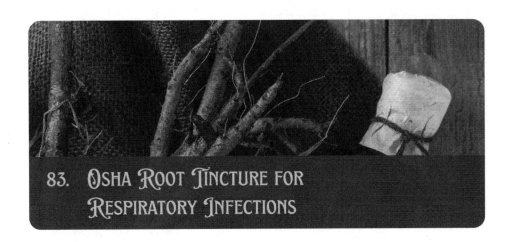

83. OSHA ROOT TINCTURE FOR RESPIRATORY INFECTIONS

Introduction:

Osha Root Tincture is a potent herbal extract celebrated for its ability to combat respiratory infections and enhance lung function. Osha root, rich in compounds like camphor and saponins, acts as a bronchodilator and expectorant, helping to clear mucus from the airways and relieve symptoms of colds, flu, and bronchitis. Utilizing vegetable glycerin as the extraction medium provides an alcohol-free option, making this tincture suitable for a wide range of users.

Ingredients and Measurements:

- 1 cup of dried osha root, finely chopped or powdered

- 2 cups of vegetable glycerin

- 1 cup of distilled water

- A clean glass jar with a tight-fitting lid
- A fine strainer or cheesecloth

Preparation:

☞ Place the dried osha root into the glass jar.

☞ Mix the vegetable glycerin and distilled water in a separate container to ensure a homogeneous solution. This blend facilitates the effective extraction of the active compounds from osha root.

☞ Pour the glycerin-water mixture over the osha root, ensuring the root is fully submerged.

☞ Seal the jar tightly and shake it well to combine the ingredients.

☞ Store the jar in a cool, dark place, shaking it daily for 4-6 weeks to promote the extraction process.

☞ After the infusion period, strain the mixture through a fine strainer or cheesecloth into another clean jar, pressing the root to extract as much liquid as possible.

☞ Transfer the strained tincture to a dropper bottle for ease of use.

How to Use:

✎ To alleviate symptoms of respiratory infections and support lung health, take 1-2 dropperfuls (about 30-60 drops) of the tincture diluted in water or juice, up to three times a day.

✎ Start with a lower dose to observe your body's response, and adjust based on your health goals and the supplement's effectiveness.

Duration:

🕐 Use the tincture regularly as part of a health regimen for respiratory support during infection periods.

🕐 Consult a healthcare professional for guidance on long-term use, especially if you have existing health conditions or are taking other medications.

🕐 Store the tincture in a cool, dark place, and it should remain effective for up to a year.

Osha Root Tincture made with vegetable glycerin is an effective way to leverage the respiratory-supporting properties of osha root, offering a natural solution to improve respiratory health and combat infections without the use of alcohol.

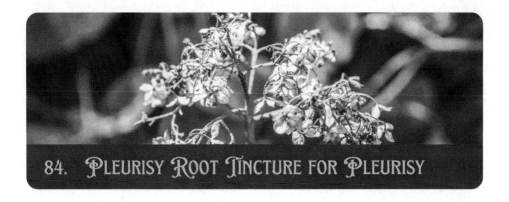

Introduction:

Pleurisy Root Tincture is an effective herbal remedy specifically formulated to address the symptoms of pleurisy, a condition where the lung's pleural layers become inflamed, causing sharp chest pain during breathing. Pleurisy root, known for its anti-inflammatory and expectorant properties, helps reduce the inflammation of the pleura and facilitates easier breathing. Using vegetable glycerin as the extraction medium makes this tincture alcohol-free, suitable for a variety of users.

Ingredients and Measurements:

- 1 cup of dried pleurisy root, finely chopped or powdered
- 2 cups of vegetable glycerin
- 1 cup of distilled water
- A clean glass jar with a tight-fitting lid
- A fine strainer or cheesecloth

Preparation:

☞ Place the dried pleurisy root into the glass jar.

☞ In a separate container, mix the vegetable glycerin and distilled water to create a consistent solution. This blend ensures efficient extraction of the active compounds from pleurisy root.

☞ Pour the glycerin-water mixture over the pleurisy root, ensuring the root is fully submerged.

☞ Seal the jar tightly and shake it well to combine the ingredients.

☞ Store the jar in a cool, dark place, shaking it daily for 4-6 weeks to promote the extraction process.

☞ After the infusion period, strain the mixture through a fine strainer or cheesecloth into another clean jar, pressing the root to extract as much liquid as possible.

☞ Transfer the strained tincture to a dropper bottle for ease of use.

How to Use:

✎ To alleviate the symptoms of pleurisy and support lung health, take 1-2 dropperfuls (about 30-60 drops) of the tincture diluted in water or juice, up to three times a day.

Begin with a lower dose to observe how your body responds, and adjust as necessary based on your health goals and reaction to the supplement.

Duration:

◎ Use the tincture regularly as part of a health regimen for respiratory support, particularly during flare-ups of pleurisy.

◎ Consult a healthcare professional for guidance on long-term use, especially if you have existing health conditions or are taking other medications.

◎ Store the tincture in a cool, dark place, and it should remain effective for up to a year.

Pleurisy Root Tincture made with vegetable glycerin is an effective way to leverage the anti-inflammatory and expectorant properties of pleurisy root, offering a natural solution to improve respiratory health and alleviate the discomfort associated with pleurisy without the use of alcohol.

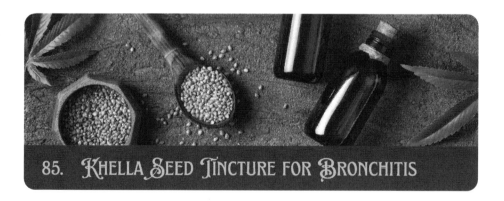

85. KHELLA SEED TINCTURE FOR BRONCHITIS

Introduction:

Khella Seed Tincture is a specialized herbal remedy known for its effectiveness in treating bronchitis and other respiratory conditions. Khella seeds, derived from the Ammi visnaga plant, contain active compounds like khellin and visnagin that help relax and widen the bronchial passages, easing breathing and reducing spasms. This tincture, made with vegetable glycerin, is an alcohol-free option suitable for various users.

Ingredients and Measurements:

- 1 cup of dried khella seeds, finely ground

- 2 cups of vegetable glycerin

- 1 cup of distilled water

- A clean glass jar with a tight-fitting lid
- A fine strainer or cheesecloth

Preparation:

☞ Place the finely ground khella seeds into the glass jar.

☞ Mix the vegetable glycerin and distilled water in a separate container to create a uniform solution. This mixture ensures efficient extraction of the active compounds from khella seeds.

☞ Pour the glycerin-water mixture over the khella seeds, ensuring they are fully submerged.

☞ Seal the jar tightly and shake it to combine the ingredients thoroughly.

☞ Store the jar in a cool, dark place, shaking it daily for 4-6 weeks to facilitate the extraction process.

☞ After the infusion period, strain the mixture through a fine strainer or cheesecloth into another clean jar, pressing the seeds to extract as much liquid as possible.

☞ Transfer the strained tincture to a dropper bottle for ease of use.

How to Use:

✎ To alleviate symptoms of bronchitis and improve respiratory function, take 1-2 dropperfuls (about 30-60 drops) of the tincture diluted in water or juice, up to three times a day.

✎ Start with a lower dose to observe your body's response and adjust as necessary based on your health goals and the supplement's effectiveness.

Duration:

☉ Use the tincture regularly as part of a health regimen for respiratory support during episodes of bronchitis.

☉ Consult a healthcare professional for guidance on long-term use, particularly if you have existing health conditions or are taking other medications.

☉ Store the tincture in a cool, dark place, and it should remain effective for up to a year.

Khella Seed Tincture made with vegetable glycerin is an effective way to harness the bronchodilatory and anti-spasmodic properties of khella seeds, offering a natural solution to improve respiratory health and manage bronchitis without the use of alcohol.

PART 04

DIGESTIVE REMEDIES (86-115)

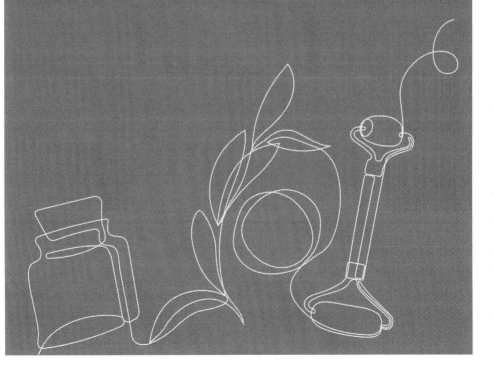

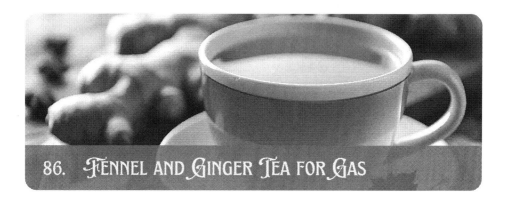

86. FENNEL AND GINGER TEA FOR GAS

Introduction:

Fennel and Ginger Tea is a soothing and effective herbal beverage designed to alleviate digestive discomfort, particularly gas and bloating. Fennel seeds are known for their antispasmodic properties that relax the digestive tract, while ginger aids in reducing inflammation and enhancing digestion. Together, they create a potent remedy for soothing upset stomachs and promoting overall digestive health.

Ingredients and Measurements:

- 1 teaspoon of fennel seeds
- 1 inch of fresh ginger root, thinly sliced or grated
- 2 cups of water
- Optional: honey or lemon to taste

Preparation:

☞ Place the fennel seeds and ginger slices in a pot.

☞ Add the water and bring the mixture to a boil.

☞ Once boiling, reduce the heat and let the tea simmer for 10-15 minutes, allowing the flavors and medicinal properties to infuse into the water.

☞ Strain the tea into a cup, removing the fennel seeds and ginger pieces.

How to Use:

✎ Drink a cup of Fennel and Ginger Tea after meals or when experiencing digestive discomfort such as gas or bloating.

✎ Enhance the flavor and additional health benefits by adding a teaspoon of honey or a squeeze of lemon, if desired.

Duration:

⊘ Fennel and Ginger Tea can be consumed regularly as part of a healthy diet to maintain digestive health and prevent discomfort.

⊘ If digestive issues persist or worsen, it is essential to consult a healthcare professional for further evaluation and treatment.

Fennel and Ginger Tea is a simple yet powerful way to incorporate the digestive benefits of fennel and ginger into your daily routine, providing a natural approach to soothing digestive discomfort and enhancing overall well-being.

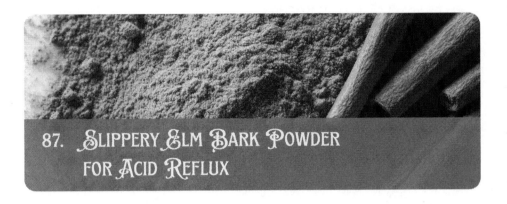

87. SLIPPERY ELM BARK POWDER FOR ACID REFLUX

Introduction:

Slippery Elm Bark Powder is a renowned natural remedy for soothing acid reflux and gastrointestinal discomfort. Slippery elm contains mucilage, a gel-like substance that coats and protects the lining of the esophagus and stomach, reducing irritation caused by stomach acid. This remedy is effective for managing symptoms of acid reflux, gastritis, and other digestive disorders.

Ingredients and Measurements:

- 1 teaspoon of slippery elm bark powder
- 1 cup of hot water
- Optional: honey or lemon to taste

Preparation:

🍵 Place the slippery elm bark powder in a cup.

🍵 Pour the hot water over the powder and stir until it is fully dissolved. The mixture will become slightly thick and gelatinous as it cools, which is normal due to the mucilage.

🍵 Allow the tea to cool to a comfortable temperature before drinking.

How to Use:

🥄 Drink this slippery elm mixture once or twice a day, especially after meals or when experiencing acid reflux symptoms.

🥄 If desired, enhance the flavor and soothing effects by adding a teaspoon of honey or a squeeze of lemon.

Duration:

- Slippery Elm Bark Powder can be used regularly as part of a routine to manage acid reflux and protect the digestive tract.

- Monitor your symptoms and adjust the frequency of use based on your body's response. If symptoms persist or worsen, consult a healthcare professional for further advice and treatment.

Slippery Elm Bark Powder provides a gentle and effective way to alleviate acid reflux and support digestive health, offering a natural and soothing solution to enhance gastrointestinal comfort and well-being.

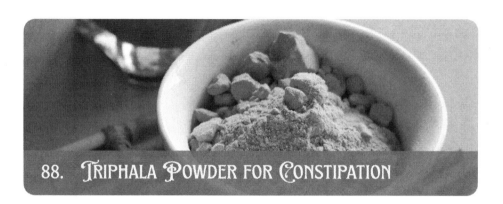

88. TRIPHALA POWDER FOR CONSTIPATION

Introduction:

Triphala Powder is a traditional Ayurvedic remedy known for its natural laxative properties and ability to promote digestive health. Composed of three dried fruits (Amalaki, Bibhitaki, and Haritaki) Triphala helps to balance the digestive system, stimulate bowel movements, and cleanse the colon. Its gentle action makes it suitable for regular use without the harsh effects of typical laxatives.

Ingredients and Measurements:

- 1 teaspoon of Triphala powder
- 1 cup of warm water
- Optional: honey or lemon to taste

Preparation:

- Dissolve the Triphala powder in a cup of warm water. Stir thoroughly to ensure the powder is fully mixed.

- Allow the mixture to sit for a few minutes, letting the components fully infuse into the water.

How to Use:

🥄 Drink the Triphala mixture once daily, preferably at night before bedtime, to aid in regular bowel movements and relieve constipation.

🥄 If needed, adjust the flavor with a teaspoon of honey or a squeeze of lemon to make it more palatable.

Duration:

⊘ Triphala Powder can be taken regularly as part of a daily routine to maintain digestive balance and prevent constipation.

⊘ If you do not notice improvement in your symptoms within a week or if you experience discomfort, it is important to consult a healthcare professional for further guidance.

Triphala Powder offers a natural, effective way to manage constipation and support overall digestive health, providing a balanced approach to enhancing regularity and digestive wellness.

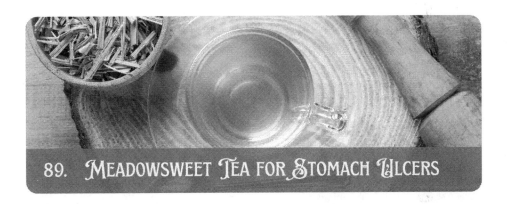

89. MEADOWSWEET TEA FOR STOMACH ULCERS

Introduction:

Meadowsweet Tea is a therapeutic herbal beverage known for its ability to soothe stomach ulcers and alleviate gastritis symptoms. Meadowsweet, rich in compounds like salicylates and tannins, has anti-inflammatory and protective properties that help heal the stomach lining and reduce acidity. Its gentle, sweet flavor makes it a pleasant remedy for digestive discomfort.

Ingredients and Measurements:

- 1-2 teaspoons of dried meadowsweet flowers and leaves

- 2 cups of boiling water

- Optional: honey to taste

Preparation:

- Place the dried meadowsweet in a teapot or heat-resistant infuser.

- Pour the boiling water over the meadowsweet and cover to preserve the essential oils and medicinal properties.

- Allow the tea to steep for 10-15 minutes, depending on the desired strength.

- Strain the tea into a cup, removing the meadowsweet plant material.

How to Use:

- Drink a cup of Meadowsweet Tea 1-2 times daily, especially after meals, to benefit from its soothing effects on the stomach and to help heal ulcers.

- If desired, add a teaspoon of honey to enhance the flavor and provide additional soothing benefits.

Duration:

- Meadowsweet Tea can be consumed regularly as part of a health-focused routine to maintain digestive health and prevent ulcer discomfort.

- If symptoms of ulcers persist or worsen, it is crucial to consult a healthcare professional for further evaluation and treatment.

Meadowsweet Tea is an effective and enjoyable way to incorporate the healing properties of meadowsweet into your daily life, offering a natural approach to soothing stomach ulcers and enhancing overall digestive well-being.

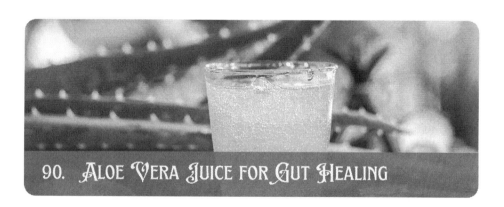

90. ALOE VERA JUICE FOR GUT HEALING

Introduction:

Aloe Vera Juice is widely recognized for its soothing and healing properties, particularly for the digestive system. Rich in vitamins, minerals, and enzymes, aloe vera helps to reduce inflammation in the gut, promote healing of ulcers and other gastrointestinal issues, and support overall digestive health. Its natural laxative effect also aids in improving bowel regularity.

Ingredients and Measurements:

- Fresh aloe vera gel from 1-2 large aloe vera leaves or pre-made pure aloe vera juice
- 2 cups of water (if extracting gel from leaves)
- Optional: honey or lemon to taste

Preparation:

- If using fresh aloe vera leaves, slice them lengthwise to extract the clear inner gel. Scoop the gel with a spoon, being careful to avoid the yellow sap near the skin, which can be irritating.

- Blend the fresh aloe vera gel with water until smooth. If using pre-made aloe vera juice, ensure it's pure and free from additives or aloin.

- Strain the mixture through a fine sieve or cheesecloth to ensure a smooth texture.

How to Use:

- Drink 1/4 to 1/2 cup of Aloe Vera Juice daily, preferably in the morning on an empty stomach, to support gut healing and improve digestive function.

- If desired, enhance the flavor and additional health benefits by adding a teaspoon of honey or a squeeze of lemon.

Duration:

- Aloe Vera Juice can be taken regularly as part of a daily regimen to maintain digestive health and aid in the healing of the gut.

- Monitor your body's response to the juice, especially if using it for specific health issues. Consult a healthcare professional if you have any underlying conditions or are taking medications, as aloe vera can interact with certain drugs.

Aloe Vera Juice provides a gentle and effective way to enhance digestive health and promote gut healing, offering a natural solution to improve gastrointestinal comfort and overall well-being.

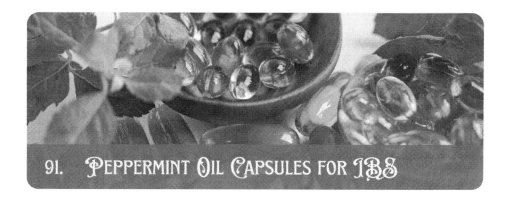

91. Peppermint Oil Capsules for IBS

Introduction:

Peppermint Oil Capsules are a widely recognized natural treatment for Irritable Bowel Syndrome (IBS). Peppermint oil contains menthol, which has antispasmodic properties that help relax the muscles in the digestive tract, alleviate cramping, and reduce bloating and gas. These capsules provide a targeted approach to relieve IBS symptoms, including abdominal pain and irregular bowel movements.

Ingredients and Measurements:

- High-quality, therapeutic-grade peppermint essential oil
- Empty gelatin or vegetarian capsules
- A small dropper or pipette

Preparation:

☞ Ensure you have high-quality, therapeutic-grade peppermint essential oil for both safety and efficacy.

☞ Take an empty capsule and carefully open it to expose the two halves.

☞ Using a dropper or pipette, fill one half of the capsule with peppermint oil. Typically, 2-4 drops are sufficient, but never exceed this amount unless directed by a healthcare professional.

☞ Once filled, reassemble the two halves of the capsule to seal the peppermint oil inside.

☞ Repeat the process for the desired number of capsules. Store the prepared capsules in a cool, dark place, ideally in an airtight container.

How to Use:

↳ For general IBS symptom relief, take 1 peppermint oil capsule 1-2 times a day, preferably 30 minutes before meals.

↳ Always take the capsules with a full glass of water to aid absorption and minimize potential digestive discomfort.

Duration:

☺ Peppermint oil capsules can be used as part of an ongoing treatment plan for IBS, especially during flare-ups or periods of increased symptoms.

Monitor your body's response to the capsules and adjust the dosage accordingly. If symptoms persist or worsen, consult a healthcare professional for further guidance.

Peppermint Oil Capsules offer a convenient and potent way to harness the natural antispasmodic properties of peppermint, providing a targeted solution to alleviate the discomfort of IBS and improve digestive health.

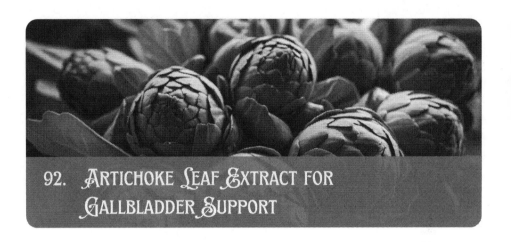

92. ARTICHOKE LEAF EXTRACT FOR GALLBLADDER SUPPORT

Introduction:

Artichoke Leaf Extract is a beneficial herbal supplement known for its ability to support gallbladder function and promote healthy bile production. Rich in cynarin and other beneficial compounds, artichoke leaf helps stimulate bile flow, aiding in fat digestion and reducing symptoms of gallbladder distress such as bloating and discomfort after meals. This extract is also known for its liver-supportive properties, enhancing overall digestive health.

Ingredients and Measurements:

- Dried artichoke leaves
- High-quality vegetable glycerin or a suitable solvent for extraction

- Distilled water
- A clean glass jar with a tight-fitting lid
- A fine strainer or cheesecloth

Preparation:

- Place the dried artichoke leaves into the glass jar.

- Mix the vegetable glycerin and distilled water in a separate container to create a consistent solution. This ensures efficient extraction of the active compounds from the artichoke leaves.

- Pour the glycerin-water mixture over the artichoke leaves, making sure they are fully submerged.

- Seal the jar tightly and shake it to mix the contents well.

- Store the jar in a cool, dark place, shaking it daily for 4-6 weeks to facilitate the extraction process.

- After the infusion period, strain the mixture through a fine strainer or cheesecloth into another clean jar, pressing the leaves to extract as much liquid as possible.

- Transfer the strained extract to a dropper bottle for ease of use.

How to Use:

- To support gallbladder health and enhance bile production, take 1-2 dropperfuls (about 30-60 drops) of the artichoke leaf extract diluted in water or juice, up to three times a day.

- Begin with a lower dose to observe how your body responds and adjust as necessary based on your health goals and reaction to the supplement.

Duration:

- Use the extract regularly as part of a health regimen for gallbladder support and liver health.

- Consult a healthcare professional for guidance on long-term use, especially if you have existing health conditions or are taking other medications.

- Store the extract in a cool, dark place, and it should remain effective for up to a year.

Artichoke Leaf Extract provides a natural and effective way to support gallbladder function and digestive health, leveraging the beneficial properties of artichoke leaves to enhance bile production and reduce gallbladder discomfort.

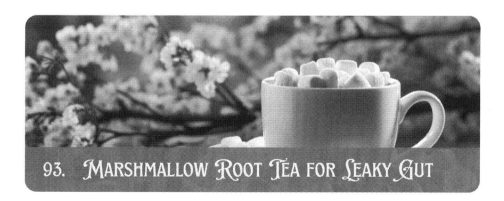

93. MARSHMALLOW ROOT TEA FOR LEAKY GUT

Introduction:

Marshmallow Root Tea is a gentle and effective herbal remedy known for its ability to soothe and repair the lining of the gastrointestinal tract, particularly beneficial for conditions like leaky gut syndrome. Marshmallow root is rich in mucilage, a gel-like substance that coats and protects the intestines, reducing inflammation and aiding in the healing of irritated mucosal layers.

Ingredients and Measurements:

- 1-2 tablespoons of dried marshmallow root
- 2 cups of water
- Optional: honey or lemon to taste

Preparation:

- Place the dried marshmallow root in a pot.
- Add the water and bring the mixture to a boil.
- Once boiling, reduce the heat and let the tea simmer for about 15-20 minutes, allowing the marshmallow root to release its mucilage and other healing compounds.
- Strain the tea into a cup, removing the marshmallow root.

How to Use:

- Drink a cup of Marshmallow Root Tea 1-2 times daily to benefit from its soothing properties and support the healing of the gut lining.
- If desired, enhance the flavor and additional health benefits by adding a teaspoon of honey or a squeeze of lemon.

Duration:

- Marshmallow Root Tea can be consumed regularly as part of a health-focused routine to maintain digestive health and alleviate symptoms of leaky gut.
- If symptoms persist or worsen, it is essential to consult a healthcare professional for further evaluation and treatment.

Marshmallow Root Tea offers a natural and comforting way to soothe digestive discomfort and enhance the healing process in the gut, providing a gentle solution to improve gastrointestinal health and well-being.

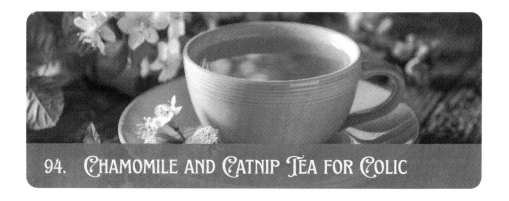

Introduction:

Chamomile and Catnip Tea is a gentle, soothing herbal remedy designed to relieve the discomfort of colic in infants and young children. Chamomile is renowned for its calming and anti-inflammatory properties, helping to ease stomach cramps and induce relaxation. Catnip, on the other hand, is a natural relaxant for the digestive system, reducing spasms and promoting a sense of calm. This combination provides a natural and effective way to soothe the symptoms of colic.

Ingredients and Measurements:

- 1 teaspoon of dried chamomile flowers
- 1 teaspoon of dried catnip leaves
- 2 cups of boiling water
- Optional: honey or lemon to taste (for older children and adults)

Preparation:

- Place the dried chamomile flowers and catnip leaves in a teapot or heat-resistant infuser.

- Pour the boiling water over the herbs and cover to keep the essential oils and medicinal properties intact.

- Allow the tea to steep for 10-15 minutes, depending on the desired strength.

- Strain the tea into a cup, removing the chamomile and catnip plant material.

How to Use:

- For infants and young children, allow the tea to cool completely and give 1-2 teaspoons at a time to help soothe colic symptoms. Always consult a pediatrician before giving any herbal remedy to an infant.

- For older children and adults, drink a cup of Chamomile and Catnip Tea 1-2 times daily to benefit from its soothing properties for digestive discomfort or stress.

- If desired, enhance the flavor with a teaspoon of honey or a slice of lemon, but only for children over one year old and adults.

Duration:

- ☼ Chamomile and Catnip Tea can be used as needed to relieve colic symptoms in infants and digestive discomfort in older children and adults.

- ☼ If symptoms persist or there is no improvement, it is crucial to consult a healthcare professional for further evaluation and treatment.

Chamomile and Catnip Tea offers a natural, gentle approach to alleviating colic and promoting digestive and overall well-being, making it a comforting solution for children and adults alike.

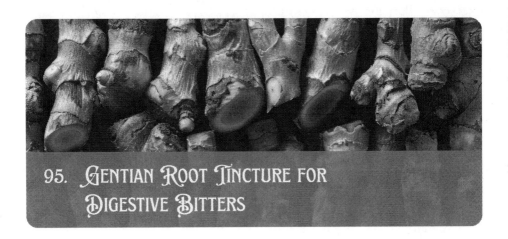

95. GENTIAN ROOT TINCTURE FOR DIGESTIVE BITTERS

Introduction:

Gentian Root Tincture is a highly effective herbal extract known for its role in stimulating digestion and enhancing overall gastrointestinal health. Gentian root, with its intensely bitter compounds, triggers the production of digestive enzymes and bile, aiding in the breakdown of food and absorption of nutrients. This tincture, made with vegetable glycerin, offers an alcohol-free alternative suitable for various users, including those who prefer to avoid alcohol.

Ingredients and Measurements:

- 1 cup of dried gentian root, finely chopped or powdered

- 2 cups of vegetable glycerin

- 1 cup of distilled water

- A clean glass jar with a tight-fitting lid

- A fine strainer or cheesecloth

Preparation:

🗑 Place the dried gentian root into the glass jar.

Mix the vegetable glycerin and distilled water in a separate container to create a consistent solution. This ensures efficient extraction of the active compounds from gentian root.

Pour the glycerin-water mixture over the gentian root, ensuring the root is fully submerged.

Seal the jar tightly and shake it well to combine the ingredients.

Store the jar in a cool, dark place, shaking it daily for 4-6 weeks to facilitate the extraction process.

After the infusion period, strain the mixture through a fine strainer or cheesecloth into another clean jar, pressing the root to extract as much liquid as possible.

Transfer the strained tincture to a dropper bottle for ease of use.

How to Use:

To stimulate digestion and relieve symptoms of indigestion, take 1-2 dropperfuls (about 30-60 drops) of the Gentian Root Tincture diluted in water or juice, 15-30 minutes before meals.

Begin with a lower dose to observe your body's response, and adjust as necessary based on your health goals and reaction to the supplement.

Duration:

Use the tincture regularly as part of a health regimen to enhance digestive function and alleviate digestive discomfort.

Consult a healthcare professional for guidance on long-term use, especially if you have existing health conditions or are taking other medications.

Store the tincture in a cool, dark place, and it should remain effective for up to a year.

Gentian Root Tincture made with vegetable glycerin is an effective way to leverage the digestive-stimulating properties of gentian root, offering a natural solution to improve digestion and overall gastrointestinal health without the use of alcohol.

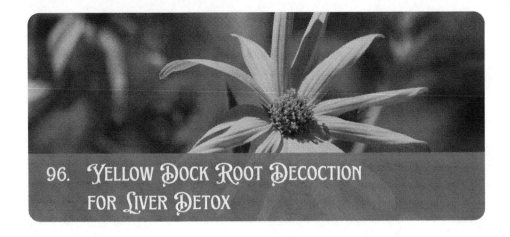

96. YELLOW DOCK ROOT DECOCTION FOR LIVER DETOX

Introduction:

Yellow Dock Root Decoction is a potent herbal remedy renowned for its ability to support liver function and promote detoxification. Yellow dock root is rich in antioxidants and bioactive compounds that stimulate bile production, enhance digestion, and facilitate the elimination of toxins from the body. This makes it an excellent choice for cleansing the liver and improving overall liver health.

Ingredients and Measurements:

- 1 tablespoon of dried yellow dock root
- 4 cups of water
- Optional: honey or lemon to taste

Preparation:

🍵 Place the dried yellow dock root in a pot.

🍵 Add the water and bring the mixture to a boil.

🍵 Once boiling, reduce the heat and let it simmer until the liquid is reduced by half, about 30-40 minutes. This slow simmer helps to extract the medicinal compounds effectively from the yellow dock root.

🍵 Strain the decoction into a cup, removing the yellow dock root.

How to Use:

🥄 Drink 1 cup of Yellow Dock Root Decoction once daily, preferably in the morning on an empty stomach, to support liver detoxification and promote healthy liver function.

🥄 If desired, enhance the flavor and additional health benefits by adding a teaspoon of honey or a squeeze of lemon.

Duration:

🕐 Yellow Dock Root Decoction can be consumed regularly as part of a health-focused routine to maintain liver health and support detoxification processes.

- If symptoms persist or worsen, it is essential to consult a healthcare professional for further evaluation and treatment.

Yellow Dock Root Decoction offers a natural and effective way to enhance liver health and detoxification, providing a gentle solution to support the body's natural cleansing processes and improve overall well-being.

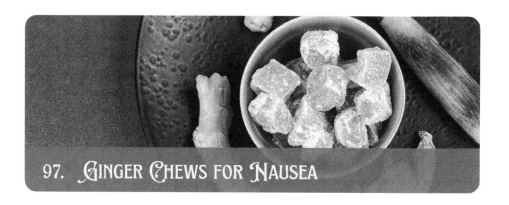

97. GINGER CHEWS FOR NAUSEA

Introduction:

Ginger Chews are a convenient and tasty remedy for combating nausea and settling an upset stomach. Ginger, known for its potent anti-nausea properties and ability to stimulate digestion, is the primary ingredient in these chews. They are particularly effective for motion sickness, morning sickness, and general gastrointestinal discomfort.

Ingredients and Measurements:

- 1 cup of fresh ginger root, peeled and finely grated
- 1 cup of sugar
- 1/2 cup of water
- Optional: additional sugar or powdered ginger for coating

Preparation:

- In a saucepan, combine the grated ginger, sugar, and water.

- Bring the mixture to a boil, then reduce the heat and simmer until it thickens into a syrupy consistency, approximately 20-30 minutes.

- Strain the mixture to remove the ginger pieces, keeping the ginger-infused syrup.

- Continue cooking the syrup until it reaches the "soft ball" stage (about 240°F on a candy thermometer).

- Pour the thickened syrup onto a tray lined with parchment paper or a silicone baking mat. Allow it to cool slightly.

- When the mixture is cool enough to handle but still pliable, roll it into small balls or cut it into chew-sized pieces.

☞ Roll the chews in additional sugar or powdered ginger to prevent sticking.

How to Use:

🥄 Consume a ginger chew as needed to relieve nausea or settle an upset stomach.

🥄 These chews are particularly useful before or during travel for motion sickness or during episodes of morning sickness.

Duration:

⏲ Ginger Chews can be stored in an airtight container at room temperature for up to 2 weeks.

⏲ If nausea persists or worsens, it is important to consult a healthcare professional for further evaluation and treatment.

⏲ Ginger Chews offer a delicious and effective way to harness the anti-nausea benefits of ginger, providing a natural solution to improve digestive comfort and well-being.

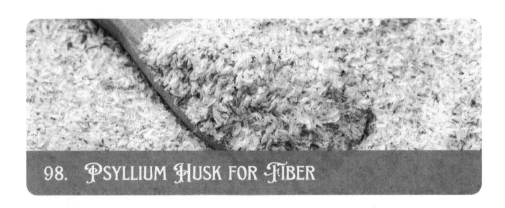

98. Psyllium Husk for Fiber

Introduction:

Psyllium Husk is a highly effective dietary supplement known for its rich fiber content, which helps improve bowel regularity, manage constipation, and support overall digestive health. Derived from the seeds of the Plantago ovata plant, psyllium absorbs water in the gut, forming a gel-like substance that aids in softening stools and promoting smooth passage through the digestive tract.

Ingredients and Measurements:

• Psyllium husk powder

• Water or any liquid of your choice (for ingestion)

Preparation:

☞ No complex preparation is needed for psyllium husk. It comes ready to use and can be easily integrated into your diet.

How to Use:

✎ Mix 1-2 teaspoons of psyllium husk powder into a glass of water, juice, or smoothie. Stir well until the psyllium is fully dissolved.

✎ Drink the mixture immediately after preparation, as psyllium thickens quickly when mixed with liquids.

✎ Follow the drink with another glass of water to ensure proper hydration and optimal fiber function.

Duration:

☺ Psyllium husk can be taken daily as part of a routine to maintain digestive health and regularity.

☺ Start with a lower dose to assess your body's response, and adjust the amount based on your dietary needs and bowel response.

☺ Consult a healthcare professional if you experience any adverse effects or if constipation persists, as ongoing issues may require further medical evaluation.

Psyllium Husk provides a simple and effective way to increase dietary fiber intake, enhancing digestive health and promoting regular bowel movements, offering a natural solution to improve gastrointestinal well-being.

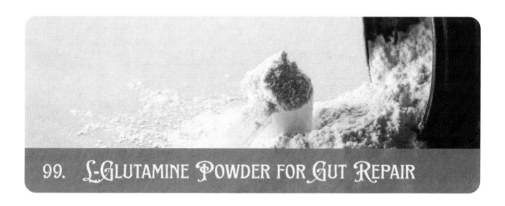

99. L-GLUTAMINE POWDER FOR GUT REPAIR

Introduction:

L-Glutamine Powder is a vital amino acid supplement known for its role in healing and maintaining the integrity of the intestinal lining. It is particularly beneficial for individuals suffering from leaky gut syndrome, inflammatory bowel diseases, and other gastrointestinal disorders. L-Glutamine aids in repairing and regenerating the gut lining,

enhancing nutrient absorption, and supporting overall digestive health.

Ingredients and Measurements:

- L-Glutamine powder

- Water or any preferred liquid for mixing

Preparation:

🗑 No complex preparation is needed for L-Glutamine powder. It is ready to use and easily dissolves in liquids.

How to Use:

⤷ Mix 1 teaspoon (approximately 5 grams) of L-Glutamine powder into a glass of water, juice, or your preferred beverage.

⤷ Stir well until the powder is fully dissolved and drink immediately.

⤷ For best results, consume this supplement once or twice daily, preferably on an empty stomach or as directed by a healthcare provider.

Duration:

🕐 L-Glutamine Powder can be taken regularly as part of a daily health regimen to support gut repair and improve overall digestive function.

🕐 Monitor your body's response to the supplement and adjust the dosage accordingly. If any adverse reactions occur or if symptoms persist, consult a healthcare professional for guidance.

L-Glutamine Powder offers a straightforward and effective way to enhance gut health, providing essential support for repairing the intestinal lining and improving the overall function of the digestive system.

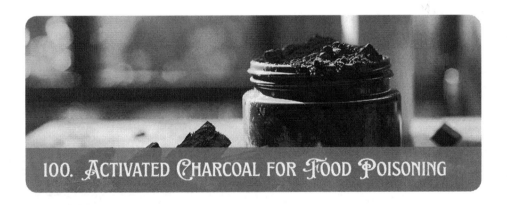

100. ACTIVATED CHARCOAL FOR FOOD POISONING

Introduction:

Activated Charcoal is a powerful and widely used remedy for treating food poisoning and detoxifying the digestive system. Its porous structure allows it to absorb toxins and chemicals, preventing them from being absorbed into the body. This makes activated charcoal particularly effective in binding and neutralizing harmful substances ingested during episodes of food poisoning.

Ingredients and Measurements:

• Activated charcoal capsules or powder

• Water or any suitable liquid for ingestion

Preparation:

⌂ No complex preparation is needed for activated charcoal. It comes ready to use in capsule form or as a loose powder.

How to Use:

↳ If using activated charcoal capsules, take 2-4 capsules with a full glass of water as soon as symptoms of food poisoning appear.

↳ If using activated charcoal powder, mix 1 teaspoon of the powder in a glass of water and drink immediately.

↳ Follow up with additional water to ensure hydration and help move the charcoal through your digestive system.

Duration:

⊘ Activated charcoal should be used only as needed in response to food poisoning symptoms and is not intended for regular use.

⊘ If symptoms of food poisoning persist for more than 24 hours or if there is severe dehydration or other complications, seek medical attention immediately.

Activated Charcoal provides an effective emergency treatment for food poisoning, helping to absorb and remove toxins from the digestive system quickly and safely.

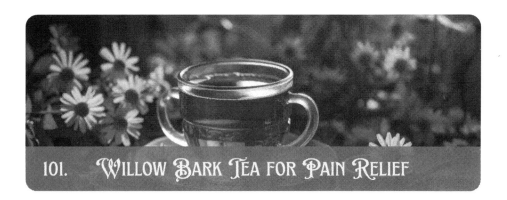

101.　WILLOW BARK TEA FOR PAIN RELIEF

Introduction:

Willow Bark Tea is a natural analgesic and anti-inflammatory remedy derived from the bark of the willow tree, known for its salicin content, which is similar to the active ingredient in aspirin. This makes it an effective treatment for reducing pain, inflammation, and fever. Willow Bark Tea is particularly beneficial for relieving headaches, arthritis pain, and lower back pain.

Ingredients and Measurements:

- 1-2 teaspoons of dried willow bark
- 2 cups of water
- Optional: honey or lemon to taste

Preparation:

- Place the dried willow bark in a pot.
- Add the water and bring the mixture to a boil.
- Once boiling, reduce the heat and let the tea simmer for about 15-20 minutes, allowing the salicin and other pain-relieving compounds to be extracted.
- Strain the tea into a cup, removing the willow bark.

How to Use:

- Drink a cup of Willow Bark Tea once or twice a day to alleviate pain and reduce inflammation.
- If desired, enhance the flavor and additional health benefits by adding a teaspoon of honey or a squeeze of lemon.

Duration:

- Willow Bark Tea can be consumed as needed for pain relief but should be used with caution over extended periods due to potential side effects similar to those of aspirin, such as stomach irritation.
- If pain persists or worsens, or if you experience any adverse effects, consult a healthcare professional for further evaluation and treatment.

Willow Bark Tea offers a natural and effective way to manage pain and inflammation, providing a gentle alternative to synthetic pain relievers.

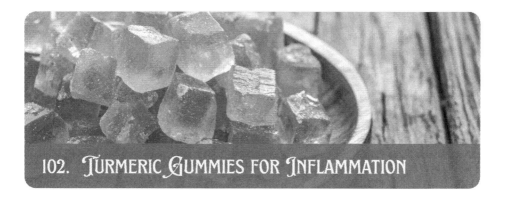

102. Turmeric Gummies for Inflammation

Introduction:

Turmeric Gummies are a flavorful and convenient way to incorporate the anti-inflammatory and antioxidant benefits of turmeric into your daily routine. Turmeric, particularly its active compound curcumin, is renowned for reducing inflammation associated with conditions like arthritis, muscle soreness, and various chronic inflammatory disorders. These gummies make it easy and enjoyable to get these benefits.

Ingredients and Measurements:

- 1/2 cup of turmeric powder
- 1 1/2 cups of fruit juice (preferably orange or pineapple for sweetness and additional vitamin C)
- 1/4 cup of gelatin powder
- 2 tablespoons of honey or another sweetener, if desired
- Optional: a pinch of black pepper to enhance curcumin absorption

Preparation:

☞ In a saucepan, mix the fruit juice and turmeric powder. Warm the mixture over medium heat but do not boil.

☞ Gradually sprinkle the gelatin powder into the warm juice while whisking constantly to avoid lumps.

☞ Continue stirring until the gelatin is completely dissolved and the mixture is smooth.

☞ Add the honey and a pinch of black pepper (if using), stirring until well combined.

☞ Pour the mixture into silicone molds or a greased baking dish.

☞ Refrigerate for 1-2 hours or until the gummies are firm.

How to Use:

✎ Consume 1-2 turmeric gummies daily to benefit from their anti-inflammatory properties.

✎ Keep the gummies stored in the refrigerator to maintain their firmness and freshness.

Duration:

- ◎ Turmeric Gummies can be a part of your daily health regimen to consistently support inflammation reduction and antioxidant protection.

- ◎ If you have specific health conditions or are on medication, especially blood thinners, consult a healthcare professional before starting a regular intake of turmeric gummies.

Turmeric Gummies provide a fun and effective way to harness the powerful anti-inflammatory benefits of turmeric, offering a tasty solution to improve overall health and reduce inflammation naturally.

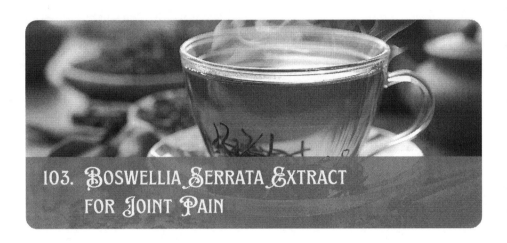

103. BOSWELLIA SERRATA EXTRACT FOR JOINT PAIN

Introduction:

Boswellia Serrata Extract is a highly regarded herbal remedy used to alleviate joint pain and reduce inflammation. Derived from the resin of the Boswellia tree, this extract contains boswellic acids, potent anti-inflammatory agents that help combat arthritis, reduce swelling, and improve mobility. It is particularly effective in managing symptoms of osteoarthritis and rheumatoid arthritis.

Ingredients and Measurements:

- Boswellia serrata resin
- High-quality vegetable glycerin or a suitable solvent for extraction
- Distilled water
- A clean glass jar with a tight-fitting lid
- A fine strainer or cheesecloth

Preparation:

🖘 Place the Boswellia serrata resin into the glass jar.

Mix the vegetable glycerin and distilled water in a separate container to create a consistent solution. This blend ensures efficient extraction of the active compounds from the resin.

Pour the glycerin-water mixture over the Boswellia serrata, ensuring the resin is fully submerged.

Seal the jar tightly and shake it well to combine the ingredients.

Store the jar in a cool, dark place, shaking it daily for 4-6 weeks to facilitate the extraction process.

After the infusion period, strain the mixture through a fine strainer or cheesecloth into another clean jar, pressing the resin to extract as much liquid as possible.

Transfer the strained extract to a dropper bottle for ease of use.

How to Use:

To alleviate joint pain and reduce inflammation, take 1-2 dropperfuls (about 30-60 drops) of the Boswellia Serrata Extract diluted in water or juice, up to three times a day.

Begin with a lower dose to observe your body's response, and adjust as necessary based on your health goals and reaction to the supplement.

Duration:

Use the extract regularly as part of a health regimen to manage joint pain and inflammation.

Consult a healthcare professional for guidance on long-term use, especially if you have existing health conditions or are taking other medications.

Store the extract in a cool, dark place, and it should remain effective for up to a year.

Boswellia Serrata Extract provides a natural and effective way to manage joint pain and inflammation, leveraging the therapeutic properties of boswellic acids to improve joint health and enhance mobility.

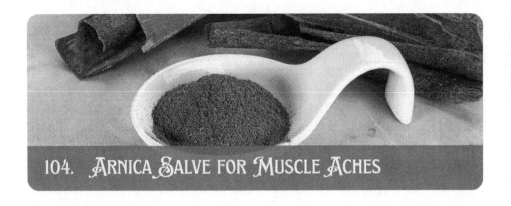

104. ARNICA SALVE FOR MUSCLE ACHES

Introduction:

Arnica Salve is a popular natural remedy used to soothe muscle aches, reduce inflammation, and accelerate healing. Derived from the arnica montana flower, this salve contains compounds that promote blood circulation and reduce pain and swelling associated with bruises, sprains, and muscle soreness. Its topical application makes it an ideal choice for athletes and those recovering from physical exertion.

Ingredients and Measurements:

- 1/4 cup of dried arnica flowers
- 1/2 cup of carrier oil (such as coconut oil or olive oil)
- 2 tablespoons of beeswax
- Optional: essential oils like lavender or peppermint for additional pain relief and scent

Preparation:

- Place the dried arnica flowers in a double boiler and cover them with the carrier oil. Heat gently for 2-3 hours to allow the arnica's active compounds to infuse into the oil.
- Strain the oil through a fine sieve or cheesecloth to remove the arnica flowers.
- Return the infused oil to the double boiler and add the beeswax. Stir until the beeswax is completely melted and the mixture is smooth.
- If using, add a few drops of essential oil and stir well.
- Pour the mixture into small tins or jars and allow it to cool and solidify.

How to Use:

- Apply a small amount of Arnica Salve to the affected area and gently massage into the skin 2-3 times a day, especially after bathing or physical activity.
- Use only on unbroken skin and avoid contact with eyes and mucous membranes.

Duration:

- Arnica Salve can be used as needed to relieve muscle aches and pains.

Store the salve in a cool, dry place, and it should remain effective for up to a year.

If symptoms persist or worsen, or if you experience any adverse reactions, consult a healthcare professional.

Arnica Salve provides a soothing and natural solution to muscle aches, enhancing recovery and offering effective pain relief through its anti-inflammatory properties.

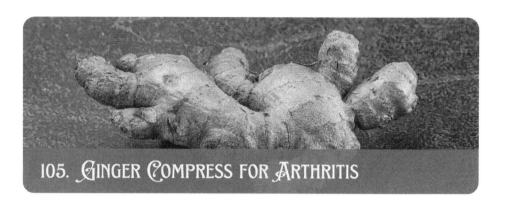

105. GINGER COMPRESS FOR ARTHRITIS

Introduction:

Ginger Compress is a traditional remedy known for its ability to alleviate pain and inflammation associated with arthritis. Ginger, rich in gingerol and other anti-inflammatory compounds, helps increase circulation, reduce stiffness, and soothe sore joints. This compress is a gentle, external treatment that offers targeted relief for arthritis symptoms.

Ingredients and Measurements:

- 1/2 cup of fresh ginger root, grated
- 4 cups of water
- A clean cloth or towel

Preparation:

Grate the fresh ginger root to maximize the surface area for extraction.

In a pot, bring the water to a boil and add the grated ginger.

Reduce the heat and simmer for 15-20 minutes to allow the ginger's medicinal properties to infuse into the water.

Remove from heat and let the mixture cool slightly to a safe, warm temperature.

How to Use:

Soak a clean cloth or towel in the warm ginger-infused water.

- Wring out the excess water and apply the compress directly to the affected area.

- Leave the compress in place for 15-30 minutes, reapplying warmth as needed.

- Repeat the process 1-2 times daily, especially after periods of increased joint stiffness or pain.

Duration:

- Use the ginger compress regularly as needed to manage arthritis symptoms and improve joint mobility.

- If symptoms persist or worsen, or if you experience any skin irritation, discontinue use and consult a healthcare professional.

Ginger Compress provides a soothing and effective way to alleviate arthritis pain and inflammation, leveraging the natural healing properties of ginger for targeted joint relief and enhanced comfort.

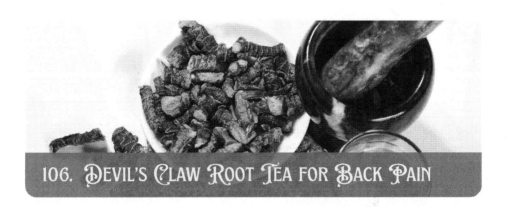

106. DEVIL'S CLAW ROOT TEA FOR BACK PAIN

Introduction:

Devil's Claw Root Tea is a natural remedy favored for its strong anti-inflammatory and analgesic properties, making it especially effective in alleviating back pain and other forms of musculoskeletal discomfort. Derived from the roots of the Devil's Claw plant, this tea contains harpagoside, a compound known to reduce inflammation and ease pain in the joints and muscles.

Ingredients and Measurements:

- 1 teaspoon of dried Devil's Claw root

- 2 cups of water

- Optional: honey or lemon to taste

Preparation:

- Place the dried Devil's Claw root in a pot.

- Add the water and bring the mixture to a boil.

- Once boiling, reduce the heat and let the tea simmer for 15-20 minutes to allow the active compounds to be extracted effectively.

- Strain the tea into a cup, removing the Devil's Claw root.

How to Use:

- Drink a cup of Devil's Claw Root Tea once or twice daily to help reduce back pain and improve overall mobility.

- If desired, enhance the flavor and additional health benefits by adding a teaspoon of honey or a squeeze of lemon.

Duration:

- Devil's Claw Root Tea can be consumed regularly as part of a routine to manage chronic back pain and other musculoskeletal issues.

- If pain persists or worsens, or if you experience any adverse effects, consult a healthcare professional for further evaluation and treatment.

Devil's Claw Root Tea offers a natural and effective approach to managing back pain, providing relief through its potent anti-inflammatory properties and improving quality of life for those suffering from musculoskeletal discomfort.

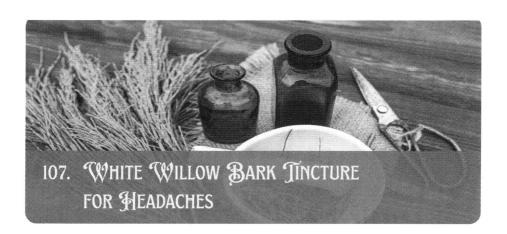

107. WHITE WILLOW BARK TINCTURE FOR HEADACHES

Introduction:

White Willow Bark Tincture is an effective herbal remedy known for its natural pain-relieving properties, particularly for treating headaches. White willow bark contains salicin, a precursor to salicylic acid, which is the active component in aspirin. This tincture, made with vegetable glycerin, offers a non-alcoholic alternative that provides the benefits of willow bark in a gentle form, making it suitable for various users, including those who avoid alcohol.

Ingredients and Measurements:

- 1 cup of dried white willow bark, finely chopped or powdered
- 2 cups of vegetable glycerin
- 1 cup of distilled water
- A clean glass jar with a tight-fitting lid
- A fine strainer or cheesecloth

Preparation:

☞ Place the dried white willow bark into the glass jar.

☞ Mix the vegetable glycerin and distilled water in a separate container to create a consistent solution. This ensures efficient extraction of the active compounds from the willow bark.

☞ Pour the glycerin-water mixture over the white willow bark, ensuring the bark is fully submerged.

☞ Seal the jar tightly and shake it well to combine the ingredients.

☞ Store the jar in a cool, dark place, shaking it daily for 4-6 weeks to facilitate the extraction process.

☞ After the infusion period, strain the mixture through a fine strainer or cheesecloth into another clean jar, pressing the bark to extract as much liquid as possible.

☞ Transfer the strained tincture to a dropper bottle for ease of use.

How to Use:

↳ To alleviate headache symptoms and reduce pain, take 1-2 dropperfuls (about 30-60 drops) of the White Willow Bark Tincture diluted in water or juice, up to three times a day.

↳ Begin with a lower dose to observe your body's response, and adjust as necessary based on your health goals and reaction to the supplement.

Duration:

⊘ Use the tincture as needed for headache relief.

⊘ Consult a healthcare professional for guidance on long-term use, especially if you have existing health conditions or are taking other medications.

⊘ Store the tincture in a cool, dark place, and it should remain effective for up to a year.

White Willow Bark Tincture made with vegetable glycerin is an effective way to harness the pain-relieving properties of white willow bark, offering a natural solution to manage headaches and enhance overall well-being.

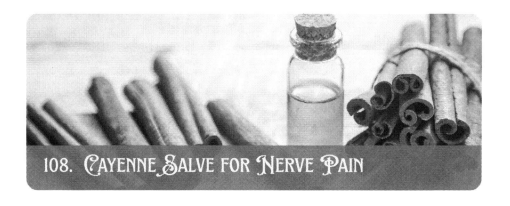

108. Cayenne Salve for Nerve Pain

Introduction:

Cayenne Salve is a potent topical remedy designed to alleviate nerve pain and discomfort. Cayenne pepper contains capsaicin, a compound that helps reduce pain by decreasing the intensity of pain signals sent to the brain. This warming salve stimulates circulation, reduces inflammation, and provides relief for conditions like neuropathy and sciatica.

Ingredients and Measurements:

- 1/4 cup of cayenne pepper powder
- 1/2 cup of carrier oil (such as coconut oil or olive oil)
- 2 tablespoons of beeswax
- Optional: a few drops of essential oils like peppermint or lavender for additional pain relief and soothing scent

Preparation:

☞ In a double boiler, gently heat the carrier oil and mix in the cayenne pepper powder. Allow this mixture to infuse for 1-2 hours over low heat, stirring occasionally.

☞ Strain the oil through a fine sieve or cheesecloth to remove the cayenne particles, retaining the infused oil.

☞ Return the infused oil to the double boiler, add the beeswax, and stir until the beeswax is completely melted and the mixture is smooth.

☞ If using, add the essential oils and stir well to combine.

☞ Pour the mixture into small tins or jars and allow it to cool and solidify.

How to Use:

↳ Apply a small amount of Cayenne Salve to the affected area, gently massaging it into the skin to help relieve nerve pain.

↳ Use caution when applying; avoid contact with eyes, mucous membranes, or broken skin.

↳ Wash hands thoroughly after application to prevent irritation to sensitive areas.

Duration:

- ⊘ Cayenne Salve can be used as needed to manage nerve pain.

- ⊘ Store the salve in a cool, dry place, and it should remain effective for up to a year.

- ⊘ If symptoms persist or worsen, or if you experience any adverse reactions, consult a healthcare professional.

Cayenne Salve provides a natural and effective way to alleviate nerve pain, leveraging the pain-relieving properties of capsaicin to improve comfort and mobility.

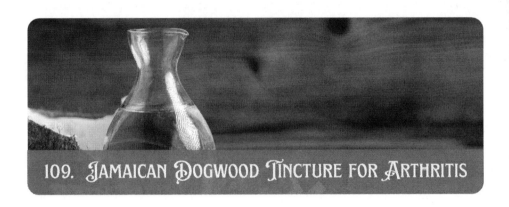

109. Jamaican Dogwood Tincture for Arthritis

Introduction:

Jamaican Dogwood Tincture is a powerful herbal extract known for its anti-inflammatory and analgesic properties, making it especially effective for managing arthritis pain and inflammation. Jamaican Dogwood contains active compounds like isoflavones that help reduce joint pain and improve mobility. Using vegetable glycerin as the extraction medium provides an alcohol-free alternative, making this tincture suitable for various users.

Ingredients and Measurements:

- 1 cup of dried Jamaican Dogwood bark, finely chopped or powdered

- 2 cups of vegetable glycerin

- 1 cup of distilled water

- A clean glass jar with a tight-fitting lid

- A fine strainer or cheesecloth

Preparation:

- ⌕ Place the dried Jamaican Dogwood bark into the glass jar.

- ⌕ Mix the vegetable glycerin and distilled water in a separate container to create a consistent solution. This ensures efficient extraction of the active compounds from the bark.

- Pour the glycerin-water mixture over the Jamaican Dogwood bark, ensuring the bark is fully submerged.

- Seal the jar tightly and shake it well to combine the ingredients.

- Store the jar in a cool, dark place, shaking it daily for 4-6 weeks to facilitate the extraction process.

- After the infusion period, strain the mixture through a fine strainer or cheesecloth into another clean jar, pressing the bark to extract as much liquid as possible.

- Transfer the strained tincture to a dropper bottle for ease of use.

How to Use:

- To alleviate arthritis pain and reduce inflammation, take 1-2 dropperfuls (about 30-60 drops) of the Jamaican Dogwood Tincture diluted in water or juice, up to three times a day.

- Begin with a lower dose to observe your body's response, and adjust as necessary based on your health goals and reaction to the supplement.

Duration:

- Use the tincture regularly as part of a health regimen to manage arthritis symptoms.

- Consult a healthcare professional for guidance on long-term use, especially if you have existing health conditions or are taking other medications.

- Store the tincture in a cool, dark place, and it should remain effective for up to a year.

Jamaican Dogwood Tincture made with vegetable glycerin is an effective way to leverage the pain-relieving properties of Jamaican Dogwood, offering a natural solution to manage arthritis pain and enhance joint mobility.

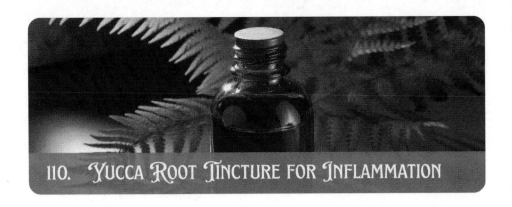

Introduction:

Yucca Root Tincture is an herbal remedy celebrated for its ability to reduce inflammation and support overall joint health. Yucca root contains saponins and polyphenolics, natural compounds that have anti-inflammatory and antioxidant properties. This makes the tincture particularly beneficial for conditions like arthritis, reducing joint pain and improving mobility. Using vegetable glycerin as the extraction medium provides an alcohol-free option for those who prefer or need to avoid alcohol.

Ingredients and Measurements:

- 1 cup of dried yucca root, finely chopped or powdered
- 2 cups of vegetable glycerin
- 1 cup of distilled water
- A clean glass jar with a tight-fitting lid
- A fine strainer or cheesecloth

Preparation:

- Place the dried yucca root into the glass jar.

- Mix the vegetable glycerin and distilled water in a separate container to ensure a uniform solution. This mixture ensures efficient extraction of the active compounds from yucca root.

- Pour the glycerin-water mixture over the yucca root, making sure the root is fully submerged.

- Seal the jar tightly and shake it well to combine the ingredients.

- Store the jar in a cool, dark place, shaking it daily for 4-6 weeks to promote the extraction process.

- After the infusion period, strain the mixture through a fine strainer or cheesecloth into another clean jar, pressing the root to extract as much liquid as possible.

- Transfer the strained tincture to a dropper bottle for ease of use.

How to Use:

- To reduce inflammation and alleviate joint pain, take 1-2 dropperfuls (about 30-60 drops) of the Yucca Root Tincture diluted in water or juice, up to three times a day.

- Begin with a lower dose to observe how your body responds, and adjust as necessary based on your health goals and the supplement's effectiveness.

Duration:

- Use the tincture regularly as part of a health regimen to manage inflammation and support joint health.

- Consult a healthcare professional for guidance on long-term use, especially if you have existing health conditions or are taking other medications.

- Store the tincture in a cool, dark place, and it should remain effective for up to a year.

Yucca Root Tincture made with vegetable glycerin is an effective way to harness the anti-inflammatory and antioxidant properties of yucca root, offering a natural solution to improve joint health and reduce inflammation.

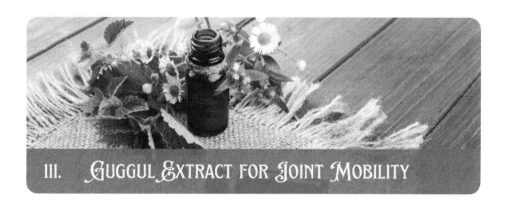

III.   GUGGUL EXTRACT FOR JOINT MOBILITY

Introduction:

Guggul Extract is a traditional Ayurvedic remedy known for its potent effects on enhancing joint mobility and reducing inflammation. Derived from the resin of the Commiphora mukul tree, guggul contains guggulsterones, compounds that help to decrease inflammation and pain associated with conditions like arthritis. This extract is particularly effective in improving flexibility and reducing stiffness in the joints.

Ingredients and Measurements:

- 1 cup of dried guggul resin
- 2 cups of vegetable glycerin
- 1 cup of distilled water
- A clean glass jar with a tight-fitting lid

- A fine strainer or cheesecloth

Preparation:

☞ Place the dried guggul resin into the glass jar.

☞ Mix the vegetable glycerin and distilled water in a separate container to create a consistent solution. This mixture ensures efficient extraction of the active compounds from the guggul resin.

☞ Pour the glycerin-water mixture over the guggul resin, ensuring it is fully submerged.

☞ Seal the jar tightly and shake it well to combine the ingredients.

☞ Store the jar in a cool, dark place, shaking it daily for 4-6 weeks to facilitate the extraction process.

☞ After the infusion period, strain the mixture through a fine strainer or cheesecloth into another clean jar, pressing the resin to extract as much liquid as possible.

☞ Transfer the strained extract to a dropper bottle for ease of use.

How to Use:

↳ To improve joint mobility and reduce inflammation, take 1-2 dropperfuls (about 30-60 drops) of the Guggul Extract diluted in water or juice, up to three times a day.

↳ Begin with a lower dose to observe your body's response, and adjust as necessary based on your health goals and reaction to the supplement.

Duration:

⊘ Use the extract regularly as part of a health regimen to manage joint pain and enhance mobility.

⊘ Consult a healthcare professional for guidance on long-term use, especially if you have existing health conditions or are taking other medications.

⊘ Store the extract in a cool, dark place, and it should remain effective for up to a year.

Guggul Extract provides a natural and effective way to harness the therapeutic properties of guggul, offering a solution to improve joint health and mobility while reducing inflammation.

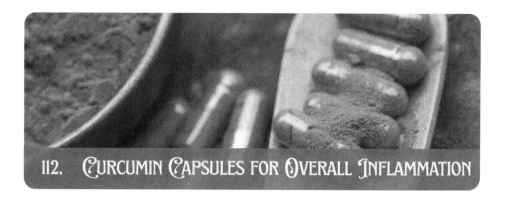

112. CURCUMIN CAPSULES FOR OVERALL INFLAMMATION

Introduction:

Curcumin Capsules are a highly effective natural supplement derived from turmeric, specifically from its active compound, curcumin. Known for its potent anti-inflammatory and antioxidant properties, curcumin helps combat systemic inflammation and oxidative stress, which are key contributors to chronic diseases and conditions like arthritis, cardiovascular disorders, and cognitive decline. These capsules offer a concentrated way to benefit from curcumin's health-promoting effects.

Ingredients and Measurements:

- Curcumin powder (extracted from turmeric)
- Empty gelatin or vegetarian capsules
- A small dropper or pipette, if needed, to fill capsules

Preparation:

☞ Ensure you have high-quality, concentrated curcumin powder. This is crucial for both safety and efficacy.

☞ Take an empty capsule and carefully open it to expose the two halves.

☞ Fill one half of the capsule with curcumin powder. A small funnel or pipette can help ensure precision and prevent spillage.

☞ Once filled, reassemble the two halves of the capsule to seal the curcumin powder inside.

☞ Repeat the process for the desired number of capsules. Store the prepared capsules in a cool, dark place, ideally in an airtight container.

How to Use:

↳ For general health and to reduce inflammation, take 1-2 curcumin capsules once or twice a day with meals.

↳ Always take the capsules with a full glass of water to aid absorption and minimize potential digestive discomfort.

↳ Including a source of healthy fats or black pepper in the meal can enhance the absorption of curcumin due to its fat-soluble nature.

Duration:

- Curcumin capsules can be used as part of an ongoing treatment plan for managing inflammation and promoting overall health.

- Monitor your body's response to the capsules and adjust the dosage accordingly. If symptoms persist or worsen, consult a healthcare professional for further guidance.

Curcumin Capsules provide a convenient and powerful way to harness the anti-inflammatory and antioxidant benefits of curcumin, offering a targeted solution to improve overall health and reduce inflammation.

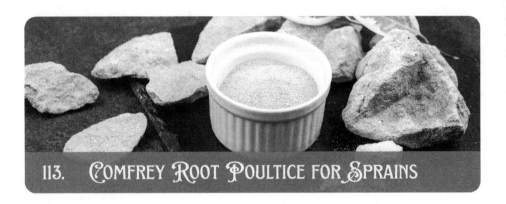

113. COMFREY ROOT POULTICE FOR SPRAINS

Introduction:

Comfrey Root Poultice is a traditional topical remedy known for its remarkable healing properties, especially in treating sprains, bruises, and other soft tissue injuries. Comfrey root contains allantoin, a compound that accelerates cell regeneration and promotes the healing of tissues. This poultice is an effective way to reduce swelling and speed up recovery from sprains.

Ingredients and Measurements:

- 1/2 cup of dried comfrey root, finely ground

- Water to create a paste
- A clean cloth or gauze

Preparation:

- Grind the dried comfrey root into a fine powder using a mortar and pestle or a coffee grinder.

- Slowly add water to the comfrey root powder in a bowl, stirring continuously, until you achieve a thick, spreadable paste.

- Spread the comfrey paste onto a clean cloth or gauze.

How to Use:

- Apply the comfrey root poultice directly to the sprained area, ensuring it covers the injured site completely.

- Wrap the area with another layer of cloth or bandage to hold the poultice in place.

- Leave the poultice on for 1-2 hours before gently removing. Wash the area with warm water after removal.

- Repeat the application once or twice daily as needed for pain relief and to support healing.

Duration:

- Use the comfrey root poultice for a few days up to a week as part of the initial treatment for sprains.

- If symptoms persist or worsen, or if there is significant pain or swelling, consult a healthcare professional for further evaluation and treatment.

Comfrey Root Poultice provides a natural and effective approach to alleviate pain, reduce inflammation, and accelerate the healing process in cases of sprains and other soft tissue injuries.

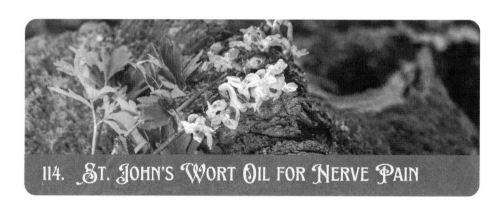

114. St. John's Wort Oil for Nerve Pain

Introduction:

St. John's Wort Oil is an effective herbal remedy known for its potent anti-inflammatory and analgesic properties, making it particularly beneficial for managing nerve pain. Derived from the flowers of the St. John's Wort plant, this oil contains hypericin and other bioactive compounds that help soothe nerve damage, reduce inflammation, and alleviate discomfort associated with conditions like neuropathy and sciatica.

Ingredients and Measurements:

- 1 cup of fresh St. John's Wort flowers

- 1 cup of carrier oil (such as olive oil or almond oil)

- A clean glass jar with a tight-fitting lid

- A fine strainer or cheesecloth

Preparation:

🫖 Place the fresh St. John's Wort flowers in the glass jar.

🫖 Pour the carrier oil over the flowers, ensuring they are completely submerged.

🫖 Seal the jar tightly and place it in a sunny window or a warm location to infuse for 4-6 weeks, shaking the jar daily to mix the contents.

🫖 After the infusion period, strain the oil through a fine strainer or cheesecloth into another clean jar, pressing the flowers to extract as much oil as possible.

How to Use:

🔸 Gently massage the St. John's Wort Oil into the affected area 2-3 times daily, focusing on areas with nerve pain or inflammation.

🔸 Use the oil consistently for several weeks to achieve the best results in pain relief and healing.

Duration:

🕑 St. John's Wort Oil can be used regularly as part of a treatment plan for nerve pain and related conditions.

🕑 Store the oil in a cool, dark place, and it should remain effective for up to a year.

🕑 If symptoms persist or worsen, or if you experience any adverse reactions, consult a healthcare professional for further guidance.

St. John's Wort Oil provides a natural and soothing solution to nerve pain, leveraging the healing properties of St. John's Wort to improve comfort and mobility effectively.

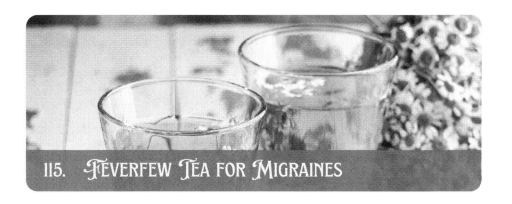

115. FEVERFEW TEA FOR MIGRAINES

Introduction:

Feverfew Tea is a traditional herbal remedy recognized for its efficacy in preventing and alleviating migraines. Feverfew contains parthenolide, a compound that helps reduce inflammation and prevent the constriction of blood vessels in the brain, key contributors to migraine pain. Regular consumption of this tea can help decrease the frequency and intensity of migraine attacks.

Ingredients and Measurements:

- 1 teaspoon of dried feverfew leaves
- 1 cup of boiling water
- Optional: honey or lemon to taste

Preparation:

- Place the dried feverfew leaves in a cup or tea infuser.
- Pour the boiling water over the leaves and cover to ensure the essential oils and active ingredients are retained.
- Allow the tea to steep for 10-15 minutes.
- Strain the tea to remove the feverfew leaves.

How to Use:

- Drink a cup of Feverfew Tea at the onset of migraine symptoms or daily as a preventive measure against migraines.
- If desired, enhance the flavor and additional health benefits by adding a teaspoon of honey or a squeeze of lemon.

Duration:

- Feverfew Tea can be consumed regularly as part of a routine to manage migraines and reduce their occurrence.
- Monitor your body's response to the tea and adjust the frequency of consumption accordingly. If migraines persist or worsen, consult a healthcare professional for further evaluation and treatment.

Feverfew Tea offers a natural and effective approach to managing migraines, providing relief from pain and improving overall quality of life for those affected by this debilitating condition.

PART 05

WOMEN'S HEALTH REMEDIES (116-130)

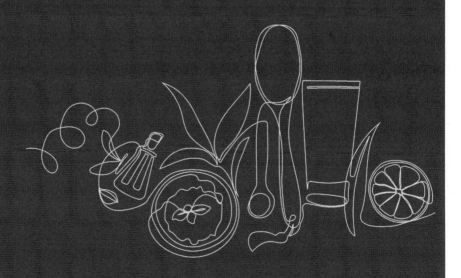

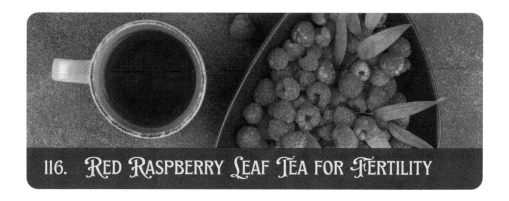

116. RED RASPBERRY LEAF TEA FOR FERTILITY

Introduction:

Red Raspberry Leaf Tea is a well-known herbal remedy often recommended to enhance fertility and support reproductive health in women. Rich in vitamins and minerals, including magnesium, potassium, and iron, red raspberry leaf helps tone the uterine muscles, improve menstrual cycle regularity, and prepare the body for pregnancy. This tea is also beneficial for overall uterine health.

Ingredients and Measurements:

- 1-2 teaspoons of dried red raspberry leaves
- 1 cup of boiling water
- Optional: honey or lemon to taste

Preparation:

- Place the dried red raspberry leaves in a cup or tea infuser.
- Pour the boiling water over the leaves and cover the cup to preserve the nutrients and essential oils.
- Allow the tea to steep for 10-15 minutes.
- Strain the tea to remove the leaves.

How to Use:

- Drink a cup of Red Raspberry Leaf Tea 1-2 times daily, particularly during the preconception period, to enhance fertility and support reproductive health.
- If desired, enhance the flavor and additional health benefits by adding a teaspoon of honey or a squeeze of lemon.

Duration:

- Red Raspberry Leaf Tea can be consumed regularly as part of a health-focused routine to support fertility and improve menstrual health.
- If there are no improvements in menstrual regularity or fertility symptoms after a few months, consult a healthcare professional for further guidance and treatment.

Red Raspberry Leaf Tea provides a natural and gentle way to support fertility and reproductive health, offering a beneficial approach to preparing the body for pregnancy and enhancing overall well-being.

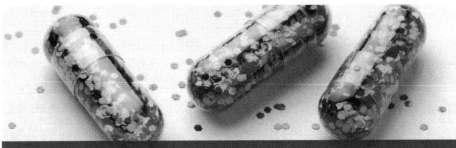

117. CHASTE TREE BERRY CAPSULES FOR PMS

Introduction:

Chaste Tree Berry, also known as Vitex, is a highly effective herbal remedy for managing symptoms of Pre-Menstrual Syndrome (PMS). The active compounds in Chaste Tree Berry help regulate hormonal balance, reducing symptoms such as mood swings, breast tenderness, and bloating. These capsules provide a convenient way to incorporate the benefits of Chaste Tree Berry into your daily routine for consistent relief.

Ingredients and Measurements:

- Chaste Tree Berry (Vitex) powder
- Empty gelatin or vegetarian capsules
- A small funnel or pipette, if needed, to fill capsules

Preparation:

☞ Ensure you have high-quality Chaste Tree Berry powder. This is crucial for both safety and efficacy.

☞ Using a small funnel or pipette, fill one half of the empty capsule with the Chaste Tree Berry powder.

☞ Once filled, reassemble the two halves of the capsule to enclose the powder.

☞ Repeat the process for the desired number of capsules. Store the prepared capsules in a cool, dark place, ideally in an airtight container.

How to Use:

✍ Take 1-2 Chaste Tree Berry capsules daily, preferably in the morning, to manage PMS symptoms effectively.

✍ Consistent use over several menstrual cycles is often necessary to observe the full benefits.

Duration:

⊘ Chaste Tree Berry Capsules can be used as part of an ongoing regimen to manage PMS symptoms.

⊘ Monitor your body's response and adjust the dosage as needed. If symptoms persist or worsen, consult a healthcare professional for further evaluation and guidance.

Chaste Tree Berry Capsules provide a straightforward and effective way to harness the hormonal balancing properties of Chaste Tree Berry, offering a targeted solution to alleviate the discomfort of PMS and enhance overall menstrual health.

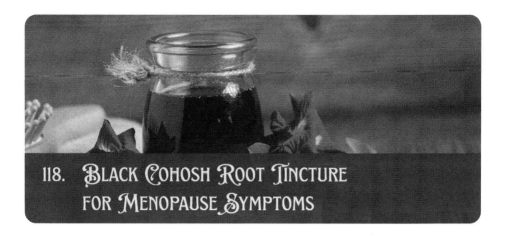

118. Black Cohosh Root Tincture for Menopause Symptoms

Introduction:

Black Cohosh Root Tincture is a well-known herbal remedy used to alleviate a range of menopause symptoms, including hot flashes, mood swings, night sweats, and sleep disturbances. Black Cohosh contains phytoestrogens that help balance hormones and provide relief from the discomfort associated with menopause. This tincture, made with vegetable glycerin, offers an alcohol-free alternative for those seeking natural menopause support.

Ingredients and Measurements:

- 1 cup of dried Black Cohosh root, finely chopped or powdered
- 2 cups of vegetable glycerin
- 1 cup of distilled water
- A clean glass jar with a tight-fitting lid
- A fine strainer or cheesecloth

Preparation:

- Place the dried Black Cohosh root into the glass jar.

- Mix the vegetable glycerin and distilled water in a separate container to create a consistent solution. This blend ensures efficient extraction of the active compounds from Black Cohosh.

- Pour the glycerin-water mixture over the Black Cohosh root, ensuring the root is fully submerged.

- Seal the jar tightly and shake it well to combine the ingredients.

- Store the jar in a cool, dark place, shaking it daily for 4-6 weeks to facilitate the extraction process.

- After the infusion period, strain the mixture through a fine strainer or cheesecloth into another clean jar, pressing the root to extract as much liquid as possible.

- Transfer the strained tincture to a dropper bottle for ease of use.

How to Use:

- To alleviate menopause symptoms, take 1-2 dropperfuls (about 30-60 drops) of the Black Cohosh Root Tincture diluted in water or juice, up to three times a day.

- Begin with a lower dose to observe your body's response, and adjust as necessary based on your health goals and reaction to the supplement.

Duration:

- Use the tincture regularly as part of a health regimen to manage menopause symptoms.

- Consult a healthcare professional for guidance on long-term use, especially if you have existing health conditions or are taking other medications.

- Store the tincture in a cool, dark place, and it should remain effective for up to a year.

- Black Cohosh Root Tincture is an effective way to leverage the hormonal balancing properties of Black Cohosh, offering a natural solution to manage menopause symptoms and enhance overall well-being.

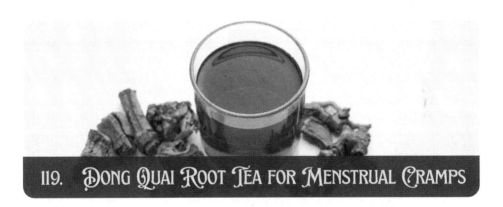

119. DONG QUAI ROOT TEA FOR MENSTRUAL CRAMPS

Introduction:

Dong Quai Root Tea is a traditional herbal remedy known for its effectiveness in alleviating menstrual cramps and promoting a healthy menstrual cycle. Dong Quai, often referred to as "female ginseng," is rich in phytoestrogens and other compounds that help relax muscle tissue, reduce inflammation, and balance hormones, making it particularly beneficial for easing menstrual discomfort.

Ingredients and Measurements:

- 1 teaspoon of dried Dong Quai root
- 1 cup of boiling water
- Optional: honey or lemon to taste

Preparation:

- Place the dried Dong Quai root in a cup or tea infuser.
- Pour the boiling water over the root and cover the cup to preserve the essential oils and active ingredients.

- Allow the tea to steep for 10-15 minutes.
- Strain the tea to remove the Dong Quai root.

How to Use:

- Drink a cup of Dong Quai Root Tea once or twice daily, starting a few days before the onset of menstruation and continuing through the menstrual period, to alleviate cramps and improve overall menstrual health.

- If desired, enhance the flavor and additional health benefits by adding a teaspoon of honey or a squeeze of lemon.

Duration:

- Dong Quai Root Tea can be consumed regularly as part of a routine to manage menstrual symptoms and promote reproductive health.

- Monitor your body's response to the tea and adjust the frequency of consumption accordingly. If symptoms persist or worsen, consult a healthcare professional for further evaluation and treatment.

Dong Quai Root Tea offers a natural and effective approach to managing menstrual cramps, providing relief from pain and improving the overall menstrual experience.

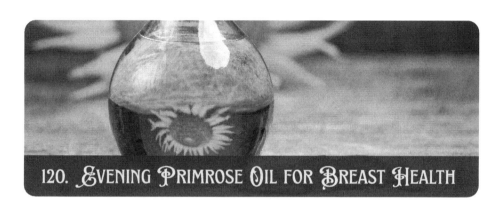

120. Evening Primrose Oil for Breast Health

Introduction:

Evening Primrose Oil is a valuable supplement recognized for its beneficial effects on breast health and hormonal balance. Rich in gamma-linolenic acid (GLA), a type of omega-6 fatty acid, Evening Primrose Oil helps reduce breast pain and tenderness associated with menstrual cycles, hormonal fluctuations, and other conditions. Its anti-inflammatory properties also contribute to overall breast wellness.

Ingredients and Measurements:

- Evening Primrose Oil capsules or liquid oil

- Optional: vitamin E for added antioxidant benefits

Preparation:

🖐 No complex preparation is needed for Evening Primrose Oil. It comes ready to use in capsule form or as a pure oil.

How to Use:

🖐 If using capsules, take 1-2 Evening Primrose Oil capsules daily with a meal, or as directed by a healthcare provider.

🖐 If using liquid oil, measure out a teaspoon and take it orally or mix it into a smoothie or salad dressing.

🖐 For topical application, especially to address localized breast tenderness, massage a small amount of oil directly onto the breast area.

Duration:

⏲ Evening Primrose Oil can be taken regularly as part of a daily routine to maintain breast health and manage symptoms of hormonal imbalance.

⏲ Monitor your body's response to the oil and adjust the dosage as necessary. If any unusual symptoms or breast changes occur, consult a healthcare professional for further evaluation and guidance.

Evening Primrose Oil provides a straightforward and effective way to support breast health, offering a natural solution to alleviate discomfort and promote hormonal balance.

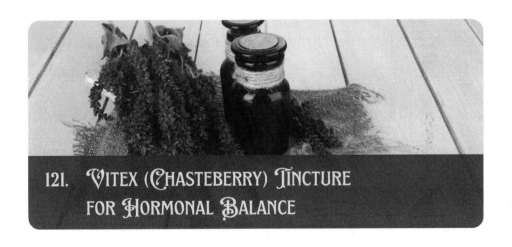

121. VITEX (CHASTEBERRY) TINCTURE FOR HORMONAL BALANCE

Introduction:

Vitex, also known as Chasteberry, is a powerful herbal remedy widely used to enhance hormonal balance and alleviate symptoms of hormonal imbalances such as PMS, menstrual irregularities, and fertility issues. The active compounds in Vitex help regulate the production of hormones like progesterone and estrogen, promoting overall reproductive health. This tincture, made with vegetable glycerin, offers an alcohol-free option suitable for various users.

Ingredients and Measurements:

- 1 cup of dried Vitex berries, finely chopped or powdered
- 2 cups of vegetable glycerin
- 1 cup of distilled water
- A clean glass jar with a tight-fitting lid
- A fine strainer or cheesecloth

Preparation:

Place the dried Vitex berries into the glass jar.

Mix the vegetable glycerin and distilled water in a separate container to create a consistent solution. This blend ensures efficient extraction of the active compounds from Vitex.

Pour the glycerin-water mixture over the Vitex berries, ensuring the berries are fully submerged.

Seal the jar tightly and shake it well to combine the ingredients.

Store the jar in a cool, dark place, shaking it daily for 4-6 weeks to facilitate the extraction process.

After the infusion period, strain the mixture through a fine strainer or cheesecloth into another clean jar, pressing the berries to extract as much liquid as possible.

Transfer the strained tincture to a dropper bottle for ease of use.

How to Use:

To support hormonal balance and alleviate symptoms of hormonal imbalances, take 1-2 dropperfuls (about 30-60 drops) of the Vitex Tincture diluted in water or juice, up to three times a day.

Begin with a lower dose to observe your body's response, and adjust as necessary based on your health goals and reaction to the supplement.

Duration:

Use the tincture regularly as part of a health regimen to manage hormonal imbalances and support reproductive health.

Consult a healthcare professional for guidance on long-term use, especially if you have existing health conditions or are taking other medications.

Store the tincture in a cool, dark place, and it should remain effective for up to a year.

Vitex Tincture made with vegetable glycerin is an effective way to harness the hormonal balancing properties of Vitex, offering a natural solution to improve reproductive health and alleviate symptoms of hormonal imbalances.

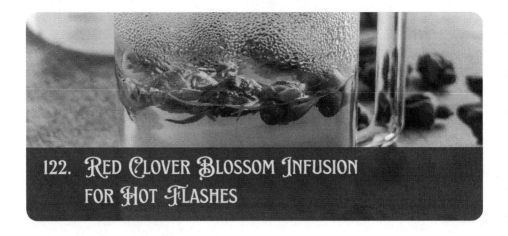

122. Red Clover Blossom Infusion for Hot Flashes

Introduction:

Red Clover Blossom Infusion is a natural herbal remedy recognized for its effectiveness in alleviating hot flashes and other menopausal symptoms. Rich in isoflavones, phytoestrogens that mimic the effects of estrogen in the body, Red Clover helps balance hormone levels, reducing the frequency and intensity of hot flashes. This infusion provides a gentle and holistic approach to managing menopause-related discomfort.

Ingredients and Measurements:

- 1-2 tablespoons of dried Red Clover blossoms
- 1 cup of boiling water
- Optional: honey or lemon to taste

Preparation:

☕ Place the dried Red Clover blossoms in a cup or tea infuser.

☕ Pour the boiling water over the blossoms and cover the cup to preserve the essential oils and active ingredients.

☕ Allow the tea to steep for 10-15 minutes.

☕ Strain the tea to remove the blossoms.

How to Use:

🥄 Drink a cup of Red Clover Blossom Infusion once or twice daily, especially during periods of increased menopausal symptoms like hot flashes.

🥄 If desired, enhance the flavor and additional health benefits by adding a teaspoon of honey or a squeeze of lemon.

Duration:

⊘ Red Clover Blossom Infusion can be consumed regularly as part of a routine to manage menopausal symptoms and promote overall hormonal balance.

⊘ Monitor your body's response to the infusion and adjust the frequency of consumption accordingly. If symptoms persist or worsen, consult a healthcare professional for further evaluation and treatment.

Red Clover Blossom Infusion offers a natural and soothing solution to manage hot flashes and other menopausal symptoms, enhancing comfort and quality of life during this transitional phase.

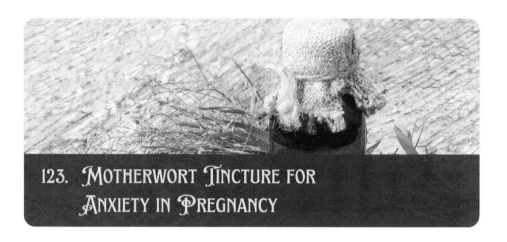

123. Motherwort Tincture for Anxiety in Pregnancy

Introduction:

Motherwort Tincture is a valuable herbal remedy used to alleviate anxiety, especially during pregnancy. Motherwort, known for its calming and heart-supportive properties, helps reduce stress and nervous tension. This tincture, made with vegetable glycerin, provides a gentle, alcohol-free option suitable for expectant mothers seeking natural ways to manage anxiety.

Ingredients and Measurements:

- 1 cup of dried Motherwort leaves and flowers
- 2 cups of vegetable glycerin
- 1 cup of distilled water

- A clean glass jar with a tight-fitting lid
- A fine strainer or cheesecloth

Preparation:

☞ Place the dried Motherwort into the glass jar.

☞ Mix the vegetable glycerin and distilled water in a separate container to create a consistent solution. This mixture ensures efficient extraction of the active compounds from Motherwort.

☞ Pour the glycerin-water mixture over the Motherwort, ensuring the herb is fully submerged.

☞ Seal the jar tightly and shake it well to combine the ingredients.

- Store the jar in a cool, dark place, shaking it daily for 4-6 weeks to facilitate the extraction process.

- After the infusion period, strain the mixture through a fine strainer or cheesecloth into another clean jar, pressing the herb to extract as much liquid as possible.

- Transfer the strained tincture to a dropper bottle for ease of use.

How to Use:

- To alleviate anxiety during pregnancy, take 1 dropperful (about 30 drops) of the Motherwort Tincture diluted in water or juice, up to twice a day.

- Consult with a healthcare provider before beginning any herbal treatment during pregnancy to ensure safety and proper dosage.

Duration:

- Use the tincture as needed to manage anxiety symptoms during pregnancy.

- Store the tincture in a cool, dark place, and it should remain effective for up to a year.

Motherwort Tincture made with vegetable glycerin is an effective way to harness the calming properties of Motherwort, offering a natural solution to manage anxiety and support emotional well-being during pregnancy.

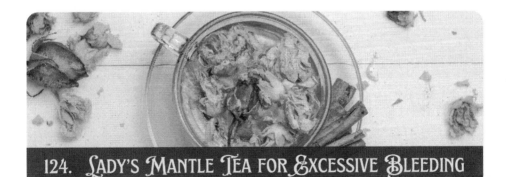

124. LADY'S MANTLE TEA FOR EXCESSIVE BLEEDING

Introduction:

Lady's Mantle Tea is an esteemed herbal remedy known for its ability to reduce excessive menstrual bleeding and enhance reproductive health. The astringent properties of Lady's Mantle help tighten tissues and blood vessels, effectively lessening heavy flow and supporting uterine health. This tea is also beneficial for overall menstrual cycle regulation.

Ingredients and Measurements:

- 1-2 teaspoons of dried Lady's Mantle leaves
- 1 cup of boiling water
- Optional: honey or lemon to taste

Preparation:

- Place the dried Lady's Mantle leaves in a cup or tea infuser.
- Pour the boiling water over the leaves and cover the cup to retain the essential oils and active ingredients.
- Allow the tea to steep for 10-15 minutes.
- Strain the tea to remove the leaves.

How to Use:

- Drink a cup of Lady's Mantle Tea 1-2 times daily, especially during the menstrual period or in the days leading up to it, to manage excessive bleeding and enhance uterine health.

- If desired, enhance the flavor and additional health benefits by adding a teaspoon of honey or a squeeze of lemon.

Duration:

- Lady's Mantle Tea can be consumed regularly as part of a routine to manage menstrual symptoms and support reproductive health.
- Monitor your body's response to the tea and adjust the frequency of consumption accordingly. If symptoms persist or worsen, consult a healthcare professional for further evaluation and treatment.

Lady's Mantle Tea offers a natural and effective way to manage excessive menstrual bleeding, providing relief and supporting overall reproductive health.

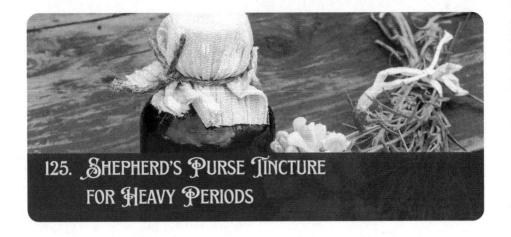

125. Shepherd's Purse Tincture for Heavy Periods

Introduction:

Shepherd's Purse Tincture is a traditional herbal remedy renowned for its effectiveness in managing heavy menstrual bleeding. Shepherd's Purse contains compounds that help constrict blood vessels and reduce uterine bleeding. Using vegetable glycerin for extraction makes this tincture an alcohol-free option, suitable for those who prefer a gentler approach to managing menstrual symptoms.

Ingredients and Measurements:

- 1 cup of dried Shepherd's Purse herb
- 2 cups of vegetable glycerin
- 1 cup of distilled water
- A clean glass jar with a tight-fitting lid
- A fine strainer or cheesecloth

Preparation:

☞ Place the dried Shepherd's Purse herb into the glass jar.

☞ Mix the vegetable glycerin and distilled water in a separate container to create a consistent solution. This mixture ensures efficient extraction of the active compounds from Shepherd's Purse.

☞ Pour the glycerin-water mixture over the Shepherd's Purse, ensuring the herb is fully submerged.

☞ Seal the jar tightly and shake it well to combine the ingredients.

☞ Store the jar in a cool, dark place, shaking it daily for 4-6 weeks to facilitate the extraction process.

☞ After the infusion period, strain the mixture through a fine strainer or cheesecloth into another clean jar, pressing the herb to extract as much liquid as possible.

☞ Transfer the strained tincture to a dropper bottle for ease of use.

How to Use:

✎ To manage heavy periods and reduce menstrual flow, take 1-2 dropperfuls (about 30-60 drops) of the Shepherd's Purse Tincture diluted in water or juice, up to three times a day during the menstrual cycle.

ꙮ Begin with a lower dose to observe your body's response, and adjust as necessary based on your health goals and reaction to the supplement.

Duration:

ꙮ Use the tincture as needed during menstrual cycles to effectively manage heavy bleeding.

ꙮ Consult a healthcare professional for guidance on long-term use, especially if you have existing health conditions or are taking other medications.

ꙮ Store the tincture in a cool, dark place, and it should remain effective for up to a year.

Shepherd's Purse Tincture made with vegetable glycerin provides a natural and effective way to manage heavy menstrual bleeding, offering a targeted solution to improve comfort and balance during menstruation

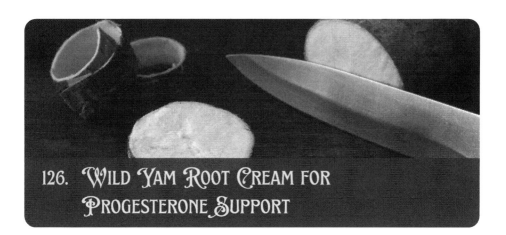

126. WILD YAM ROOT CREAM FOR PROGESTERONE SUPPORT

Introduction:

Wild Yam Root Cream is a popular natural remedy used to support hormonal balance, particularly by enhancing progesterone levels. Wild yam contains diosgenin, a compound that is believed to support the body's production of progesterone. This cream is often used to alleviate symptoms of hormonal imbalances such as PMS, menopause, and conditions related to low progesterone levels.

Ingredients and Measurements:

- 1/4 cup of wild yam root powder

- 1/2 cup of carrier oil (such as almond oil or coconut oil)

- 1/4 cup of distilled water

- 2 tablespoons of beeswax

- Optional: essential oils like lavender or clary sage for additional therapeutic benefits

Preparation:

- In a double boiler, combine the carrier oil and wild yam root powder. Gently heat the mixture, stirring occasionally, to infuse the oil with the active compounds for about 1-2 hours.

- Strain the oil through a fine sieve or cheesecloth to remove the wild yam particles, retaining the infused oil.

- Return the infused oil to the double boiler, add the beeswax, and stir until the beeswax is completely melted and the mixture is smooth.

- Gradually add the distilled water, stirring continuously to create an emulsion.

- If using, add a few drops of essential oil and stir well to combine.

- Pour the mixture into small jars or tins and allow it to cool and solidify.

How to Use:

- Apply a small amount of Wild Yam Root Cream to the skin, focusing on areas with good blood flow such as the wrists, inner arms, or abdomen, 1-2 times daily.

- Massage the cream into the skin until fully absorbed, particularly during times when progesterone support is needed.

Duration:

Wild Yam Root Cream can be used regularly as part of a daily routine to support hormonal balance and alleviate related symptoms.

Monitor your body's response to the cream and adjust usage as needed. If any adverse reactions occur or if symptoms persist, consult a healthcare professional.

Wild Yam Root Cream offers a natural and effective way to support hormonal balance and progesterone levels, providing relief from symptoms of hormonal imbalance and enhancing overall well-being.

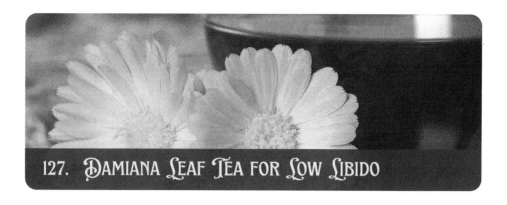

127. Damiana Leaf Tea for Low Libido

Introduction:

Damiana Leaf Tea is an herbal remedy celebrated for its aphrodisiac properties, commonly used to enhance libido and improve sexual health. Damiana leaves contain compounds that stimulate blood flow and increase sensitivity, which can help alleviate low libido and promote overall sexual wellness.

Ingredients and Measurements:

- 1-2 teaspoons of dried Damiana leaves
- 1 cup of boiling water
- Optional: honey or lemon to taste

Preparation:

☕ Place the dried Damiana leaves in a cup or tea infuser.

☕ Pour the boiling water over the leaves and cover the cup to preserve the essential oils and active ingredients.

☕ Allow the tea to steep for 10-15 minutes.

☕ Strain the tea to remove the leaves.

How to Use:

🍵 Drink a cup of Damiana Leaf Tea once or twice daily, particularly when seeking to boost libido and enhance sexual health.

🍵 If desired, enhance the flavor and additional health benefits by adding a teaspoon of honey or a squeeze of lemon.

Duration:

⊘ Damiana Leaf Tea can be consumed regularly as part of a routine to support sexual health and manage symptoms of low libido.

⊘ Monitor your body's response to the tea and adjust the frequency of consumption accordingly. If symptoms persist or worsen, consult a healthcare professional for further evaluation and treatment.

Damiana Leaf Tea provides a natural and effective way to enhance libido and improve sexual well-being, offering a holistic approach to boosting vitality and passion.

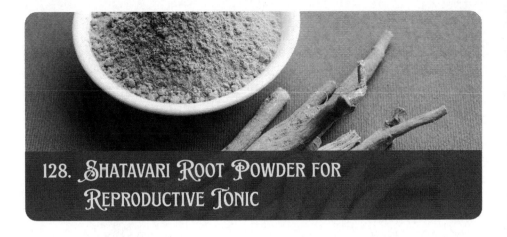

128. Shatavari Root Powder for Reproductive Tonic

Introduction:

Shatavari Root Powder is a revered herbal supplement in Ayurvedic medicine, known for its nourishing and rejuvenating effects on the female reproductive system. Rich in saponins and phytoestrogens, Shatavari enhances fertility, regulates menstrual cycles, and supports overall reproductive health. This powder is particularly beneficial for women at various stages of life, from enhancing fertility to easing menopausal symptoms.

Ingredients and Measurements:

- Shatavari root powder
- Water, milk, or a smoothie for mixing

Preparation:

☞ No complex preparation is needed for Shatavari root powder. It is ready to use and easily dissolves in liquids.

How to Use:

✎ Mix 1 teaspoon of Shatavari root powder into a glass of water, milk, or your favorite smoothie.

✎ Drink this mixture once or twice daily to benefit from its reproductive health-supporting properties.

Duration:

◎ Shatavari root powder can be taken regularly as part of a daily health regimen to support reproductive health and hormonal balance.

◎ Monitor your body's response to the supplement and adjust the dosage as needed. If any unusual symptoms occur or if there is no improvement in reproductive health symptoms, consult a healthcare professional for further guidance.

Shatavari Root Powder provides a straightforward and effective way to support reproductive health, offering a natural solution to enhance fertility and balance hormones.

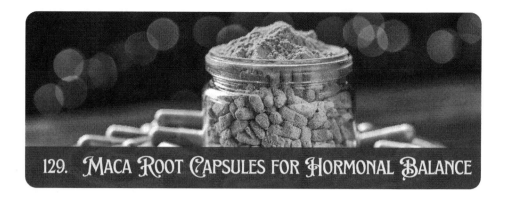

129. MACA ROOT CAPSULES FOR HORMONAL BALANCE

Introduction:

Maca Root Capsules are a popular natural supplement derived from the maca plant, known for its remarkable ability to support hormonal balance and enhance overall vitality. Rich in vitamins, minerals, and phytonutrients, maca root helps regulate and stabilize hormonal levels, improve mood, and boost energy. This makes it particularly beneficial for both men and women experiencing hormonal imbalances or seeking a natural boost in their daily wellness.

Ingredients and Measurements:

- Maca root powder
- Empty gelatin or vegetarian capsules
- A small funnel or pipette, if needed, to fill capsules

Preparation:

☞ Ensure you have high-quality maca root powder. This is essential for both safety and efficacy.

☞ Using a small funnel or pipette, carefully fill one half of the empty capsule with maca root powder.

☞ Once filled, reassemble the two halves of the capsule to seal the maca powder inside.

☞ Repeat the process for the desired number of capsules. Store the prepared capsules in a cool, dark place, ideally in an airtight container.

How to Use:

✎ Take 1-2 Maca Root Capsules daily, preferably with a meal, to support hormonal balance and enhance overall energy and mood.

✎ Consistent use over several weeks is often necessary to observe the full benefits.

Duration:

☺ Maca Root Capsules can be used as part of an ongoing regimen to manage hormonal imbalances and promote general health.

Monitor your body's response to the capsules and adjust the dosage as necessary. If symptoms persist or worsen, consult a healthcare professional for further evaluation and guidance.

Maca Root Capsules provide a convenient and effective way to harness the hormonal balancing and energy-boosting properties of maca, offering a targeted solution to improve well-being and support hormonal health.

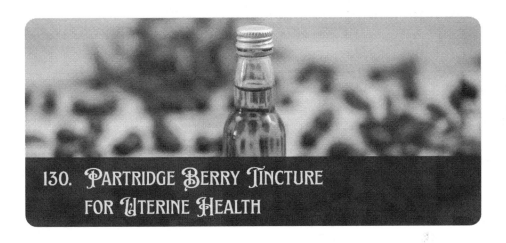

130. PARTRIDGE BERRY TINCTURE FOR UTERINE HEALTH

Introduction:

Partridge Berry Tincture is an esteemed herbal remedy known for its supportive effects on uterine health. Partridge Berry, often recommended for women, aids in strengthening and toning the uterus, which can enhance fertility, support pregnancy, and alleviate menstrual discomfort. This tincture, made with vegetable glycerin, provides a non-alcoholic means to harness the benefits of Partridge Berry in a gentle and effective manner.

Ingredients and Measurements:

- 1 cup of dried Partridge Berry leaves and berries
- 2 cups of vegetable glycerin

- 1 cup of distilled water
- A clean glass jar with a tight-fitting lid
- A fine strainer or cheesecloth

Preparation:

🥣 Place the dried Partridge Berry leaves and berries into the glass jar.

🥣 Mix the vegetable glycerin and distilled water in a separate container to create a consistent solution. This mixture ensures efficient extraction of the active compounds from Partridge Berry.

🥣 Pour the glycerin-water mixture over the Partridge Berry, ensuring the herb is fully submerged.

🥣 Seal the jar tightly and shake it well to combine the ingredients.

- Store the jar in a cool, dark place, shaking it daily for 4-6 weeks to facilitate the extraction process.

- After the infusion period, strain the mixture through a fine strainer or cheesecloth into another clean jar, pressing the herb to extract as much liquid as possible.

- Transfer the strained tincture to a dropper bottle for ease of use.

How to Use:

- To support uterine health and alleviate menstrual discomfort, take 1-2 dropperfuls (about 30-60 drops) of the Partridge Berry Tincture diluted in water or juice, up to three times a day.

- Begin with a lower dose to observe your body's response, and adjust as necessary based on your health goals and reaction to the supplement.

Duration:

- Use the tincture regularly as part of a health regimen to support uterine health and manage menstrual symptoms.

- Consult a healthcare professional for guidance on long-term use, especially if you have existing health conditions or are taking other medications.

- Store the tincture in a cool, dark place, and it should remain effective for up to a year.

Partridge Berry Tincture made with vegetable glycerin is an effective way to leverage the uterine-supportive properties of Partridge Berry, offering a natural solution to enhance reproductive health and alleviate menstrual discomfort.

PART 06

IMMUNE-BOOSTING
REMEDIES (131-160)

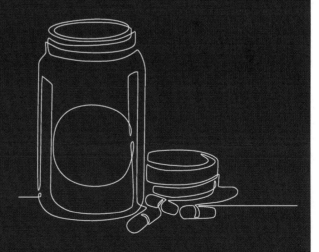

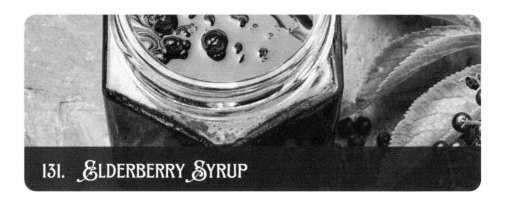

131. ELDERBERRY SYRUP

Introduction:

Elderberry Syrup is a well-known natural remedy celebrated for its immune-boosting properties. Rich in vitamins and antioxidants, elderberries help strengthen the immune system, combat viral infections, and reduce the duration and severity of colds and flu. This syrup is a tasty and effective way to incorporate the health benefits of elderberries into your daily routine.

Ingredients and Measurements:

- 1 cup of dried elderberries
- 4 cups of water
- 1 cup of honey
- Optional: a stick of cinnamon or a few cloves for additional flavor and benefits

Preparation:

In a saucepan, combine the dried elderberries and water. If using, add the cinnamon stick or cloves.

Bring the mixture to a boil, then reduce the heat and let it simmer until the liquid is reduced by half, about 45 minutes.

Strain the mixture through a fine sieve or cheesecloth to remove the elderberries and any spices, retaining the liquid.

Allow the liquid to cool to lukewarm before stirring in the honey to preserve its natural enzymes and benefits.

Pour the syrup into a clean glass bottle or jar and seal tightly.

How to Use:

Take 1-2 tablespoons of Elderberry Syrup daily during cold and flu season to boost your immune system.

If you are already experiencing cold or flu symptoms, increase the dosage to 1 tablespoon every 3-4 hours until symptoms subside.

Duration:

Elderberry Syrup can be stored in the refrigerator and used as part of your regular health regimen during the cold and flu season.

Monitor your body's response to the syrup and adjust the dosage as necessary. If any adverse reactions occur or if symptoms persist, consult a healthcare professional for further guidance.

Elderberry Syrup provides a natural and delicious way to enhance immune function, offering a preventative and therapeutic solution to support overall health and resilience against infections.

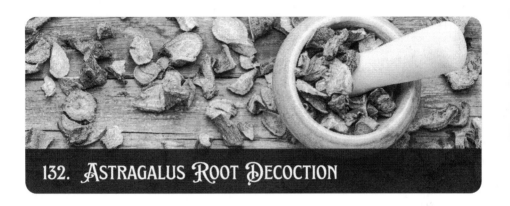

132. ASTRAGALUS ROOT DECOCTION

Introduction:

Astragalus Root Decoction is a potent herbal remedy known for its immune-boosting and vitalizing properties. Astragalus root, rich in polysaccharides, saponins, and flavonoids, strengthens the immune system, enhances energy levels, and supports overall health. This decoction is particularly effective in preventing illness and speeding recovery from sickness.

Ingredients and Measurements:

- 1-2 tablespoons of dried Astragalus root slices
- 4 cups of water
- Optional: ginger or honey to enhance flavor and add extra health benefits

Preparation:

🖾 Place the dried Astragalus root slices in a pot.

🖾 Add the water and bring the mixture to a boil.

🖾 Once boiling, reduce the heat and let it simmer until the liquid is reduced by half, about 30-40 minutes. This slow simmer helps to extract the medicinal compounds effectively.

🖾 Strain the decoction into a cup, removing the Astragalus root.

How to Use:

✎ Drink 1 cup of Astragalus Root Decoction daily, especially during times when your immune system needs a boost, such as the cold and flu season or periods of stress.

✎ If desired, enhance the flavor and additional health benefits by adding a slice of ginger during the simmering process or a teaspoon of honey just before drinking.

Duration:

⊘ Astragalus Root Decoction can be consumed regularly as part of a health-focused routine to maintain immune function and overall vitality.

⊘ If any adverse effects occur or if symptoms of illness persist, consult a healthcare professional for further evaluation and treatment.

Astragalus Root Decoction provides a straightforward and effective way to harness the immune-boosting properties of Astragalus, offering a natural solution to enhance well-being and prevent illness.

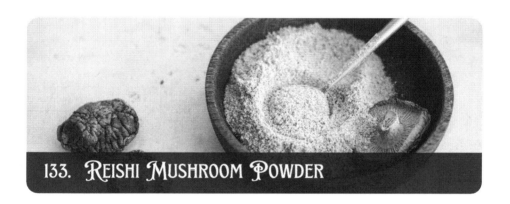

133. REISHI MUSHROOM POWDER

Introduction:

Reishi Mushroom Powder is derived from the Reishi mushroom, a medicinal fungus highly esteemed for its immune-enhancing and health-promoting properties. Reishi contains polysaccharides, triterpenoids, and peptides that support immune function, reduce stress, and promote longevity. This powder is an easy way to incorporate the benefits of Reishi into your daily wellness routine.

Ingredients and Measurements:

• Reishi mushroom powder

• Water, juice, or a smoothie for mixing

Preparation:

📋 No complex preparation is needed for Reishi mushroom powder. It comes ready to use and easily blends into various liquids.

How to Use:

🥄 Mix 1 teaspoon of Reishi mushroom powder into a glass of water, juice, or your favorite smoothie.

🥄 Drink this mixture once or twice daily to benefit from its immune-boosting and health-enhancing properties.

Duration:

🕐 Reishi mushroom powder can be taken regularly as part of a daily health regimen to support immune function and overall well-being.

🕐 Monitor your body's response to the supplement and adjust the dosage as necessary. If any unusual symptoms occur or if there is no improvement in health, consult a healthcare professional for further guidance.

Reishi Mushroom Powder provides a convenient and effective way to harness the powerful immune-supporting and health-promoting benefits of Reishi mushrooms, offering a targeted solution to improve well-being and resilience.

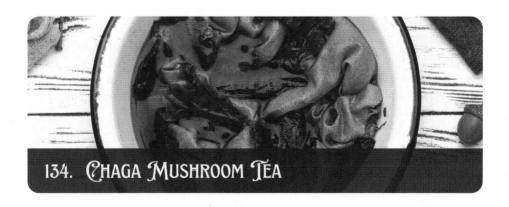

134. Chaga Mushroom Tea

Introduction:

Chaga Mushroom Tea is a potent herbal beverage known for its high antioxidant content and immune-supporting properties. Chaga mushrooms grow on birch trees and are rich in betulinic acid, melanin, and a variety of vitamins and minerals. These compounds help fight inflammation, support the immune system, and potentially reduce the risk of chronic diseases. Chaga Tea is a great way to integrate the health benefits of this medicinal mushroom into your daily routine.

Ingredients and Measurements:

- 1-2 teaspoons of dried Chaga mushroom chunks or powder
- 2 cups of water
- Optional: honey or lemon to taste

Preparation:

☞ If using Chaga chunks, place them in a pot. If using powder, you may prefer to steep it like loose leaf tea.

☞ Add the water and bring the mixture to a boil.

☞ Reduce the heat and let the Chaga simmer for about 30-60 minutes if using chunks, or steep for 10-15 minutes if using powder, to extract its medicinal properties.

☞ Strain the tea into a cup to remove any mushroom pieces or sediment.

How to Use:

✑ Drink a cup of Chaga Mushroom Tea once or twice daily to harness its immune-boosting and antioxidant benefits.

✑ If desired, enhance the flavor and additional health benefits by adding a teaspoon of honey or a squeeze of lemon.

Duration:

Chaga Mushroom Tea can be consumed regularly as part of a health-focused routine to maintain immune function and overall vitality.

Monitor your body's response to the tea and adjust the frequency of consumption accordingly. If symptoms persist or worsen, consult a healthcare professional for further evaluation and treatment.

Chaga Mushroom Tea offers a natural and effective way to boost immune function and promote overall health, leveraging the rich antioxidant properties of Chaga mushrooms for improved well-being.

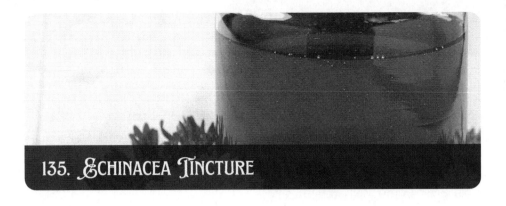

135. ECHINACEA TINCTURE

Introduction:

Echinacea Tincture is a renowned herbal remedy used to enhance immune function and prevent infections. Echinacea is rich in alkamides, polysaccharides, and flavonoids, which support the immune system, reduce inflammation, and help the body fight off colds, flu, and other infections. Using vegetable glycerin as the extraction medium provides a non-alcoholic alternative suitable for all ages.

Ingredients and Measurements:

- 1 cup of dried Echinacea flowers, leaves, and roots
- 2 cups of vegetable glycerin
- 1 cup of distilled water
- A clean glass jar with a tight-fitting lid
- A fine strainer or cheesecloth

Preparation:

- Place the dried Echinacea into the glass jar.
- Mix the vegetable glycerin and distilled water in a separate container

to create a consistent solution. This mixture ensures efficient extraction of the active compounds from Echinacea.

- Pour the glycerin-water mixture over the Echinacea, ensuring the plant material is fully submerged.
- Seal the jar tightly and shake it well to combine the ingredients.
- Store the jar in a cool, dark place, shaking it daily for 4-6 weeks to facilitate the extraction process.
- After the infusion period, strain the mixture through a fine strainer or cheesecloth into another clean jar, pressing the plant material to extract as much liquid as possible.
- Transfer the strained tincture to a dropper bottle for ease of use.

How to Use:

- To boost the immune system and help prevent infections, take 1-2 dropperfuls (about 30-60 drops) of the Echinacea Tincture diluted in water or juice, up to three times a day, especially during cold and flu season or when feeling the onset of illness.

- Begin with a lower dose to observe your body's response, and adjust as necessary based on your health goals and reaction to the supplement.

Duration:

- Use the tincture regularly as part of a health regimen to maintain immune function and support overall health.

- Consult a healthcare professional for guidance on long-term use, especially if you have existing health conditions or are taking other medications.

- Store the tincture in a cool, dark place, and it should remain effective for up to a year.

Echinacea Tincture made with vegetable glycerin is an effective way to harness the immune-supporting properties of Echinacea, offering a natural solution to enhance well-being and protect against infections.

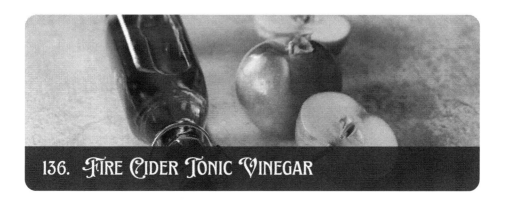

136. Fire Cider Tonic Vinegar

Introduction:

Fire Cider Tonic Vinegar is a potent herbal concoction renowned for its ability to boost the immune system, clear congestion, and stimulate digestion. This spicy, tangy tonic combines various ingredients like garlic, ginger, and hot peppers, all steeped in apple cider vinegar. The resulting blend is rich in vitamins, minerals, and antioxidants, making it a powerful remedy for colds, flu, and overall health enhancement.

Ingredients and Measurements:

- 1/2 cup of grated fresh ginger root
- 1/2 cup of grated fresh horseradish root
- 1/2 cup of chopped onion
- 1/4 cup of minced garlic
- 1/4 cup of chopped jalapeno or cayenne peppers

- 2 tablespoons of turmeric powder or grated fresh turmeric
- 4 cups of apple cider vinegar
- 1/4 cup of honey, or to taste
- Optional: a few sprigs of fresh rosemary or thyme for added flavor

Preparation:

☞ Combine the ginger, horseradish, onion, garlic, peppers, and turmeric in a large glass jar.

☞ Pour the apple cider vinegar over the ingredients until they are completely submerged.

☞ If using, add the fresh herbs.

☞ Seal the jar with a tight-fitting lid and shake well to mix the ingredients.

☞ Store the jar in a cool, dark place for 4-6 weeks, shaking it daily to ensure thorough infusion.

☞ After the infusion period, strain the mixture through a fine sieve or cheesecloth into another clean jar, pressing the solids to extract all the liquid.

☞ Stir in the honey to the strained tonic until fully dissolved.

How to Use:

☟ Take 1-2 tablespoons of Fire Cider Tonic Vinegar daily, either straight or diluted in water, to boost immunity and support overall health.

☟ It can also be used as a salad dressing or marinade for an extra health kick.

Duration:

🕐 Fire Cider Tonic Vinegar can be consumed regularly, especially during the cold and flu season, to maintain immune function and overall vitality.

🕐 Store the tonic in the refrigerator, and it should remain potent for up to a year.

🕐 If any adverse reactions occur or if symptoms of illness persist, consult a healthcare professional for further guidance.

Fire Cider Tonic Vinegar offers a flavorful and effective way to boost the immune system and promote health, harnessing the natural power of its spicy and tangy ingredients.

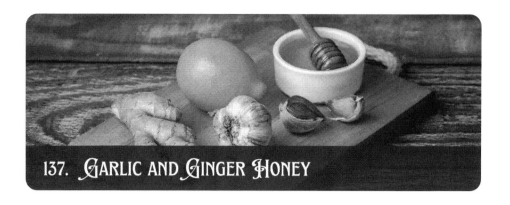

137. GARLIC AND GINGER HONEY

Introduction:

Garlic and Ginger Honey is a natural remedy celebrated for its immune-boosting and anti-inflammatory properties. Combining the potent benefits of garlic and ginger with the soothing and antimicrobial qualities of honey, this concoction is excellent for fighting infections, soothing sore throats, and enhancing overall health.

Ingredients and Measurements:

- 1/2 cup of fresh garlic cloves, peeled and finely minced
- 1/2 cup of fresh ginger root, peeled and finely grated
- 1 cup of raw, organic honey

Preparation:

- In a clean jar, combine the minced garlic and grated ginger.
- Pour the honey over the garlic and ginger, ensuring the ingredients are fully submerged.
- Stir the mixture thoroughly to ensure the garlic and ginger are evenly distributed throughout the honey.
- Seal the jar with a tight-fitting lid and allow it to sit at room temperature for 1-2 weeks, stirring occasionally to mix the ingredients.

How to Use:

- Take 1-2 teaspoons of Garlic and Ginger Honey daily, especially during cold and flu season, to boost the immune system and prevent infections.
- For a soothing throat remedy, mix a teaspoon of the honey into a cup of warm water or tea and drink as needed.

Duration:

- Garlic and Ginger Honey can be stored in a cool, dark place and consumed regularly as part of a health-focused routine to maintain immune function and overall vitality.
- If symptoms of illness persist or if any adverse reactions occur, consult a healthcare professional for further evaluation and treatment.

Garlic and Ginger Honey provides a delicious and potent way to harness the health benefits of garlic, ginger, and honey, offering a natural solution to boost immunity and soothe symptoms of colds and flu.

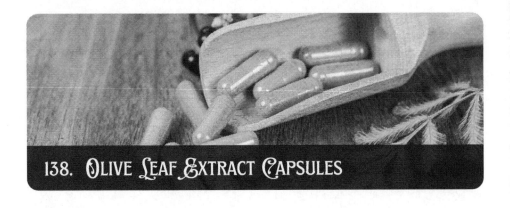

138. OLIVE LEAF EXTRACT CAPSULES

Introduction:

Olive Leaf Extract Capsules are a powerful natural supplement known for their robust antioxidant and antimicrobial properties. Derived from the leaves of the olive tree, these capsules contain oleuropein, a compound that supports the immune system, reduces inflammation, and helps protect against various pathogens. Olive Leaf Extract is particularly beneficial for cardiovascular health and fighting off viral and bacterial infections.

Ingredients and Measurements:

- Olive leaf extract powder
- Empty gelatin or vegetarian capsules
- A small funnel or pipette, if needed, to fill capsules

Preparation:

☞ Ensure you have high-quality olive leaf extract powder. This is crucial for both safety and efficacy.

☞ Using a small funnel or pipette, carefully fill one half of the empty capsule with the olive leaf extract powder.

☞ Once filled, reassemble the two halves of the capsule to seal the extract inside.

☞ Repeat the process for the desired number of capsules. Store the prepared capsules in a cool, dark place, ideally in an airtight container.

How to Use:

✎ Take 1-2 Olive Leaf Extract Capsules daily, preferably with a meal, to support the immune system and promote overall health.

✎ Consistent use over several weeks is often necessary to observe the full benefits.

Duration:

◔ Olive Leaf Extract Capsules can be used as part of an ongoing regimen to maintain immune function and support cardiovascular health.

◔ Monitor your body's response to the capsules and adjust the dosage as necessary. If symptoms persist or worsen, consult a healthcare professional for further evaluation and guidance.

Olive Leaf Extract Capsules provide a convenient and effective way to harness the health benefits of olive leaf, offering a targeted solution to enhance immune function and support overall well-being.

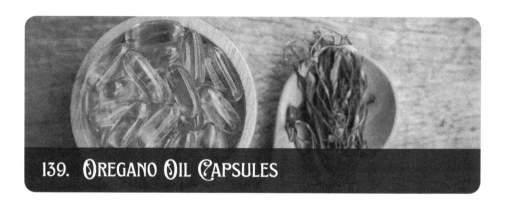

139. OREGANO OIL CAPSULES

Introduction:

Oregano Oil Capsules are a potent natural supplement known for their strong antimicrobial, antiviral, and antifungal properties. Oregano oil, derived from the leaves of the oregano plant, contains carvacrol and thymol, compounds that help fight infections and boost the immune system. These capsules are an excellent choice for targeting intestinal parasites, respiratory infections, and even skin conditions.

Ingredients and Measurements:

- Oregano essential oil (high-quality, therapeutic grade)
- Empty gelatin or vegetarian capsules
- A small dropper or pipette

Preparation:

☞ Ensure you have high-quality, therapeutic-grade oregano essential oil. This is crucial for both safety and efficacy.

☞ Take an empty capsule and carefully open it to expose the two halves.

☞ Using a dropper or pipette, fill one half of the capsule with oregano oil. Typically, 2-4 drops are sufficient, but never exceed this amount unless directed by a healthcare professional.

☞ Once filled, reassemble the two halves of the capsule to seal the oregano oil inside.

☞ Repeat the process for the desired number of capsules. Store the prepared capsules in a cool, dark place, ideally in an airtight container.

How to Use:

✎ For general immune support or to address minor infections, take 1 oregano oil capsule once or twice a day with meals.

✎ In the case of more severe infections or outbreaks, you may increase the dosage to 1 capsule three times a day, but only for short-term use (7-10 days).

✎ Always take the capsules with a full glass of water to aid absorption and minimize any potential digestive discomfort.

Duration:

⊘ Oregano oil capsules should typically be used for short-term treatment due to their potency. A usual course lasts 7-10 days.

⊘ For preventive measures or milder conditions, limit use to one capsule per day for up to two weeks.

⊘ If symptoms persist or worsen, it is essential to consult a healthcare professional for further guidance.

⊘ Oregano Oil Capsules are a convenient and potent way to harness the natural antibiotic properties of oregano. They offer a targeted approach to combatting various infections and boosting overall health without the side effects often associated with synthetic antibiotics.

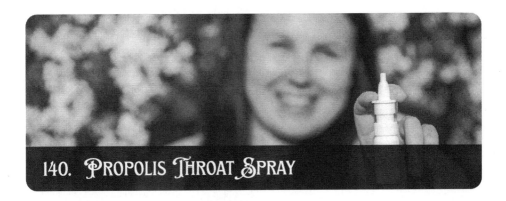

140. ℗ROPOLIS 𝒯HROAT 𝒮PRAY

Introduction:

Propolis Throat Spray is a natural remedy highly effective for soothing sore throats, reducing inflammation, and protecting against bacterial and viral infections. Propolis, a resinous substance collected by bees, is rich in antimicrobial compounds and has been used for centuries for its healing properties. This spray provides immediate relief and supports the body's natural defenses, especially during cold and flu season.

Ingredients and Measurements:

- 1/4 cup of propolis extract
- 3/4 cup of distilled water
- 1 tablespoon of raw honey (optional, for added soothing effect)
- A small spray bottle

Preparation:

- In a small bowl or container, mix the propolis extract and distilled water until thoroughly combined.
- If using honey, add it to the mixture and stir until it is fully dissolved to enhance the soothing properties.
- Using a funnel, pour the mixture into the spray bottle.
- Ensure the spray bottle is securely closed.

How to Use:

- Shake the bottle well before each use.
- Spray 2-3 spritzes directly into the throat 3-4 times a day, or as needed to relieve sore throat discomfort and irritation.
- Allow the spray to coat the throat for maximum effectiveness.

Duration:

- Use Propolis Throat Spray as needed for symptom relief during times of throat discomfort or susceptibility to respiratory infections.
- The spray can be stored in a cool, dark place, preferably refrigerated, and should remain effective for up to 6 months.
- If symptoms persist or worsen, or if any adverse reactions occur, consult a healthcare professional for further evaluation and treatment.

Propolis Throat Spray offers a natural and effective way to soothe sore throats, reduce inflammation, and bolster the immune system, leveraging the potent healing properties of propolis for quick and reliable relief.

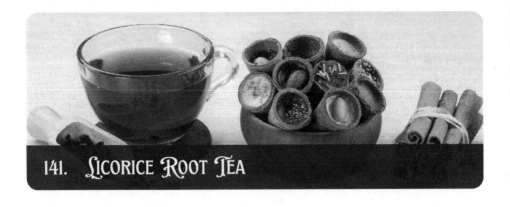

141. Licorice Root Tea

Introduction:

Licorice Root Tea is a traditional herbal beverage known for its sweet flavor and therapeutic benefits. Rich in glycyrrhizin, licorice root helps soothe gastrointestinal issues, reduce inflammation, and support respiratory health. This tea is particularly beneficial for those dealing with stomach ulcers, acid reflux, and sore throats, as it coats and protects mucous membranes.

Ingredients and Measurements:

- 1-2 teaspoons of dried licorice root
- 1 cup of boiling water
- Optional: honey or lemon to taste

Preparation:

☕ Place the dried licorice root in a cup or tea infuser.

☕ Pour the boiling water over the licorice root and cover the cup to preserve the essential oils and active ingredients.

☕ Allow the tea to steep for 10-15 minutes.

☕ Strain the tea to remove the licorice root.

How to Use:

✎ Drink a cup of Licorice Root Tea once or twice daily, particularly when experiencing gastrointestinal discomfort or respiratory issues.

✎ If desired, enhance the flavor and additional health benefits by adding a teaspoon of honey or a squeeze of lemon.

Duration:

◎ Licorice Root Tea can be consumed regularly as part of a routine to manage symptoms of stomach ulcers, acid reflux, and sore throats.

◎ Monitor your body's response to the tea and adjust the frequency of consumption accordingly. If symptoms persist or worsen, consult a healthcare professional for further evaluation and treatment.

Licorice Root Tea offers a natural and soothing solution to gastrointestinal and respiratory issues, providing relief from discomfort and enhancing overall health with its sweet and potent properties.

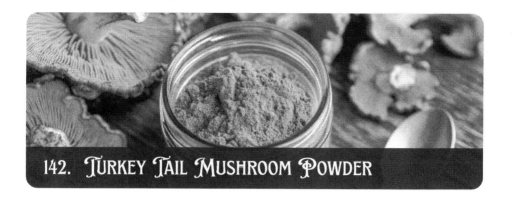

142. TURKEY TAIL MUSHROOM POWDER

Introduction:

Turkey Tail Mushroom Powder is derived from the Turkey Tail mushroom, celebrated for its exceptional immune-boosting properties. This mushroom is abundant in polysaccharides and beta-glucans, which enhance the body's immune response and support overall health. Turkey Tail is often used to fortify the immune system, especially for those recovering from illness or seeking to prevent infections.

Ingredients and Measurements:

- Turkey Tail mushroom powder
- Water, juice, or a smoothie for mixing

Preparation:

🍽 No complex preparation is needed for Turkey Tail mushroom powder. It comes ready to use and easily dissolves in various liquids.

How to Use:

🥄 Mix 1 teaspoon of Turkey Tail mushroom powder into a glass of water, juice, or your favorite smoothie.

🥄 Drink this mixture once or twice daily to benefit from its immune-boosting and health-enhancing properties.

Duration:

⊘ Turkey Tail mushroom powder can be taken regularly as part of a daily health regimen to support immune function and overall well-being.

⊘ Monitor your body's response to the supplement and adjust the dosage as necessary. If any unusual symptoms occur or if there is no improvement in health, consult a healthcare professional for further guidance.

Turkey Tail Mushroom Powder provides a convenient and effective way to harness the powerful immune-supporting benefits of Turkey Tail mushrooms, offering a targeted solution to enhance well-being and resilience.

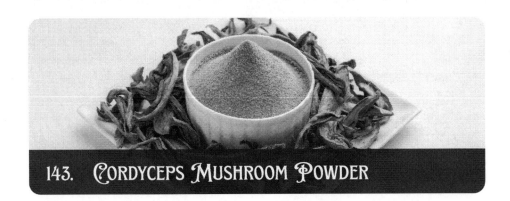

143. CORDYCEPS MUSHROOM POWDER

Introduction:

Cordyceps Mushroom Powder is a renowned supplement derived from the Cordyceps mushroom, known for its energy-boosting and performance-enhancing properties. Cordyceps is rich in adenosine and cordycepin, compounds that improve oxygen utilization, boost stamina, and support overall vitality. This powder is especially popular among athletes and those looking to enhance their physical and mental energy levels.

Ingredients and Measurements:

- Cordyceps mushroom powder
- Water, juice, or a smoothie for mixing

Preparation:

☞ No complex preparation is needed for Cordyceps mushroom powder. It comes ready to use and easily blends into various liquids.

How to Use:

↳ Mix 1 teaspoon of Cordyceps mushroom powder into a glass of water, juice, or your favorite smoothie.

↳ Drink this mixture once or twice daily, especially before physical activities or during times of increased mental demand, to benefit from its energy-boosting and health-enhancing properties.

Duration:

⊘ Cordyceps mushroom powder can be taken regularly as part of a daily health regimen to enhance energy levels, improve physical performance, and support overall well-being.

⊘ Monitor your body's response to the supplement and adjust the dosage as necessary. If any unusual symptoms occur or if there is no improvement in energy levels, consult a healthcare professional for further guidance.

Cordyceps Mushroom Powder provides a convenient and effective way to harness the energy-enhancing and performance-boosting benefits of Cordyceps, offering a natural solution to improve stamina and vitality.

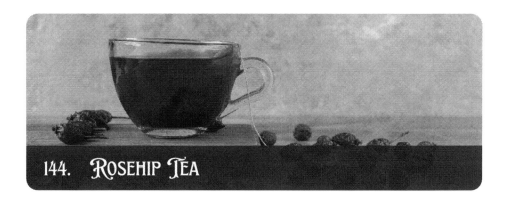

144. ROSEHIP TEA

Introduction:

Rosehip Tea is a delightful and nutritious beverage made from the fruit of the rose plant. Known for its high vitamin C content and array of antioxidants, rosehips help boost the immune system, promote skin health, and reduce inflammation. This tea is a tasty way to enjoy the benefits of rosehips while hydrating and supporting overall health.

Ingredients and Measurements:

- 1-2 teaspoons of dried rosehips
- 1 cup of boiling water
- Optional: honey or lemon to taste

Preparation:

☞ Place the dried rosehips in a cup or tea infuser.

☞ Pour the boiling water over the rosehips and cover the cup to preserve the essential oils and active ingredients.

☞ Allow the tea to steep for 10-15 minutes.

☞ Strain the tea to remove the rosehips.

How to Use:

↳ Drink a cup of Rosehip Tea once or twice daily to benefit from its immune-boosting and health-promoting properties.

↳ If desired, enhance the flavor and additional health benefits by adding a teaspoon of honey or a squeeze of lemon.

Duration:

⊘ Rosehip Tea can be consumed regularly as part of a routine to support immune function, skin health, and overall well-being.

⊘ Monitor your body's response to the tea and adjust the frequency of consumption accordingly. If symptoms persist or worsen, consult a healthcare professional for further evaluation and treatment.

Rosehip Tea offers a natural and flavorful way to enhance health, leveraging the rich vitamin C and antioxidant properties of rosehips for improved immunity and vitality.

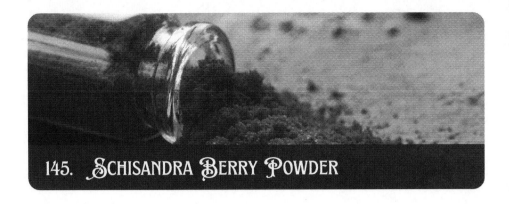

145. Schisandra Berry Powder

Introduction:

Schisandra Berry Powder is derived from the Schisandra chinensis fruit, celebrated for its adaptogenic properties that help the body resist physical, chemical, and biological stress. Rich in lignans and other bioactive compounds, Schisandra enhances liver function, boosts energy levels, and improves mental clarity. This powder is an excellent way to incorporate the benefits of Schisandra into your daily wellness routine.

Ingredients and Measurements:

- Schisandra berry powder
- Water, juice, or a smoothie for mixing

Preparation:

☞ No complex preparation is needed for Schisandra berry powder. It comes ready to use and easily dissolves in various liquids.

How to Use:

✎ Mix 1 teaspoon of Schisandra berry powder into a glass of water, juice, or your favorite smoothie.

✎ Drink this mixture once or twice daily, especially during times of increased stress or when seeking to enhance mental and physical performance.

Duration:

◎ Schisandra berry powder can be taken regularly as part of a daily health regimen to support stress resistance, liver health, and overall vitality.

◎ Monitor your body's response to the supplement and adjust the dosage as necessary. If any unusual symptoms occur or if there is no improvement in health, consult a healthcare professional for further guidance.

Schisandra Berry Powder provides a convenient and effective way to harness the adaptogenic and health-promoting benefits of Schisandra, offering a natural solution to enhance resilience and improve well-being.

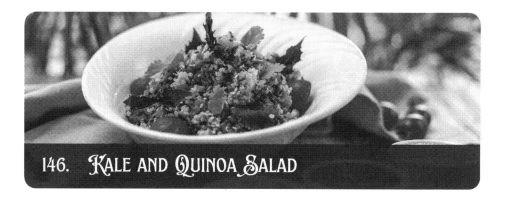

146. KALE AND QUINOA SALAD

Introduction:

Kale and Quinoa Salad is a powerhouse dish packed with nutrient-dense superfoods that provide a range of health benefits. Kale is rich in vitamins A, C, and K, along with minerals and antioxidants, while quinoa offers high-quality protein and all essential amino acids. This salad is an excellent choice for boosting energy, supporting overall health, and maintaining a balanced diet.

Ingredients and Measurements:

- 2 cups of fresh kale, washed and chopped
- 1 cup of cooked quinoa
- 1/2 cup of cherry tomatoes, halved
- 1/4 cup of sliced cucumbers
- 1/4 cup of red onion, thinly sliced
- 2 tablespoons of olive oil
- 1 tablespoon of lemon juice
- Salt and pepper to taste
- Optional: nuts, seeds, or dried fruits for extra texture and flavor

Preparation:

- In a large salad bowl, combine the chopped kale, cooked quinoa, cherry tomatoes, cucumbers, and red onion.
- In a small bowl, whisk together the olive oil and lemon juice to create a simple dressing.
- Pour the dressing over the salad and toss well to ensure all ingredients are evenly coated.
- Season with salt and pepper to taste.
- If desired, sprinkle with nuts, seeds, or dried fruits for added nutrition and flavor.

How to Use:

- Serve the Kale and Quinoa Salad as a main dish or as a side to complement other meals.
- Enjoy this salad fresh for the best flavor and nutritional benefits.

Duration:

- This salad is best consumed fresh but can be stored in the refrigerator for up to 2 days in an airtight container.

For longer-lasting freshness, add the dressing just before serving.

Kale and Quinoa Salad is a delicious and healthy option that combines essential nutrients and flavors, making it a perfect addition to any meal plan for enhanced well-being and vitality.

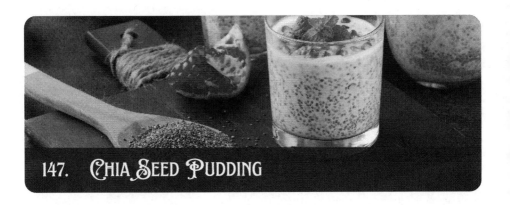

147.   CHIA SEED PUDDING

Introduction:

Chia Seed Pudding is a nutritious and versatile dish that offers a wealth of health benefits. Chia seeds are a superfood loaded with omega-3 fatty acids, fiber, protein, and essential minerals. This pudding is easy to prepare and can be customized with various flavors and toppings, making it an ideal breakfast or snack to boost energy and support digestive health.

Ingredients and Measurements:

- 1/4 cup of chia seeds
- 1 cup of milk (dairy or plant-based)
- 1 tablespoon of honey or maple syrup (optional for sweetness)
- Optional: vanilla extract, fruits, nuts, or spices for flavor and garnish

Preparation:

In a bowl or mason jar, mix the chia seeds with the milk.

Add honey or maple syrup and a splash of vanilla extract if desired for additional sweetness and flavor.

Stir the mixture well to ensure the chia seeds are evenly distributed.

Cover the bowl or jar and refrigerate for at least 4 hours, preferably overnight, allowing the chia seeds to absorb the liquid and form a gel-like pudding.

How to Use:

Once the pudding has set, stir it again to break up any clumps.

Top with fresh fruits, nuts, or spices like cinnamon before serving to enhance flavor and add extra nutrients.

Duration:

- Chia Seed Pudding can be stored in the refrigerator for up to 5 days in an airtight container.

- Prepare in batches to enjoy as a quick and healthy breakfast or snack throughout the week.

Chia Seed Pudding is a simple yet powerful way to incorporate more superfoods into your diet, offering sustained energy, improved digestion, and a delicious taste that can be customized to suit any preference.

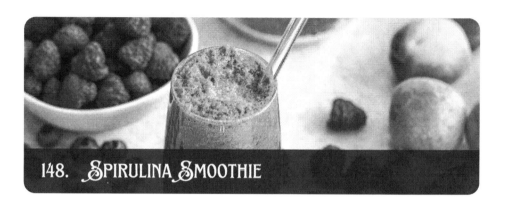

148. SPIRULINA SMOOTHIE

Introduction:

Spirulina Smoothie is a vibrant and nutritious beverage packed with the benefits of spirulina, a blue-green algae known for its high protein content, vitamins, minerals, and antioxidants. This smoothie is an excellent way to boost energy, support immune function, and detoxify the body. The addition of fruits and vegetables enhances its flavor and nutritional profile, making it a perfect choice for a healthy, energizing meal or snack.

Ingredients and Measurements:

- 1 tablespoon of spirulina powder
- 1 cup of fresh spinach or kale
- 1 banana, peeled
- 1/2 cup of mixed berries (such as blueberries, strawberries, or raspberries)
- 1 cup of almond milk, coconut milk, or water
- Optional: honey, agave syrup, or a pitted date for sweetness

Preparation:

- In a blender, combine the spirulina powder, fresh spinach or kale, banana, and mixed berries.

- Add the almond milk, coconut milk, or water to help blend the ingredients smoothly.

- Blend on high until the mixture is creamy and smooth.

🍵 Taste and add honey, agave syrup, or a date if additional sweetness is desired. Blend again to incorporate the sweetener evenly.

How to Use:

🥄 Pour the Spirulina Smoothie into a glass and enjoy immediately for the freshest flavor and most potent nutritional benefits.

🥄 Drink this smoothie in the morning for a nutrient-rich start to your day or as a post-workout recovery beverage to replenish and rehydrate.

Duration:

⏱ Spirulina Smoothie is best enjoyed fresh but can be stored in the refrigerator for up to 24 hours. Shake or stir well before drinking if stored.

Spirulina Smoothie offers a delightful and powerful way to incorporate a superfood into your diet, enhancing overall health with its rich array of nutrients and energizing properties.

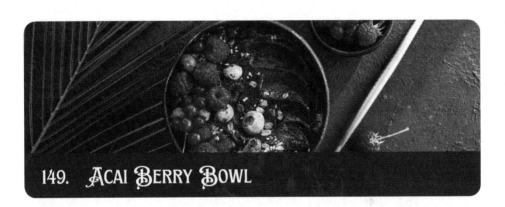

149. Acai Berry Bowl

Introduction:

An Acai Berry Bowl is a vibrant and delicious dish packed with the nutritional power of acai berries, known for their high antioxidant content and heart-healthy fats. This bowl combines acai with various fruits, nuts, and seeds for a balanced meal that energizes, supports immune function, and promotes skin health.

Ingredients and Measurements:

- 2 packets of frozen acai berry puree (about 200 grams)

- 1 banana, sliced

- 1/2 cup of mixed berries (such as blueberries, strawberries, or raspberries)

- 1/4 cup of granola

- 1 tablespoon of chia seeds

- 1 tablespoon of honey or maple syrup (optional)
- Additional toppings: sliced almonds, coconut flakes, or fresh fruit slices

Preparation:

🖐 Blend the frozen acai berry puree and half of the banana until smooth.

🖐 Pour the acai mixture into a bowl.

🖐 Arrange the sliced banana, mixed berries, and granola over the acai mixture.

🖐 Sprinkle chia seeds and other chosen toppings over the bowl.

🖐 Drizzle with honey or maple syrup for added sweetness if desired.

How to Use:

🖐 Enjoy the Acai Berry Bowl as a nutritious breakfast, snack, or light meal.

🖐 Customize the bowl with your favorite fruits and toppings for variety and added nutrients.

Duration:

🕙 Acai Berry Bowl is best enjoyed fresh to maximize the benefits of its ingredients.

🕙 If needed, prepare the base mixture ahead of time and store it in the freezer, adding toppings just before serving.

The Acai Berry Bowl is an energizing and wholesome way to start your day or refuel your body, offering a delightful mix of flavors and a boost of essential nutrients.

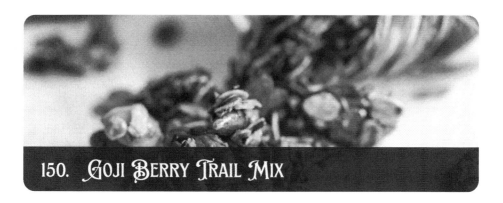

150. GOJI BERRY TRAIL MIX

Introduction:

Goji Berry Trail Mix is a dynamic and nutrient-rich snack that combines the health benefits of goji berries with nuts and seeds. Goji berries are famed for their high antioxidant content, vitamins, and minerals that support vision, immune function, and overall well-being. This trail mix is an excellent portable snack that provides energy, satisfies hunger, and offers a variety of textures and flavors.

Ingredients and Measurements:

- 1 cup of goji berries
- 1/2 cup of almonds
- 1/2 cup of walnuts
- 1/2 cup of pumpkin seeds
- 1/4 cup of sunflower seeds
- Optional: dried fruits like raisins or cranberries, and a sprinkle of dark chocolate chips for added sweetness

Preparation:

- In a large bowl, combine the goji berries, almonds, walnuts, pumpkin seeds, and sunflower seeds.
- If using, add dried fruits and dark chocolate chips to the mix for additional flavor and sweetness.
- Toss the ingredients together until well mixed.

How to Use:

- Store the Goji Berry Trail Mix in an airtight container and keep it handy for a quick snack.
- Enjoy a handful as an energy-boosting snack during outdoor activities, work breaks, or any time you need a nutritious pick-me-up.

Duration:

- Goji Berry Trail Mix can be stored at room temperature in an airtight container for up to a month.
- Ensure the mix is kept dry and cool to maintain freshness and prevent spoilage.
- Goji Berry Trail Mix is a convenient and delicious way to incorporate a superfood into your diet, enhancing your energy levels and providing a mix of essential nutrients for optimal health.

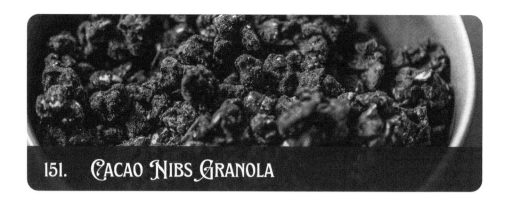

151. CACAO NIBS GRANOLA

Introduction:

Cacao Nibs Granola is a delightful and healthful treat that combines the rich flavor of cacao nibs with the crunch and nourishment of granola. Cacao nibs are packed with antioxidants, magnesium, and flavonoids, which can enhance mood, improve heart health, and support overall well-being. This granola is perfect for a nutritious breakfast or a tasty snack that satisfies both your taste buds and nutritional needs.

Ingredients and Measurements:

- 2 cups of rolled oats
- 1 cup of mixed nuts (such as almonds, walnuts, and pecans), chopped
- 1/2 cup of cacao nibs
- 1/4 cup of coconut flakes
- 1/4 cup of honey or maple syrup
- 1/4 cup of coconut oil, melted
- 1 teaspoon of vanilla extract
- 1/2 teaspoon of salt
- Optional: cinnamon or nutmeg for added flavor

Preparation:

- Preheat your oven to 300°F (150°C).
- In a large bowl, mix the rolled oats, chopped nuts, cacao nibs, and coconut flakes.
- In a separate small bowl, combine the honey or maple syrup, melted coconut oil, and vanilla extract.
- Pour the wet ingredients over the dry ingredients and stir until everything is evenly coated. Sprinkle with salt and optional spices like cinnamon or nutmeg.
- Spread the mixture evenly on a baking sheet lined with parchment paper.
- Bake for 25-30 minutes, stirring halfway through, until the granola is golden and toasted.
- Allow the granola to cool completely on the baking sheet. It will become crispier as it cools.

How to Use:

⮳ Serve the Cacao Nibs Granola over yogurt, with milk, or as a standalone snack.

⮳ Store in an airtight container at room temperature to maintain its crunch and freshness.

Duration:

⏲ Cacao Nibs Granola can be stored for up to 3 weeks in an airtight container.

⏲ Ensure it is kept in a cool, dry place to preserve its quality and flavor.

Cacao Nibs Granola offers a tasty and nutritious way to start your day or energize your afternoon, delivering a blend of wholesome ingredients and the rich, chocolatey goodness of cacao nibs.

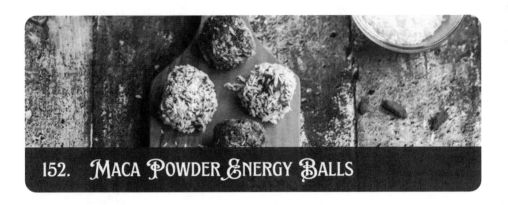

152. Maca Powder Energy Balls

Introduction:

Maca Powder Energy Balls are a convenient and tasty snack packed with the benefits of maca powder, known for its ability to boost energy, enhance stamina, and support hormonal balance. Combined with nuts and seeds, these energy balls provide a balanced blend of protein, healthy fats, and carbohydrates, making them perfect for a pre-workout boost or an afternoon pick-me-up.

Ingredients and Measurements:

- 1 cup of dates, pitted
- 1/2 cup of almonds
- 1/2 cup of cashews
- 1/4 cup of maca powder
- 1 tablespoon of chia seeds
- 1 tablespoon of flaxseeds
- 2 tablespoons of coconut oil
- Optional: shredded coconut or cocoa powder for coating

Preparation:

- ☞ In a food processor, blend the dates until they form a sticky paste.

- ☞ Add the almonds and cashews to the processor and pulse until finely chopped and mixed with the date paste.

- ☞ Add the maca powder, chia seeds, flaxseeds, and coconut oil. Blend until the mixture is well combined and sticks together when pressed.

- ☞ Take small portions of the mixture and roll them into balls, about the size of a walnut.

- ☞ If desired, roll the energy balls in shredded coconut or cocoa powder for an extra layer of flavor and texture.

- ☞ Place the energy balls on a tray or plate lined with parchment paper.

How to Use:

- ✎ Store the Maca Powder Energy Balls in an airtight container in the refrigerator for up to two weeks.

- ✎ Enjoy one or two balls as needed for a quick energy boost or as a healthy snack throughout the day.

Duration:

- ⊘ Maca Powder Energy Balls are best kept refrigerated and consumed within two weeks for optimal freshness and nutritional value.

Maca Powder Energy Balls are a delicious and healthful way to enjoy the benefits of maca, providing sustained energy and essential nutrients in a portable and satisfying form.

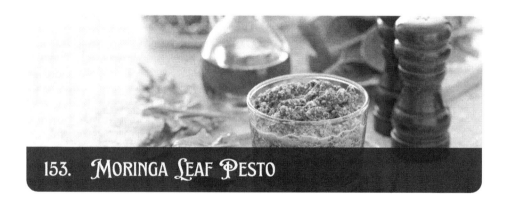

153. MORINGA LEAF PESTO

Introduction:

Moringa Leaf Pesto is a vibrant and nutritious twist on traditional pesto, using moringa leaves known for their rich content of vitamins, minerals, and antioxidants. Moringa enhances energy levels, supports immune function, and offers anti-inflammatory benefits. This pesto is perfect for adding a health boost to pasta, sandwiches, or as a dip.

Ingredients and Measurements:

- 2 cups of fresh moringa leaves, washed and dried
- 1/2 cup of Parmesan cheese, grated
- 1/3 cup of pine nuts or walnuts
- 2-3 garlic cloves, peeled
- 1/2 cup of olive oil
- Salt and pepper to taste
- Optional: lemon juice for added zest

Preparation:

- In a food processor, combine the moringa leaves, Parmesan cheese, nuts, and garlic cloves.
- Pulse until the ingredients are coarsely chopped.
- While the processor is running, gradually add the olive oil until the mixture forms a smooth paste.
- Season with salt and pepper, and add a squeeze of lemon juice if desired for extra freshness.
- Adjust the consistency by adding more olive oil if needed.

How to Use:

- Spread the Moringa Leaf Pesto on sandwiches, mix into pasta, or use it as a dip for vegetables and crackers.
- It's a versatile condiment that can elevate the nutritional profile of many dishes.

Duration:

- Store Moringa Leaf Pesto in an airtight container in the refrigerator for up to a week.
- For longer storage, you can freeze the pesto in ice cube trays and then transfer the cubes to a freezer bag, where they can be kept for up to 3 months.

Moringa Leaf Pesto offers a delightful way to incorporate a superfood into your diet, enhancing meals with its unique flavor and impressive range of health benefits.

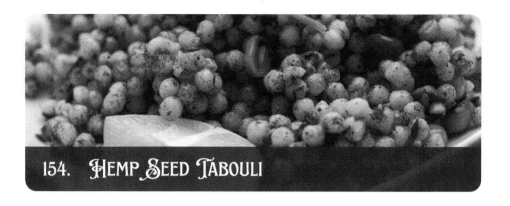

154. Hemp Seed Tabouli

Introduction:

Hemp Seed Tabouli is a modern twist on the classic Middle Eastern salad, incorporating hemp seeds for their exceptional nutritional value. Rich in protein, omega-3 and omega-6 fatty acids, and essential minerals, hemp seeds add a nutty flavor and extra health benefits to the refreshing mix of parsley, tomatoes, and bulgur. This dish is perfect for a light meal or a nutritious side that supports heart health and digestion.

Ingredients and Measurements:

- 1 cup of bulgur wheat
- 1 1/2 cups of boiling water
- 1 cup of fresh parsley, finely chopped
- 1/2 cup of fresh mint, finely chopped
- 2 medium tomatoes, diced
- 1 cucumber, diced
- 1/4 cup of hemp seeds
- 1/4 cup of lemon juice
- 1/3 cup of olive oil
- Salt and pepper to taste

Preparation:

- Place the bulgur in a large bowl and pour the boiling water over it. Cover and let sit for 30 minutes until the water is absorbed and the bulgur is tender.

- Fluff the bulgur with a fork and allow it to cool to room temperature.

- Once cooled, add the chopped parsley, mint, tomatoes, cucumber, and hemp seeds to the bulgur.

- In a small bowl, whisk together the lemon juice, olive oil, salt, and pepper.

- Pour the dressing over the tabouli and toss well to combine all the ingredients.

How to Use:

- Serve the Hemp Seed Tabouli immediately, or refrigerate for an hour to allow the flavors to meld.

- Enjoy this dish as a standalone salad, a side with grilled meats, or as part of a larger Mediterranean meal.

Duration:

🕐 Hemp Seed Tabouli can be stored in an airtight container in the refrigerator and is best enjoyed within 2-3 days for optimal freshness and flavor.

Hemp Seed Tabouli is a delicious and healthful way to enjoy a classic dish with a nutritional boost from hemp seeds, offering a balance of flavors and essential nutrients for overall wellness.

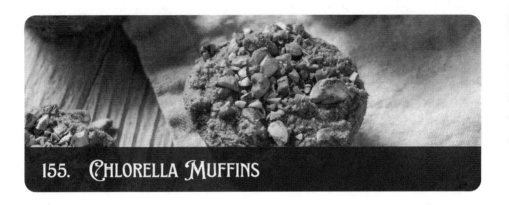

155. CHLORELLA MUFFINS

Introduction:

Chlorella Muffins incorporate the superfood chlorella, known for its high content of proteins, vitamins, minerals, and chlorophyll, into a tasty and nutritious baked treat. These muffins are an excellent way to boost detoxification, support immune health, and increase energy levels while enjoying a delightful snack or breakfast option.

Ingredients and Measurements:

- 1 1/2 cups of whole wheat flour or all-purpose flour
- 1/2 cup of sugar or a sugar alternative
- 1 tablespoon of chlorella powder
- 1 teaspoon of baking powder
- 1/2 teaspoon of baking soda
- 1/2 teaspoon of salt
- 1 cup of milk (dairy or plant-based)
- 1/3 cup of vegetable oil or melted coconut oil
- 1 large egg
- 1 teaspoon of vanilla extract
- Optional: 1/2 cup of mix-ins like blueberries, chopped nuts, or chocolate chips

Preparation:

🍽 Preheat the oven to 375°F (190°C). Line a muffin tin with paper liners or grease the cups.

🍽 In a large bowl, whisk together the flour, sugar, chlorella powder, baking powder, baking soda, and salt.

🍽 In another bowl, mix the milk, oil, egg, and vanilla extract until well combined.

- Pour the wet ingredients into the dry ingredients and stir until just combined, being careful not to overmix. If using, fold in your chosen mix-ins like blueberries or nuts.

- Divide the batter evenly among the muffin cups, filling each about 3/4 full.

- Bake for 18-20 minutes, or until a toothpick inserted into the center of a muffin comes out clean.

- Allow the muffins to cool in the pan for a few minutes before transferring them to a wire rack to cool completely.

How to Use:

- Enjoy Chlorella Muffins as a part of a healthy breakfast or as a snack throughout the day.

- Store muffins in an airtight container at room temperature for up to 3 days, or freeze for longer storage.

Duration:

- Chlorella Muffins can be kept at room temperature for up to 3 days or frozen for up to 3 months for best quality.

Chlorella Muffins are a creative and delicious way to incorporate the health benefits of chlorella into your diet, offering a nutritious boost in a familiar and enjoyable form.

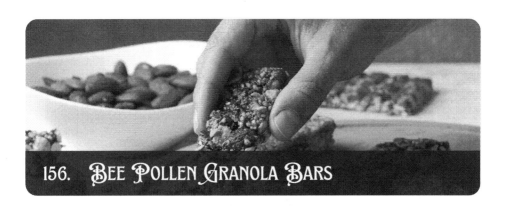

156.   BEE POLLEN GRANOLA BARS

Introduction:

Bee Pollen Granola Bars are a nutrient-packed snack that combines the natural benefits of bee pollen with the wholesome goodness of oats and nuts. Bee pollen is rich in proteins, vitamins, minerals, and antioxidants, making these bars an excellent choice for enhancing energy, supporting immunity, and promoting overall wellness.

Ingredients and Measurements:

- 2 cups of rolled oats

- 1 cup of mixed nuts (such as almonds, walnuts, and pecans), chopped

- 1/2 cup of bee pollen
- 1/4 cup of honey or maple syrup
- 1/4 cup of coconut oil, melted
- 1/2 cup of dried fruits (such as cranberries or raisins)
- 1 teaspoon of vanilla extract
- 1/2 teaspoon of salt
- Optional: a sprinkle of cinnamon or nutmeg for extra flavor

Preparation:

- Preheat the oven to 350°F (175°C). Line a baking dish or tray with parchment paper.

- In a large bowl, combine the rolled oats, chopped nuts, and bee pollen.

- In a separate bowl, mix the honey or maple syrup, melted coconut oil, and vanilla extract.

- Pour the wet ingredients over the dry ingredients and stir until well combined. Ensure all the oats and nuts are coated evenly.

- Fold in the dried fruits and add a sprinkle of cinnamon or nutmeg if desired.

- Spread the mixture evenly in the prepared baking dish, pressing down firmly to compact the ingredients.

- Bake for 20-25 minutes or until the edges are golden brown.

- Allow the granola bars to cool completely in the dish before cutting them into bars or squares.

How to Use:

- Enjoy Bee Pollen Granola Bars as a nutritious snack during the day or as a quick breakfast on the go.

- Store the bars in an airtight container at room temperature for up to a week or in the refrigerator for extended freshness.

Duration:

- Bee Pollen Granola Bars can be stored at room temperature for up to a week or refrigerated for up to two weeks.

- Bee Pollen Granola Bars offer a delicious and healthful way to enjoy the benefits of bee pollen, delivering a satisfying snack packed with energy and essential nutrients.

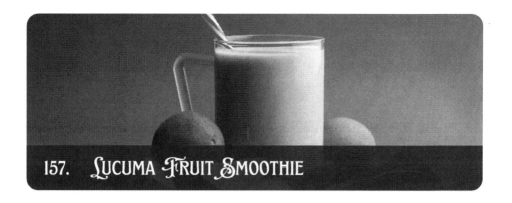

157. LUCUMA FRUIT SMOOTHIE

Introduction:

Lucuma Fruit Smoothie is a creamy and delightful beverage that highlights the sweet, caramel-like flavor of lucuma, a nutritious fruit from South America. Rich in antioxidants, fiber, vitamins, and minerals, lucuma enhances this smoothie's health benefits, supporting skin health, digestion, and energy levels. This smoothie is perfect for a refreshing treat or a nutrient-packed start to your day.

Ingredients and Measurements:

- 1 cup of milk (dairy or plant-based)
- 1/2 cup of plain yogurt or a dairy-free alternative
- 2 tablespoons of lucuma powder
- 1 banana, sliced and frozen
- 1 tablespoon of honey or maple syrup (optional for added sweetness)
- Ice cubes (optional)

Preparation:

- In a blender, combine the milk, yogurt, lucuma powder, frozen banana, and honey or maple syrup if using.

- Blend on high until the mixture is smooth and creamy.

- Add a few ice cubes if you prefer a colder and thicker smoothie. Blend again until smooth.

- Taste and adjust sweetness if necessary by adding a little more honey or syrup.

How to Use:

- Pour the Lucuma Fruit Smoothie into a glass and enjoy immediately for the best taste and nutrient content.

- Garnish with a sprinkle of lucuma powder or sliced fruit for an extra touch of flavor and visual appeal.

Duration:

- Lucuma Fruit Smoothie is best enjoyed fresh, but you can store it in the refrigerator for up to 24 hours. Shake or stir well before drinking if stored.

Lucuma Fruit Smoothie offers a delicious and healthful way to incorporate the unique benefits of lucuma into your diet, providing a satisfying and energizing beverage full of essential nutrients.

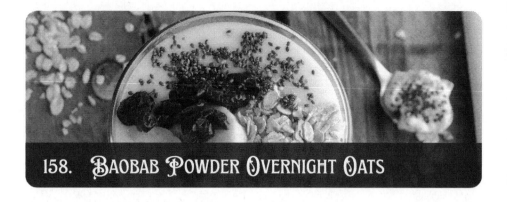

158. BAOBAB POWDER OVERNIGHT OATS

Introduction:

Baobab Powder Overnight Oats is a nutritious and convenient breakfast option that combines the health benefits of baobab powder with the sustained energy of oats. Baobab is high in vitamin C, fiber, and antioxidants, which help boost immunity, improve digestion, and support overall wellness. This overnight oats recipe is an easy way to start your day with a meal that is both filling and rich in essential nutrients.

Ingredients and Measurements:

- 1 cup of rolled oats
- 1 tablespoon of baobab powder
- 1 cup of almond milk or any plant-based milk
- 1/2 cup of Greek yogurt or a dairy-free yogurt alternative
- 1 tablespoon of chia seeds
- 1 tablespoon of honey or maple syrup (optional for sweetness)
- Toppings: fresh fruits, nuts, or seeds for extra flavor and texture

Preparation:

- In a mason jar or bowl, combine the rolled oats, baobab powder, almond milk, Greek yogurt, and chia seeds.
- Stir in the honey or maple syrup if desired for added sweetness.
- Mix well until all ingredients are thoroughly combined.
- Cover the jar or bowl and place it in the refrigerator overnight or for at least 6 hours.

How to Use:

- In the morning, stir the mixture to ensure the oats are well soaked and the baobab powder is evenly distributed.
- Add your favorite toppings, such as fresh fruits, nuts, or seeds, to enhance the flavor and nutritional value.

Duration:

- Baobab Powder Overnight Oats can be stored in the refrigerator for up to 5 days.

Enjoy this meal as a quick and healthy breakfast option throughout the week.

Baobab Powder Overnight Oats provide a wholesome and delicious start to your day, delivering a balance of slow-releasing energy and vital nutrients from baobab and other superfood ingredients.

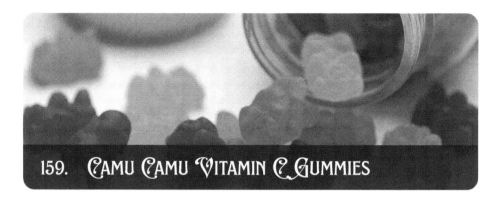

159. Camu Camu Vitamin C Gummies

Introduction:

Camu Camu Vitamin C Gummies are a tasty and fun way to boost your intake of vitamin C, essential for immune support, skin health, and antioxidant protection. Camu camu is a superfruit from the Amazon rainforest, known for its extraordinarily high vitamin C content, along with bioflavonoids that enhance the body's absorption of the vitamin. These gummies are a great alternative to traditional supplements, especially for those who prefer a flavorful approach to health.

Ingredients and Measurements:

- 1/2 cup of camu camu powder
- 1 cup of fresh orange juice or any citrus juice
- 1/4 cup of honey or agave syrup
- 3 tablespoons of gelatin (or agar agar for a vegan option)
- Silicone molds or an ice cube tray

Preparation:

In a small saucepan, whisk together the camu camu powder, orange juice, and honey or agave syrup.

Heat the mixture over medium heat until it is warm but not boiling.

Gradually sprinkle the gelatin or agar agar over the warm liquid, whisking constantly to prevent lumps.

Continue to whisk until the gelatin is fully dissolved and the mixture is smooth.

Remove from heat and let the mixture cool slightly.

- 🥄 Carefully pour the mixture into silicone molds or an ice cube tray.
- 🥄 Place the molds in the refrigerator and chill until the gummies are firm, about 1-2 hours.

How to Use:

- 🥄 Enjoy 1-2 Camu Camu Vitamin C Gummies daily to support your immune system and increase your vitamin C intake.
- 🥄 Store the gummies in an airtight container in the refrigerator.

Duration:

- 🕐 Camu Camu Vitamin C Gummies can be stored in the refrigerator for up to 2 weeks.

Camu Camu Vitamin C Gummies offer a delightful and effective way to supplement your diet with high levels of vitamin C, providing a boost to your immune function and overall health in a delicious form.

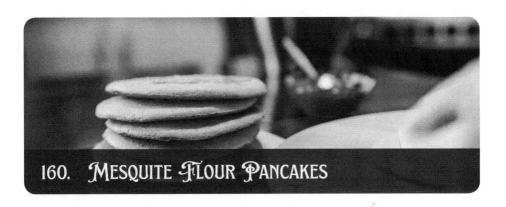

160. MESQUITE FLOUR PANCAKES

Introduction:

Mesquite Flour Pancakes are a wholesome and flavorful alternative to traditional pancakes, utilizing the unique taste and nutritional benefits of mesquite flour. Mesquite flour is derived from the pods of the mesquite tree and is known for its low glycemic index, high fiber content, and rich mineral profile, including calcium and magnesium. These pancakes are a great way to start your day with a meal that is both energizing and supportive of healthy blood sugar levels.

Ingredients and Measurements:

- 1 cup of mesquite flour
- 1 cup of all-purpose flour (or use gluten-free flour if preferred)
- 2 teaspoons of baking powder
- 1/2 teaspoon of salt

- 2 tablespoons of sugar or a sugar alternative
- 1 1/4 cups of milk (dairy or plant-based)
- 1 large egg
- 2 tablespoons of melted butter or vegetable oil
- Optional: vanilla extract for added flavor

Preparation:

In a large mixing bowl, whisk together the mesquite flour, all-purpose flour, baking powder, salt, and sugar.

In a separate bowl, combine the milk, egg, melted butter or oil, and vanilla extract if using.

Pour the wet ingredients into the dry ingredients and stir until just combined, being careful not to overmix. Some lumps are okay.

Heat a non-stick skillet or griddle over medium heat. Lightly grease with butter or oil.

Pour about 1/4 cup of batter for each pancake onto the hot skillet. Cook until bubbles form on the surface, then flip and cook for another 1-2 minutes until golden brown.

Repeat with the remaining batter.

How to Use:

Serve the Mesquite Flour Pancakes warm with your favorite toppings, such as maple syrup, fresh fruits, or a dollop of yogurt.

Duration:

Mesquite Flour Pancakes are best enjoyed fresh but can be stored in the refrigerator for up to 3 days or frozen for up to a month. Reheat in a toaster or microwave before serving.

Mesquite Flour Pancakes offer a delicious and nutritious way to enjoy a classic breakfast dish, with the added benefits of mesquite flour for a hearty and healthful start to your day.

PART 07

ANTI-INFLAMMATORY DISHES (161-175)

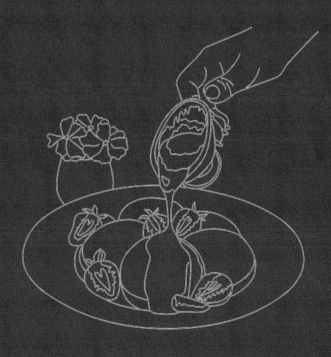

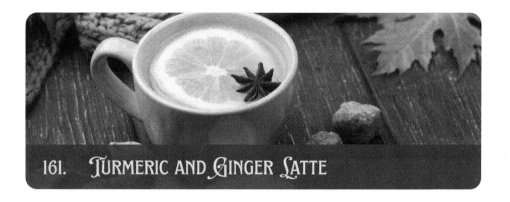

161. TURMERIC AND GINGER LATTE

Introduction:

Turmeric and Ginger Latte, often known as "Golden Milk," is a soothing and anti-inflammatory beverage that combines the powerful health benefits of turmeric and ginger. Both spices are renowned for their ability to reduce inflammation, boost immune function, and support digestive health. This warm, spiced drink is perfect for relaxing evenings or as a healthful start to your day.

Ingredients and Measurements:

- 1 teaspoon of turmeric powder
- 1/2 teaspoon of grated fresh ginger or ginger powder
- 1 cup of milk (dairy or plant-based)
- 1 tablespoon of honey or maple syrup (optional, for sweetness)
- A pinch of black pepper (to enhance turmeric absorption)
- Optional: a pinch of cinnamon or cardamom for added flavor

Preparation:

- In a small saucepan, combine the milk, turmeric powder, ginger, and black pepper.
- Warm the mixture over medium heat, stirring constantly, until it is hot but not boiling.
- Remove from heat and stir in the honey or maple syrup if using, and any additional spices like cinnamon or cardamom.
- Use a frother or whisk vigorously to create a light froth.

How to Use:

- Pour the Turmeric and Ginger Latte into a mug and enjoy immediately while warm.
- This latte can be enjoyed in the morning for an energizing start or in the evening for a calming end to the day.

Duration:

- Turmeric and Ginger Latte is best enjoyed fresh, but you can store any leftovers in the refrigerator for up to 24 hours. Reheat gently before serving.

Turmeric and Ginger Latte offers a delicious and healthful way to incorporate anti-inflammatory spices into your diet, providing a comforting and beneficial drink that supports overall well-being.

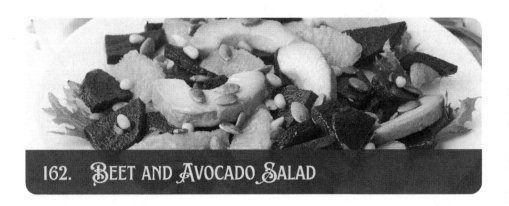

162. Beet and Avocado Salad

Introduction:

Beet and Avocado Salad is a vibrant and nutrient-rich dish that combines the earthy sweetness of beets with the creamy texture of avocado. Beets are high in fiber, vitamins, and minerals, and are known for their detoxifying properties. Avocado adds healthy fats and additional fiber, making this salad not only delicious but also beneficial for heart health and inflammation reduction.

Ingredients and Measurements:

- 2 medium beets, roasted, peeled, and diced
- 1 ripe avocado, peeled, pitted, and diced
- 1/2 cup of mixed greens like arugula or spinach
- 1/4 cup of crumbled feta cheese or goat cheese
- 2 tablespoons of chopped walnuts or almonds
- 2 tablespoons of olive oil
- 1 tablespoon of balsamic vinegar
- Salt and pepper to taste
- Optional: a squeeze of lemon juice or orange segments for extra zest

Preparation:

- If using raw beets, wrap them in foil and roast in a preheated oven at 400°F (200°C) for about 45-60 minutes until tender. Once cooled, peel and dice them.
- In a salad bowl, arrange the mixed greens as the base.
- Add the diced beets and avocado on top of the greens.
- Sprinkle with crumbled feta or goat cheese and chopped nuts.

- In a small bowl, whisk together the olive oil, balsamic vinegar, salt, and pepper to create the dressing.

- Drizzle the dressing over the salad and gently toss to combine all ingredients.

- If desired, add a squeeze of lemon juice or a few orange segments for additional flavor.

How to Use:

- Serve the Beet and Avocado Salad immediately as a fresh, standalone meal or as a side to complement other dishes.

Duration:

- This salad is best enjoyed fresh due to the avocado's tendency to brown. However, you can prepare the beets ahead of time and assemble the salad just before serving.

Beet and Avocado Salad is a delightful and healthful choice, offering a combination of flavors and textures that enhance its nutritional benefits and appeal.

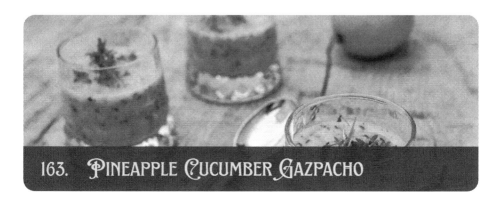

163. PINEAPPLE CUCUMBER GAZPACHO

Introduction:

Pineapple Cucumber Gazpacho is a refreshing and cooling soup, perfect for warm weather or as a light starter to any meal. This dish combines the sweetness of pineapple with the crispness of cucumber, enhanced by the tang of lime and the heat of jalapeño. Rich in vitamins, antioxidants, and hydration, this gazpacho helps reduce inflammation and supports digestive health.

Ingredients and Measurements:

- 2 cups of fresh pineapple, diced
- 1 large cucumber, peeled and diced
- 1 small red onion, finely chopped
- 1 jalapeño pepper, seeded and minced (adjust based on heat preference)
- 1 red bell pepper, diced
- 1/4 cup of fresh cilantro, chopped
- Juice of 2 limes

- 1 tablespoon of olive oil
- Salt and pepper to taste
- Optional: a splash of coconut water or vegetable broth for a thinner consistency

Preparation:

In a blender or food processor, combine the pineapple, half of the cucumber, half of the red onion, and the jalapeño pepper. Blend until smooth.

Transfer the blended mixture to a large bowl.

Stir in the remaining diced cucumber, red onion, red bell pepper, and cilantro.

Add the lime juice and olive oil, mixing well to combine all the flavors.

Season with salt and pepper to taste. Adjust the consistency with coconut water or vegetable broth if desired.

Chill in the refrigerator for at least 1 hour before serving to allow the flavors to meld.

How to Use:

Serve the Pineapple Cucumber Gazpacho chilled, garnished with extra cilantro or a lime wedge.

Enjoy this gazpacho as a standalone refreshing soup or as a part of a larger meal with grilled seafood or a light salad.

Duration:

Pineapple Cucumber Gazpacho can be stored in an airtight container in the refrigerator and is best consumed within 2-3 days for optimal freshness and flavor.

Pineapple Cucumber Gazpacho offers a delightful blend of flavors and nutrients, making it a perfect choice for a hydrating, anti-inflammatory, and deliciously light meal.

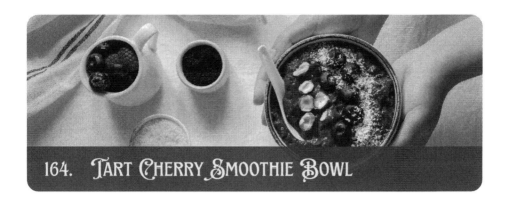

164. Tart Cherry Smoothie Bowl

Introduction:

Tart Cherry Smoothie Bowl is a nutrient-rich and visually appealing dish that harnesses the anti-inflammatory and antioxidant benefits of tart cherries. Known for their ability to reduce muscle soreness and improve sleep quality, tart cherries make this smoothie bowl not only a treat for the taste buds but also a boost for health. Combined with other fruits and superfoods, it's an excellent way to start your day or recover after a workout.

Ingredients and Measurements:

- 1 cup of frozen tart cherries
- 1 banana, frozen
- 1/2 cup of Greek yogurt or a dairy-free alternative
- 1/2 cup of almond milk or another plant-based milk
- 1 tablespoon of chia seeds
- 1 tablespoon of honey or maple syrup (optional, for sweetness)
- Toppings: sliced fresh fruits, granola, nuts, seeds, or a drizzle of honey

Preparation:

- In a blender, combine the frozen tart cherries, frozen banana, Greek yogurt, almond milk, and chia seeds.
- Blend until the mixture is smooth and creamy. Add a bit more milk if needed to adjust the consistency.
- Taste and add honey or maple syrup if additional sweetness is desired. Blend again to incorporate.
- Pour the smoothie mixture into a bowl.

How to Use:

- Arrange your chosen toppings over the smoothie bowl for added texture, flavor, and nutrients.
- Serve immediately to enjoy the full flavor and benefits of the ingredients.

Duration:

- Tart Cherry Smoothie Bowl is best enjoyed fresh. However, you can prepare the smoothie mixture and store it in the refrigerator for up to 24 hours if needed. Stir well before adding toppings and serving.

Tart Cherry Smoothie Bowl offers a delightful and healthful experience, combining the powerful benefits of tart cherries with the pleasure of a creamy, customizable smoothie bowl.

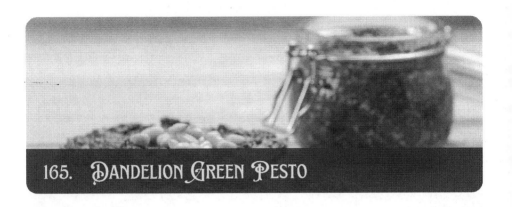

165. DANDELION GREEN PESTO

Introduction:

Dandelion Green Pesto is an innovative and healthful twist on traditional pesto, using the nutritious leaves of the dandelion plant. Rich in vitamins A, C, and K, as well as iron and antioxidants, dandelion greens offer a slightly bitter, earthy flavor that complements the other ingredients beautifully. This pesto is perfect for enhancing pasta dishes, spreading on sandwiches, or as a dip for a variety of snacks.

Ingredients and Measurements:

- 2 cups of dandelion greens, washed and roughly chopped
- 1/2 cup of Parmesan cheese, grated
- 1/3 cup of pine nuts or walnuts
- 2-3 garlic cloves, peeled
- 1/2 cup of olive oil
- Salt and pepper to taste
- Optional: lemon juice for added zest

Preparation:

- In a food processor, combine the dandelion greens, Parmesan cheese, nuts, and garlic cloves.
- Pulse until the ingredients are coarsely chopped.
- While the processor is running, gradually add the olive oil until the mixture forms a smooth paste.
- Season with salt and pepper, and add a squeeze of lemon juice if desired for extra freshness.
- Adjust the consistency by adding more olive oil if needed.

How to Use:

- Serve the Dandelion Green Pesto with pasta, as a spread on sandwiches, or as a flavorful addition to salads and roasted vegetables.
- It can also be used as a dip for bread or fresh vegetables.

Duration:

- Store Dandelion Green Pesto in an airtight container in the refrigerator for up to a week.

- For longer storage, you can freeze the pesto in ice cube trays and then transfer the cubes to a freezer bag, where they can be kept for up to 3 months.

Dandelion Green Pesto offers a unique and nutritious way to enjoy the health benefits of dandelion greens, providing a versatile and delicious enhancement to a variety of dishes.

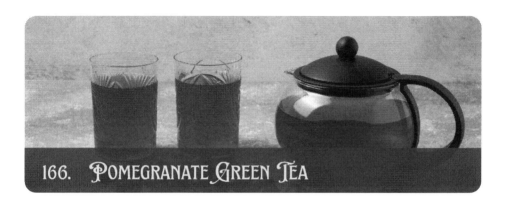

166. POMEGRANATE GREEN TEA

Introduction:

Pomegranate Green Tea is a refreshing and healthful beverage that combines the antioxidant-rich qualities of green tea with the vibrant, nutrient-packed pomegranate. This tea is excellent for heart health, improving digestion, and boosting the immune system. Its delightful blend of flavors makes it a perfect drink for hydration and overall wellness.

Ingredients and Measurements:

- 2 teaspoons of green tea leaves or 2 green tea bags
- 1 cup of pomegranate juice

- 2 cups of water
- Optional: honey or lemon slices for added sweetness and zest

Preparation:

- Boil the water in a kettle or saucepan. Once boiling, remove from heat and let it cool slightly to about 175°F (80°C) to prevent the green tea from becoming bitter.

- Steep the green tea leaves or tea bags in the hot water for about 3 minutes.

- Remove the tea leaves or bags and let the tea cool to room temperature.

- In a large pitcher, mix the cooled green tea with the pomegranate juice.

Stir well to combine the flavors. If desired, sweeten with honey or add lemon slices for a tangy twist.

How to Use:

Serve the Pomegranate Green Tea chilled over ice for a refreshing drink, or enjoy it at room temperature.

This tea can be enjoyed any time of the day for a healthful boost.

Duration:

Pomegranate Green Tea can be stored in the refrigerator in an airtight container for up to 5 days.

Pomegranate Green Tea offers a delicious and nutritious way to stay hydrated and reap the benefits of both green tea and pomegranate, enhancing your health with its rich antioxidants and pleasing taste.

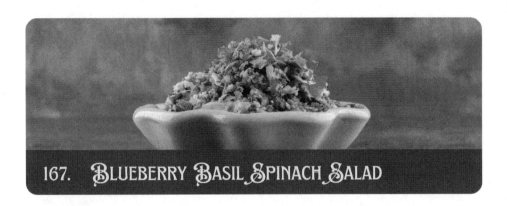

167. BLUEBERRY BASIL SPINACH SALAD

Introduction:

Blueberry Basil Spinach Salad is a vibrant and nutritious dish that combines the sweet, antioxidant-rich blueberries with the fresh, aromatic basil and the iron-packed spinach. This salad is perfect for a light meal or as a side, offering a blend of flavors and textures that support overall health, particularly heart health and immune function.

Ingredients and Measurements:

• 3 cups of fresh spinach leaves, washed and dried

• 1 cup of fresh blueberries

• 1/2 cup of crumbled feta or goat cheese

• 1/4 cup of toasted slivered almonds or walnuts

• 1/4 cup of fresh basil leaves, chopped

• 2 tablespoons of olive oil

• 1 tablespoon of balsamic vinegar

• 1 teaspoon of honey or maple syrup

• Salt and pepper to taste

Preparation:

☞ In a large salad bowl, combine the spinach, blueberries, feta or goat cheese, and toasted nuts.

☞ In a small bowl, whisk together the olive oil, balsamic vinegar, honey or maple syrup, salt, and pepper to create the dressing.

☞ Drizzle the dressing over the salad and gently toss to coat all the ingredients evenly.

☞ Sprinkle the chopped basil over the top for a fresh, herbal finish.

How to Use:

⤷ Serve the Blueberry Basil Spinach Salad immediately to enjoy the fresh flavors and crisp textures.

⤷ This salad is ideal as a standalone meal or paired with a protein source like grilled chicken or salmon for a more substantial dish.

Duration:

⟳ Blueberry Basil Spinach Salad is best enjoyed fresh but can be refrigerated for a few hours if needed. Keep the dressing separate until ready to serve to maintain the best texture and flavor.

Blueberry Basil Spinach Salad is a delightful and healthful choice, providing a mix of essential nutrients and flavors that enhance your well-being and culinary experience.

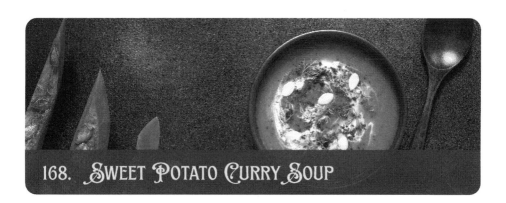

168. SWEET POTATO CURRY SOUP

Introduction:

Sweet Potato Curry Soup is a warm, comforting dish that combines the natural sweetness of sweet potatoes with the robust flavors of curry spices. This soup is rich in vitamins A and C, fiber, and antioxidants, providing a nutritious boost to the immune system and aiding in digestion. Its creamy texture and depth of flavor make it a perfect meal for colder days or as a nourishing starter.

Ingredients and Measurements:

- 2 large sweet potatoes, peeled and diced
- 1 onion, chopped
- 2 garlic cloves, minced
- 1 tablespoon of curry powder
- 1 teaspoon of ground ginger or 1 tablespoon of fresh ginger, minced
- 4 cups of vegetable broth
- 1 can (14 oz) of coconut milk
- 2 tablespoons of olive oil
- Salt and pepper to taste
- Optional: cilantro or parsley for garnish

Preparation:

- In a large pot, heat the olive oil over medium heat. Add the chopped onion and sauté until translucent.
- Add the minced garlic and ginger, cooking for another minute until fragrant.
- Stir in the curry powder and let it cook for a minute to release its flavors.
- Add the diced sweet potatoes to the pot and stir to coat them with the spices.
- Pour in the vegetable broth and bring the mixture to a boil. Reduce the heat and let it simmer until the sweet potatoes are tender, about 20 minutes.
- Use an immersion blender to puree the soup in the pot until smooth. Alternatively, carefully transfer the soup to a blender and puree in batches.
- Stir in the coconut milk and season with salt and pepper. Heat through.
- Taste and adjust the seasoning as needed.

How to Use:

- Serve the Sweet Potato Curry Soup hot, garnished with chopped cilantro or parsley if desired.
- Accompany this soup with crusty bread or a side salad for a complete meal.

Duration:

- Sweet Potato Curry Soup can be stored in the refrigerator in an airtight container for up to 5 days.
- It can also be frozen for up to 3 months. Thaw and reheat gently before serving.

Sweet Potato Curry Soup offers a delightful and healthful experience, blending the creaminess of sweet potatoes with the aromatic spices of curry for a dish that's both satisfying and beneficial for your health.

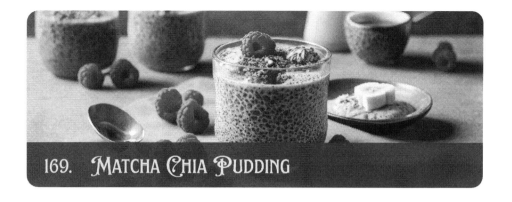

169. MATCHA CHIA PUDDING

Introduction:

Matcha Chia Pudding is a delicious and energizing treat that combines the antioxidant-rich matcha green tea with the fiber and omega-3 fatty acids of chia seeds. This pudding is ideal for a healthy breakfast or a refreshing snack, offering a steady release of energy and supporting overall wellness with its nutrient-packed ingredients.

Ingredients and Measurements:

- 2 tablespoons of matcha green tea powder
- 1 cup of milk (dairy or plant-based)
- 1/2 cup of chia seeds
- 1 tablespoon of honey or maple syrup (optional, for sweetness)
- Optional: fresh fruits, nuts, or coconut flakes for topping

Preparation:

- In a bowl, whisk together the matcha powder and a small amount of milk until smooth and free of lumps.

- Add the remaining milk and honey or maple syrup, stirring to combine thoroughly.

- Stir in the chia seeds until evenly distributed.

- Divide the mixture into serving glasses or a container, cover, and refrigerate overnight or for at least 4 hours until the pudding has thickened.

How to Use:

- Serve the Matcha Chia Pudding chilled, topped with fresh fruits, nuts, or coconut flakes for added texture and flavor.

- Enjoy this as a nutritious start to your day or as a revitalizing snack.

Duration:

- Matcha Chia Pudding can be stored in the refrigerator for up to 5 days.

- Ensure it is kept in an airtight container to maintain freshness and prevent any odors from affecting its taste.

Matcha Chia Pudding is a perfect blend of health and taste, providing a vibrant and nourishing option that benefits both mind and body with its superfood ingredients.

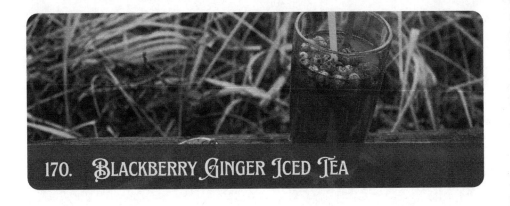

170. BLACKBERRY GINGER ICED TEA

Introduction:

Blackberry Ginger Iced Tea is a refreshing and flavorful beverage that combines the tart sweetness of blackberries with the spicy warmth of ginger. This iced tea is perfect for cooling down on a hot day or as a healthful alternative to sugary drinks, offering a delightful mix of antioxidants from blackberries and digestive benefits from ginger.

Ingredients and Measurements:

- 4 cups of water
- 2 tablespoons of loose black tea or 4 black tea bags
- 1 cup of fresh blackberries
- 1-inch piece of fresh ginger, thinly sliced
- 1/3 cup of honey or to taste
- Ice cubes
- Additional blackberries and mint leaves for garnish

Preparation:

- In a medium saucepan, bring water to a boil. Remove from heat and add the black tea or tea bags. Steep for 3-4 minutes, then remove the tea or bags.

- In a blender, combine the fresh blackberries and ginger slices. Blend until smooth.

- Strain the blackberry and ginger mixture through a fine mesh sieve into a large pitcher, pressing to extract as much liquid as possible.

- Add the brewed tea to the pitcher with the blackberry ginger juice. Stir in the honey until dissolved.

- Chill the tea in the refrigerator until cold, or for at least 1 hour.

- Serve over ice, garnished with extra blackberries and mint leaves for a touch of elegance.

How to Use:

- Enjoy Blackberry Ginger Iced Tea as a revitalizing drink throughout the day or serve it at gatherings for a unique and healthy beverage option that guests will love.

Duration:

🕐 Blackberry Ginger Iced Tea can be stored in the refrigerator for up to 5 days. Keep it in an airtight container to preserve the flavors and freshness.

Blackberry Ginger Iced Tea is not just a thirst quencher but a vibrant blend of natural tastes and health benefits, making it a perfect addition to any daily routine or special occasion.

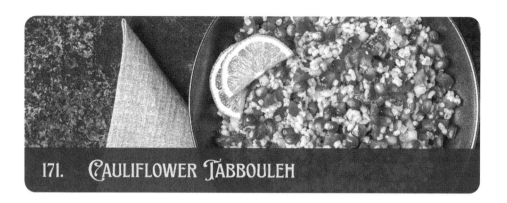

171. CAULIFLOWER TABBOULEH

Introduction:

Cauliflower Tabbouleh is a fresh and vibrant twist on the traditional Middle Eastern salad. By using cauliflower rice instead of bulgur wheat, this dish becomes a low-carb, nutrient-dense option suitable for various dietary needs. Packed with herbs, vegetables, and a zesty dressing, this salad is perfect for a light lunch or as a side dish that complements any meal.

Ingredients and Measurements:

- 1 large head of cauliflower, grated or processed into rice-sized pieces
- 1 cup of fresh parsley, finely chopped
- 1/2 cup of fresh mint, finely chopped
- 1 cup of cherry tomatoes, halved

- 1 cucumber, diced
- 3 green onions, thinly sliced
- Juice of 2 lemons
- 1/4 cup of extra virgin olive oil
- Salt and pepper to taste
- Optional: 1 clove of garlic, minced, for extra flavor

Preparation:

🍴 In a large mixing bowl, combine the grated cauliflower, chopped parsley, mint, tomatoes, cucumber, and green onions.

🍴 In a smaller bowl, whisk together the lemon juice, olive oil, salt, pepper, and minced garlic (if using) to create the dressing.

🍴 Pour the dressing over the cauliflower mixture and toss thoroughly to ensure all ingredients are well-coated.

Allow the tabbouleh to sit in the refrigerator for at least 30 minutes before serving. This resting time lets the flavors meld together beautifully.

How to Use:

Serve the Cauliflower Tabbouleh chilled as a refreshing side dish with grilled meats or as part of a mezze platter.

It's also great as a standalone meal for a light and healthy lunch option.

Duration:

Cauliflower Tabbouleh can be stored in the refrigerator in an airtight container for up to 3 days. It's best enjoyed fresh to maintain the crispness and vibrant flavors of the ingredients.

Cauliflower Tabbouleh is not just a delightful dish but also a testament to how simple substitutions can transform traditional recipes into new, health-focused favorites.

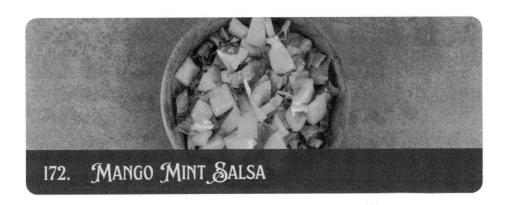

172. MANGO MINT SALSA

Introduction:

Mango Mint Salsa is a delightful mix of sweet and zesty flavors, combining ripe mangoes with refreshing mint, crisp red onion, and a hint of spice from jalapeño. This salsa is perfect for adding a tropical flair to dishes, making it an ideal complement to grilled meats, seafood, or as a vibrant dip for chips.

Ingredients and Measurements:

- 2 ripe mangoes, peeled and diced

- 1/2 cup of fresh mint leaves, finely chopped

- 1/2 red onion, finely diced

- 1 jalapeño, seeded and minced

- Juice of 1 lime

- Salt and pepper to taste

Preparation:

In a medium bowl, mix the diced mangoes, chopped mint, diced red onion, and minced jalapeño.

- Drizzle the lime juice over the mixture and toss gently to combine.
- Season with salt and pepper to your liking.
- Let the salsa rest for about 10 minutes to allow the flavors to blend.

How to Use:

- Serve Mango Mint Salsa as a fresh accompaniment to grilled fish, chicken, or use it to elevate the taste of tacos and wraps. It's also excellent as a standalone snack with tortilla chips.

Duration:

- Mango Mint Salsa is best enjoyed fresh but can be stored in the refrigerator for up to 2 days in an airtight container.

Mango Mint Salsa is not just a recipe but a celebration of flavors that brings a touch of the tropics to any meal, making it a perfect choice for those looking to refresh their palate with something vibrant and nourishing.

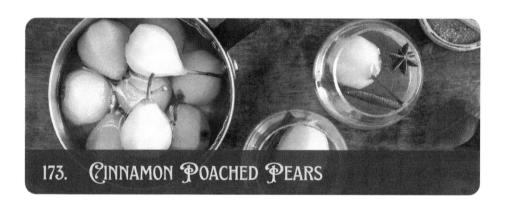

173. CINNAMON POACHED PEARS

Introduction:

Cinnamon Poached Pears are an elegant and simple dessert that showcases the natural sweetness of pears infused with the warm spice of cinnamon. This dish is perfect for a sophisticated end to a meal or as a comforting treat on a chilly evening, offering a light yet flavorful option that appeals to all ages.

Ingredients and Measurements:

- 4 ripe but firm pears, peeled, halved, and cored
- 4 cups of water
- 1 cup of sugar
- 2 cinnamon sticks
- 1 teaspoon of vanilla extract

Preparation:

- In a large saucepan, combine water, sugar, cinnamon sticks, and vanilla extract, bringing the mixture to a simmer over medium heat until the sugar is fully dissolved.
- Add the pear halves to the simmering liquid, ensuring they are submerged.
- Reduce the heat and let the pears simmer gently for 15-20 minutes, or until they are tender but not falling apart.
- Carefully remove the pears from the liquid and set them aside to cool.
- Continue to simmer the liquid until it reduces by half and thickens into a syrup.
- Pour the syrup over the pears before serving.

How to Use:

- Serve the Cinnamon Poached Pears with a drizzle of the reduced cinnamon syrup. They can be paired with vanilla ice cream, a dollop of whipped cream, or enjoyed on their own for a lighter dessert option.

Duration:

- Cinnamon Poached Pears can be stored in the refrigerator in an airtight container for up to 5 days, making them a convenient make-ahead dessert.

Cinnamon Poached Pears are a testament to the beauty of simplicity in cooking, offering a dessert that is as delightful to look at as it is to eat, enriching your dining experience with minimal effort.

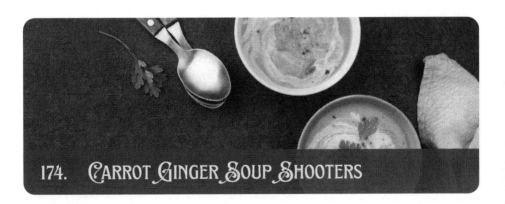

174. CARROT GINGER SOUP SHOOTERS

Introduction:

Carrot Ginger Soup Shooters are a vibrant and zesty appetizer that combines the sweetness of carrots with the spicy kick of ginger. These shooters are perfect for serving at parties or gatherings as a unique and flavorful starter. Their smooth texture and rich taste provide a warming sensation, making them ideal for both casual and elegant occasions.

Ingredients and Measurements:

- 1 pound of carrots, peeled and chopped
- 2 tablespoons of olive oil
- 1 onion, chopped
- 2 cloves of garlic, minced
- 2 tablespoons of fresh ginger, grated
- 4 cups of vegetable broth
- Salt and pepper to taste
- Optional garnish: fresh parsley or a swirl of cream

Preparation:

In a large pot, heat the olive oil over medium heat. Add the onion and sauté until translucent.

Add the garlic and ginger, cooking for an additional minute until fragrant.

Stir in the chopped carrots and cook for 3-4 minutes, allowing them to slightly soften.

Pour in the vegetable broth, bring to a boil, then reduce to a simmer. Cook until the carrots are tender, about 20 minutes.

Use an immersion blender or transfer the mixture to a regular blender to purée the soup until smooth.

Season with salt and pepper to taste. Adjust the consistency by adding more broth if needed.

How to Use:

Pour the soup into small shot glasses and garnish with a sprinkle of fresh parsley or a swirl of cream for an added touch of elegance. Serve these shooters warm or at room temperature as a delightful appetizer.

Duration:

Carrot Ginger Soup Shooters can be stored in the refrigerator for up to 4 days in an airtight container. Reheat gently before serving to preserve the smooth texture and vibrant flavors.

Carrot Ginger Soup Shooters are more than just a dish; they are an experience that combines the comfort of soup with the novelty of an appetizer, enhancing any meal with their bright color and engaging flavors.

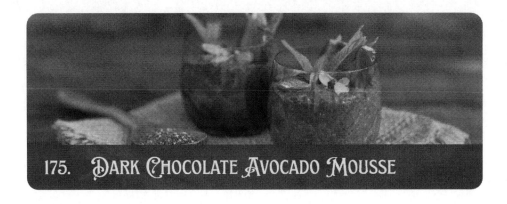

175. DARK CHOCOLATE AVOCADO MOUSSE

Introduction:

Dark Chocolate Avocado Mousse is a rich and creamy dessert that merges the health benefits of avocado with the indulgence of dark chocolate. This mousse is not only delicious but also a healthier alternative to traditional mousse, offering a blend of good fats, antioxidants, and a smooth, velvety texture that satisfies any sweet tooth.

Ingredients and Measurements:

- 2 ripe avocados, pitted and scooped
- 1/2 cup of high-quality dark chocolate, melted
- 1/4 cup of cocoa powder
- 1/4 cup of honey or maple syrup
- 1 teaspoon of vanilla extract
- A pinch of salt

Preparation:

- In a blender or food processor, combine the avocados, melted dark chocolate, cocoa powder, honey or maple syrup, vanilla extract, and salt.

- Blend until the mixture is completely smooth and creamy, stopping to scrape down the sides as necessary.
- Taste and adjust the sweetness if needed by adding a little more honey or maple syrup.
- Transfer the mousse into small serving dishes or ramekins and chill in the refrigerator for at least an hour before serving.

How to Use:

- Serve the Dark Chocolate Avocado Mousse chilled, garnished with fresh berries, a sprinkle of cocoa powder, or a few shavings of dark chocolate for an extra touch of elegance.

Duration:

- This mousse can be stored in the refrigerator in an airtight container for up to 3 days. It's best to cover the surface with plastic wrap to prevent browning.

Dark Chocolate Avocado Mousse is an exemplary dessert that combines simplicity and sophistication, offering a guilt-free way to indulge in the rich flavors of chocolate while benefiting from the nutritious properties of avocado.

PART 08

GUT-HEALING
RECIPES (176-190)

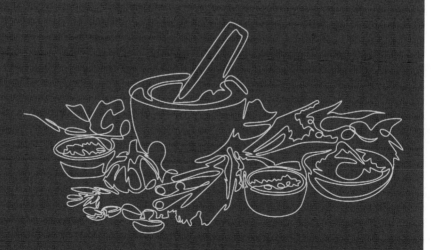

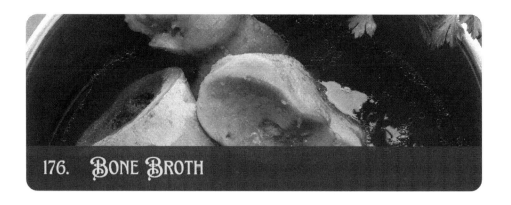

176. Bone Broth

Introduction:

Bone Broth is a nutrient-rich liquid made by simmering bones and connective tissues of animals. It's renowned for its healing properties, especially for the gut, due to its high collagen content, which can help repair intestinal lining and support overall digestive health. This broth is also a great source of minerals and amino acids essential for immunity and joint health.

Ingredients and Measurements:

- 2 pounds of mixed bones (beef, chicken, or turkey), preferably from grass-fed or organic sources
- 2 carrots, chopped
- 2 celery stalks, chopped
- 1 onion, quartered
- 4 garlic cloves, peeled
- 2 tablespoons of apple cider vinegar
- 1 teaspoon of salt
- 1/2 teaspoon of whole peppercorns
- Optional: herbs like parsley, thyme, or bay leaves

Preparation:

- If using beef bones, roast them in a preheated oven at 400°F for 30 minutes to enhance their flavor. For chicken or turkey bones, this step can be skipped.

- Place the bones in a large stockpot and cover them with cold water. Add the apple cider vinegar; this helps to extract the minerals from the bones.

- Add the carrots, celery, onion, garlic, salt, peppercorns, and any optional herbs to the pot.

- Bring the mixture to a boil, then reduce the heat to a low simmer. Skim off any foam or impurities that rise to the surface.

- Simmer the broth for 12-24 hours for chicken bones or up to 48 hours for beef bones. The longer it simmers, the more nutrients are extracted.

- Strain the broth through a fine-mesh sieve, discarding the solids. Allow the broth to cool, and then store it in the refrigerator or freezer.

How to Use:

🥄 Bone Broth can be consumed on its own, seasoned with additional salt and pepper, or used as a base for soups, stews, and sauces. It's also an excellent addition to rice or pasta dishes for extra flavor and nutrients.

Duration:

🕐 Bone Broth will keep in the refrigerator for up to 5 days and can be frozen for up to 6 months for long-term storage.

Bone Broth is a versatile and essential component of a gut-healing diet, offering deep nourishment and support for the body's foundational health needs.

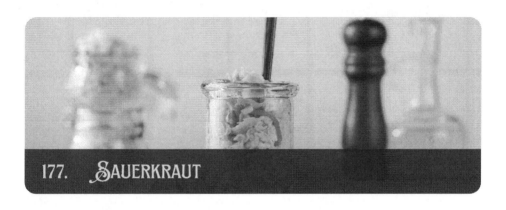

177. SAUERKRAUT

Introduction:

Sauerkraut is a traditional fermented cabbage dish known for its tangy flavor and numerous health benefits, particularly for the gut. Rich in probiotics, vitamins, and fiber, sauerkraut aids in digestion, boosts the immune system, and contributes to a healthy gut flora. This simple, age-old preparation is a staple in many cultures and a must-have for anyone looking to improve their digestive health.

Ingredients and Measurements:

- 1 medium head of cabbage (about 2 pounds), finely shredded

- 1 tablespoon of sea salt
- Optional: caraway seeds or other spices for additional flavor

Preparation:

☞ In a large bowl, combine the shredded cabbage and sea salt. Massage the salt into the cabbage with your hands for about 10 minutes, or until the cabbage releases its liquid and begins to soften.

☞ If using, sprinkle caraway seeds or your chosen spices over the cabbage and mix thoroughly.

☞ Pack the cabbage into a clean, large glass jar or a fermenting crock, pressing it down firmly until the liquid rises above the cabbage. It is crucial that the cabbage is submerged in its brine to prevent mold.

- Cover the jar with a clean cloth or coffee filter and secure it with a rubber band. This allows gases to escape while keeping contaminants out.

- Let the sauerkraut ferment at room temperature, away from direct sunlight, for at least 1 week and up to 4 weeks. Check regularly to ensure the cabbage remains submerged, pressing it down if needed.

- Taste the sauerkraut after 1 week. Once it reaches your desired flavor and tanginess, seal the jar with a lid and store it in the refrigerator.

How to Use:

- Sauerkraut can be served as a side dish, added to salads, sandwiches, or used as a topping for sausages and other meats. Its crisp texture and sour taste complement a wide range of dishes and enhance their nutritional value.

Duration:

- Sauerkraut can be kept in the refrigerator for several months, maintaining its taste and probiotic benefits when stored properly in an airtight container.

Sauerkraut is more than just a condiment; it's a functional food that promotes gut health and adds a lively flavor to any meal, making it a valuable addition to a health-conscious diet.

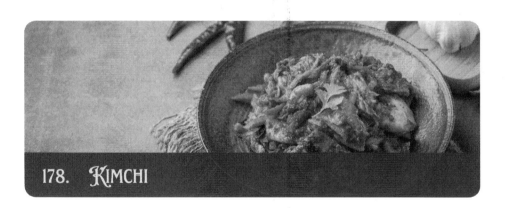

178. KIMCHI

Introduction:

Kimchi is a vibrant and spicy fermented vegetable dish originating from Korea. This staple of Korean cuisine combines the benefits of fermentation with the potent flavors of chili, garlic, and ginger. Known for its probiotic qualities, kimchi aids in digestion and boosts the immune system while providing a unique and robust taste experience.

Ingredients and Measurements:

- 1 medium Napa cabbage, cut into 2-inch pieces
- 1/4 cup of sea salt
- Water to cover the cabbage
- 4 tablespoons of Korean red pepper flakes (gochugaru)
- 1 tablespoon of grated ginger
- 4 cloves of garlic, minced
- 1 small Asian pear or apple, grated
- 4 green onions, chopped
- 1 daikon radish, peeled and julienned
- 1 tablespoon of fish sauce or soy sauce (for a vegan option)

Preparation:

- Place the cut Napa cabbage in a large bowl and sprinkle with sea salt. Toss to coat evenly, then cover with water. Let sit for 1-2 hours until the cabbage is softened.

- Rinse the cabbage under cold water, drain, and set aside.

- In a separate bowl, mix the Korean red pepper flakes, grated ginger, minced garlic, grated pear or apple, green onions, and daikon radish. Add the fish sauce or soy sauce and stir until well combined.

- Add the salted and drained cabbage to the spice mixture. Wearing gloves to protect your hands from the chili, thoroughly mix and massage the cabbage with the seasoning until fully coated.

- Pack the kimchi into a clean, airtight container or a fermenting jar, pressing down firmly to eliminate air pockets and ensure the vegetables are submerged in their own liquid.

- Seal the container and let it ferment at room temperature for 1-5 days, depending on your taste preferences and the room temperature. Check daily, pressing the vegetables down if they rise above the liquid.

- Once fermented to your liking, store the kimchi in the refrigerator.

How to Use:

- Kimchi can be enjoyed on its own, as a side dish with rice, in stews, or as an ingredient in various recipes like pancakes or scrambled eggs, adding depth and spice to every meal.

Duration:

- Kimchi will continue to ferment and develop in flavor over time. It can be stored in the refrigerator for up to several months, becoming more sour as it ages.

Kimchi is not just a dish; it's a celebration of flavors and health benefits, making it a must-have for those seeking to enhance their meals with both taste and nutritional value.

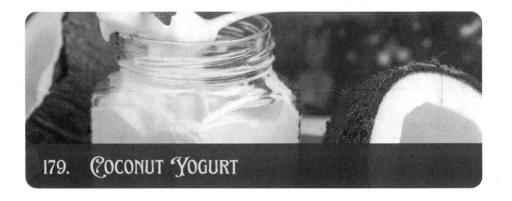

179. Coconut Yogurt

Introduction:

Coconut Yogurt is a creamy, dairy-free alternative to traditional yogurt, made from the rich milk of coconuts. This vegan-friendly option is not only delicious but also packed with probiotics that support digestive health. Its mild sweetness and smooth texture make it an excellent base for a variety of dishes or a delightful treat on its own.

Ingredients and Measurements:

- 4 cups of full-fat coconut milk
- 2 probiotic capsules or 1 tablespoon of store-bought coconut yogurt with live cultures
- 1 tablespoon of maple syrup or agave syrup (optional, for sweetness)

Preparation:

- Pour the coconut milk into a clean, heat-safe bowl. If using canned coconut milk, stir well to combine the cream and liquid.
- Warm the coconut milk gently in a saucepan or microwave just until it's lukewarm, not exceeding 110°F to preserve the live cultures.
- If using probiotic capsules, open them and pour the powder into the warm coconut milk. If using store-bought coconut yogurt, stir it in directly. Mix thoroughly to ensure even distribution of the probiotics.
- Cover the bowl with a clean cloth or coffee filter and secure it with a rubber band. Place the bowl in a warm, draft-free area, such as an oven with the light on (but not heated) or a yogurt maker, for 24-48 hours.
- After fermentation, check the yogurt for a tangy flavor and thickened consistency. Stir in the maple syrup or agave syrup if desired for added sweetness.
- Transfer the yogurt to airtight containers and refrigerate.

How to Use:

- Serve the Coconut Yogurt with fresh fruits, granola, or honey for a nutritious breakfast or snack. It can also be used in smoothies, as a base for dressings, or in baking as a substitute for dairy yogurt.

Duration:

🕐 Coconut Yogurt can be stored in the refrigerator for up to 7 days. Keep it sealed tightly to maintain its freshness and probiotic benefits.

Coconut Yogurt is a versatile and healthful addition to any diet, offering a plant-based option that enriches meals with flavor and functional benefits, ensuring a delightful culinary experience for those avoiding dairy or seeking a lighter alternative.

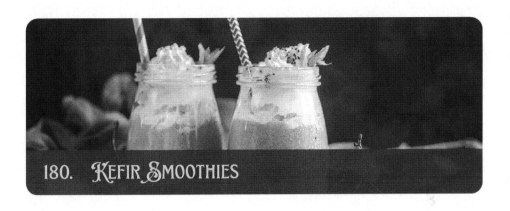

180. KEFIR SMOOTHIES

Introduction:

Kefir Smoothies are a delicious way to enjoy the probiotic benefits of kefir, a fermented milk drink similar to yogurt but with a thinner consistency and more potent probiotic profile. Blended with fruits, these smoothies are a refreshing and nutritious option, perfect for boosting gut health, enhancing immunity, and providing a quick, energizing meal or snack.

Ingredients and Measurements:

- 1 cup of kefir (dairy or water-based for a non-dairy option)
- 1 banana, sliced

- 1/2 cup of mixed berries (such as strawberries, blueberries, and raspberries)
- 1 tablespoon of honey or agave syrup (optional, for sweetness)
- A handful of spinach or kale (optional, for added nutrients)

Preparation:

🍽 In a blender, combine the kefir, banana, mixed berries, and optional honey or agave syrup.

🍽 If using, add the spinach or kale to incorporate extra vitamins and minerals.

🍽 Blend the ingredients until smooth and creamy, adjusting the consistency by adding more kefir or a little water if needed.

Taste and adjust the sweetness by adding more honey or agave syrup if desired.

How to Use:

Pour the Kefir Smoothie into a glass and enjoy immediately for the best flavor and nutrient content. It's perfect as a quick breakfast, a post-workout refreshment, or a healthy snack throughout the day.

Duration:

Kefir Smoothies are best enjoyed fresh but can be stored in the refrigerator for up to 24 hours. Shake or stir well before drinking if separated.

Kefir Smoothies are more than just a treat; they're a functional beverage that combines the pleasure of fruity flavors with the health benefits of kefir, making them an ideal choice for anyone looking to maintain a balanced and vibrant lifestyle.

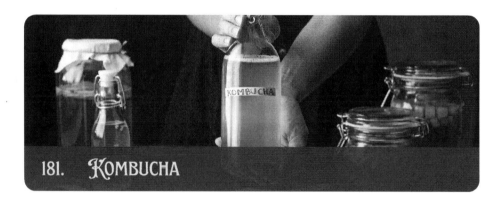

181. KOMBUCHA

Introduction:

Kombucha is a fermented tea beverage known for its tangy flavor and numerous health benefits, including improved digestion, enhanced immune function, and detoxification. Made from sweetened tea fermented by a symbiotic colony of bacteria and yeast (SCOBY), kombucha is a probiotic-rich drink that supports gut health and offers a refreshing alternative to sugary sodas.

Ingredients and Measurements:

- 1 SCOBY (symbiotic culture of bacteria and yeast)
- 4 cups of water
- 4 tea bags (black or green tea)
- 1 cup of sugar
- 1 cup of starter kombucha (from a previous batch or store-bought unpasteurized kombucha)

Preparation:

- Bring the water to a boil in a large pot. Remove from heat and add the tea bags, steeping them for about 15 minutes.

- Remove the tea bags and stir in the sugar until it is completely dissolved.

- Allow the sweetened tea to cool to room temperature. It's crucial that the tea is not hot, as high temperatures can harm the SCOBY.

- Pour the cooled tea into a large glass jar and add the starter kombucha. Gently place the SCOBY on top of the liquid. The SCOBY should float, but if it sinks, it's still fine.

- Cover the jar with a clean cloth or coffee filter and secure it with a rubber band. This setup allows air in but keeps contaminants out.

- Place the jar in a warm, dark place away from direct sunlight for 7-14 days. The longer it ferments, the less sweet and more vinegary it will taste.

- Taste the kombucha after 7 days to decide if you prefer it sweeter or more tart. Once it reaches your desired flavor, remove the SCOBY and reserve some kombucha as a starter for your next batch.

- Bottle the kombucha in clean glass bottles, leaving some headspace for carbonation. Seal the bottles and let them ferment at room temperature for 2-3 more days for added fizziness.

- Refrigerate to halt fermentation and enjoy chilled.

How to Use:

- Drink kombucha as is for a revitalizing and health-promoting beverage, or mix it into smoothies, cocktails, or other drinks for a probiotic boost.

Duration:

- Bottled kombucha can be stored in the refrigerator for up to a month. The flavor will continue to develop but at a much slower rate due to the cold temperature.

Kombucha is a dynamic and beneficial drink that combines the art of fermentation with the pleasure of a naturally effervescent beverage, enriching your health regimen with its distinct taste and probiotic power.

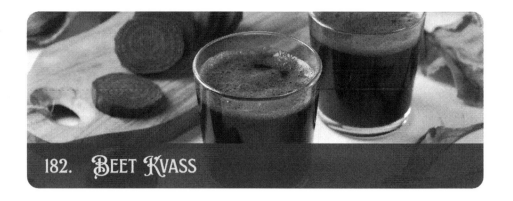

182. BEET KVASS

Introduction:

Beet Kvass is a traditional Eastern European fermented drink celebrated for its deep, earthy flavor and remarkable health benefits. Made from fermented beets, this tonic is rich in nutrients, enzymes, and probiotics, aiding in digestion, liver detoxification, and boosting overall vitality. Its vibrant color and unique tang make it a standout addition to any health-conscious diet.

Ingredients and Measurements:

- 2 medium beets, scrubbed and chopped into large cubes (do not peel to retain beneficial bacteria)

- 1 tablespoon of sea salt

- 4 cups of filtered water

- Optional: garlic cloves, mustard seeds, or herbs like dill or parsley for added flavor

Preparation:

☞ Place the chopped beets in a clean, quart-sized glass jar, filling it about one-third of the way.

☞ If using, add the optional flavorings like garlic, mustard seeds, or herbs.

☞ Dissolve the sea salt in the filtered water and pour this brine over the beets, ensuring they are completely submerged. Leave about an inch of space at the top of the jar.

☞ Cover the jar with a cloth or coffee filter and secure it with a rubber band to allow gases to escape while keeping out dust and insects.

☞ Place the jar in a cool, dark place for 5-7 days. Check daily to ensure the beets remain submerged, pressing them down if they rise above the brine.

☞ Taste the kvass after 5 days; it should be tangy with a slight sweetness. If a deeper flavor is desired, allow it to ferment for a couple more days.

☞ Strain out the beets and transfer the kvass to a clean bottle. Refrigerate to slow further fermentation.

How to Use:

☙ Drink a small glass (about 4 ounces) of Beet Kvass each morning on an empty stomach or use it in salad dressings or as a vibrant base for soups.

Duration:

🕐 Stored in the refrigerator, Beet Kvass can last for up to a month. Its flavors will continue to mature, becoming more complex over time.

Beet Kvass is not just a beverage but a potent health elixir, offering a simple yet effective way to enhance wellness with its blend of flavor, tradition, and nutritional benefits.

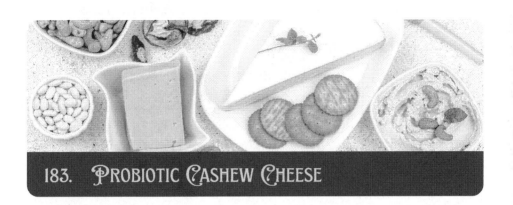

183. PROBIOTIC CASHEW CHEESE

Introduction:

Probiotic Cashew Cheese is a creamy, dairy-free alternative to traditional cheese, crafted from fermented cashews to yield a rich texture and tangy flavor. This vegan cheese is loaded with probiotics, enhancing gut health while offering a versatile, nutritious option for cheese lovers seeking plant-based alternatives.

Ingredients and Measurements:

- 2 cups of raw cashews, soaked overnight and drained
- 1/4 cup of rejuvelac or water kefir for fermentation
- 1 tablespoon of nutritional yeast for a cheesy flavor
- 1 teaspoon of sea salt

- Optional: herbs, garlic, or spices for additional flavor

Preparation:

🥄 After soaking, rinse the cashews under cold water and drain them thoroughly.

🥄 In a high-speed blender, combine the soaked cashews, rejuvelac or water kefir, nutritional yeast, and sea salt. Blend until smooth and creamy.

🥄 If desired, mix in herbs, garlic, or spices at this stage for extra flavor.

🥄 Transfer the mixture to a clean, airtight container. Cover and let it ferment at room temperature for 24-48 hours, depending on the desired level of tanginess.

- After fermentation, stir the cheese to incorporate any separation and adjust the seasoning if needed.

- Refrigerate the cheese to firm up before serving. It can be shaped into a block or used as a spread.

How to Use:

- Enjoy Probiotic Cashew Cheese spread on crackers, stirred into pasta dishes, or as a flavorful addition to sandwiches and salads.

Duration:

- This cheese can be stored in the refrigerator for up to 2 weeks. Keep it in an airtight container to maintain freshness and probiotic activity.

Probiotic Cashew Cheese enriches your diet with beneficial bacteria and a delightful taste, making it an excellent choice for enhancing meals with both flavor and health benefits.

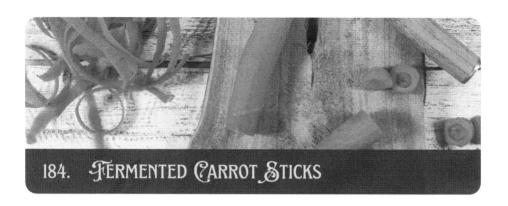

184. FERMENTED CARROT STICKS

Introduction:

Fermented Carrot Sticks are a crunchy, tangy snack that combines the natural sweetness of carrots with the gut-friendly benefits of fermentation. This easy-to-make treat is perfect for adding a probiotic boost to your diet, supporting digestion and immune health with every bite.

Ingredients and Measurements:

- 1 pound of organic carrots, peeled and cut into sticks

- 2 cups of filtered water
- 1 tablespoon of sea salt
- Optional: garlic cloves, dill, or mustard seeds for extra flavor

Preparation:

- In a large bowl, dissolve the sea salt in the filtered water to create a brine.

- Place the carrot sticks in a clean, quart-sized glass jar. If using, add the optional flavorings like garlic, dill, or mustard seeds.

- Pour the brine over the carrots, ensuring they are completely submerged. Leave about an inch of space at the top of the jar.

- Cover the jar with a cloth or coffee filter and secure it with a rubber band to allow gases to escape while keeping out contaminants.

- Let the jar sit at room temperature in a cool, dark place for 5-7 days. Check daily to ensure the carrots remain submerged, pressing them down if they rise above the brine.

- Taste the carrots after 5 days; they should be tangy with a firm texture. If a more robust flavor is desired, allow them to ferment for a couple more days.

- Once fermented to your liking, seal the jar with a lid and refrigerate.

How to Use:

- Serve Fermented Carrot Sticks as a healthy snack, add them to salads for extra crunch and flavor, or use them as a zesty accompaniment to meals.

Duration:

- Stored in the refrigerator, Fermented Carrot Sticks can last for up to a month, providing a convenient and healthful snack option that enhances meals with both taste and nutritional benefits.

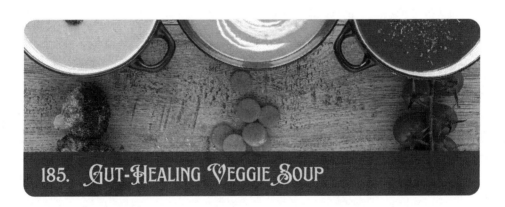

185. GUT-HEALING VEGGIE SOUP

Introduction:

Gut-Healing Veggie Soup is a nourishing blend of vegetables, herbs, and bone broth designed to support digestive health and soothe the gut. Packed with fiber, vitamins, and minerals, this soup helps reduce inflammation, promote healing, and restore balance to the digestive system.

Ingredients and Measurements:

- 2 tablespoons of olive oil
- 1 onion, chopped

- 2 cloves of garlic, minced
- 2 carrots, peeled and diced
- 2 celery stalks, diced
- 1 zucchini, diced
- 1 cup of chopped kale or spinach
- 4 cups of bone broth or vegetable broth for a vegan option
- 1 teaspoon of turmeric powder
- 1/2 teaspoon of ginger powder
- Salt and pepper to taste
- Optional: fresh herbs like parsley or thyme for garnish

Preparation:

- In a large pot, heat the olive oil over medium heat. Add the onion and sauté until translucent.

- Add the garlic, carrots, and celery, cooking for 3-4 minutes until they begin to soften.

- Stir in the zucchini and continue to cook for another 2 minutes.

- Pour in the bone broth or vegetable broth and bring the mixture to a boil.

- Reduce the heat to a simmer and add the turmeric and ginger powder. Season with salt and pepper to taste.

- Simmer the soup for 20-25 minutes, or until all vegetables are tender.

- Add the chopped kale or spinach and cook for an additional 5 minutes until the greens are wilted and tender.

- Adjust seasoning as needed and serve hot, garnished with fresh herbs if desired.

How to Use:

- Enjoy Gut-Healing Veggie Soup as a main course or a side dish. It's ideal for meal prep and can be a comforting part of a health-focused diet.

Duration:

- This soup can be stored in the refrigerator in an airtight container for up to 5 days or frozen for up to 3 months, making it a convenient and effective way to incorporate gut-friendly nutrients into your diet regularly.

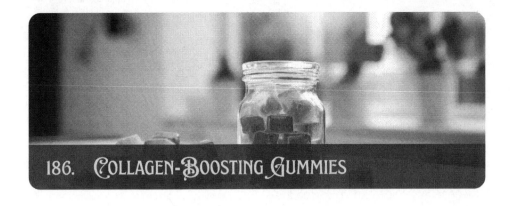

186. COLLAGEN-BOOSTING GUMMIES

Introduction:

Collagen-Boosting Gummies are a delightful and effective way to support skin, joint, and bone health. These tasty treats combine the benefits of collagen with the natural sweetness of fruit juice, providing a fun and convenient method to increase your collagen intake. Rich in protein and essential nutrients, these gummies help improve skin elasticity, strengthen joints, and enhance overall well-being.

Ingredients and Measurements:

- 1/2 cup of fruit juice (preferably high in vitamin C like orange or pomegranate)
- 2 tablespoons of honey or agave syrup
- 4 tablespoons of unflavored gelatin or agar-agar for a vegan option
- 2 scoops of collagen powder (ensure it's suitable for your dietary preferences)
- Optional: A few drops of natural food coloring or additional flavor extracts

Preparation:

- In a small saucepan, gently warm the fruit juice over low heat. Do not boil to preserve the nutrients.

- Add the honey or agave syrup to the warm juice and stir until completely dissolved.

- Sprinkle the gelatin or agar-agar over the liquid and let it sit for a minute to "bloom." Then, stir continuously until the gelatin or agar-agar is fully dissolved.

- Remove the saucepan from heat and whisk in the collagen powder until there are no lumps.

- If using, add natural food coloring or flavor extracts at this stage and mix well.

- Pour the mixture into silicone molds or a shallow dish lined with parchment paper.

- Refrigerate the gummies for at least 1 hour or until they are firm.

- Once set, pop the gummies out of the molds or cut them into bite-sized pieces if using a dish.

How to Use:

🥄 Enjoy Collagen-Boosting Gummies as a daily snack to supplement your collagen intake. They are perfect for on-the-go nutrition or a quick treat that benefits your health.

Duration:

🕐 These gummies can be stored in an airtight container in the refrigerator for up to 2 weeks, ensuring you have a steady supply of collagen-rich snacks ready at all times.

Collagen-Boosting Gummies are an enjoyable and practical solution for maintaining youthful skin, healthy joints, and overall vitality, offering a flavorful and nutritious addition to any wellness routine.

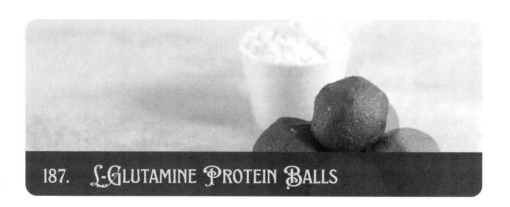

187. L-GLUTAMINE PROTEIN BALLS

Introduction:

L-Glutamine Protein Balls are a powerhouse snack designed to support muscle recovery and gut health. Infused with L-glutamine, an essential amino acid known for its role in gut and immune function, these protein balls are a great way to boost your energy levels and aid in recovery after workouts. Packed with nuts, seeds, and protein powder, they provide a balanced blend of nutrients in a convenient, bite-sized format.

Ingredients and Measurements:

- 1 cup of rolled oats
- 1/2 cup of protein powder (your choice of flavor)
- 1/4 cup of L-glutamine powder
- 1/2 cup of nut butter (such as almond, peanut, or cashew)
- 1/4 cup of honey or maple syrup
- 1/4 cup of seeds (chia, flax, or hemp)

- Optional: dark chocolate chips, dried fruit, or coconut flakes for extra flavor and texture

Preparation:

🖮 In a large bowl, mix the rolled oats, protein powder, L-glutamine powder, and seeds until well combined.

🖮 Stir in the nut butter and honey or maple syrup. Mix thoroughly until the ingredients form a sticky, cohesive dough. If the mixture is too dry, add a little more nut butter or syrup.

🖮 Fold in any optional ingredients like chocolate chips, dried fruit, or coconut flakes at this stage.

🖮 Using your hands, roll the mixture into small balls, about the size of a walnut.

🖮 Place the protein balls on a baking sheet lined with parchment paper and refrigerate for at least 30 minutes to set.

How to Use:

🖐 Grab L-Glutamine Protein Balls as a quick snack before or after workouts, or enjoy them as a healthy treat throughout the day to keep your energy levels up and support your nutritional goals.

Duration:

⊘ These protein balls can be stored in an airtight container in the refrigerator for up to 2 weeks or frozen for longer shelf life, ensuring you always have a nutritious snack on hand.

L-Glutamine Protein Balls are a smart and tasty way to incorporate essential nutrients into your daily routine, supporting both your physical and digestive health with every bite.

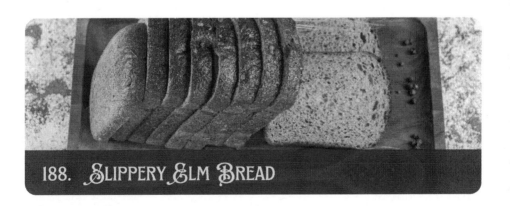

188. SLIPPERY ELM BREAD

Introduction:

Slippery Elm Bread is a wholesome and healing food that leverages the soothing properties of slippery elm bark. Known for its ability to calm the digestive tract and ease inflammation, slippery elm is a fantastic addition to this nutritious bread. This recipe creates a moist, tender loaf that's perfect for anyone seeking a gentle, gut-friendly option.

Ingredients and Measurements:

- 1 1/2 cups of whole wheat flour
- 1/2 cup of all-purpose flour
- 2 tablespoons of slippery elm powder
- 1 teaspoon of baking soda
- 1/2 teaspoon of salt
- 1/3 cup of vegetable oil or melted coconut oil
- 3/4 cup of honey or maple syrup
- 2 eggs, beaten
- 1 cup of buttermilk or a dairy-free alternative with 1 tablespoon of vinegar or lemon juice
- Optional: 1/2 cup of nuts or dried fruits for added texture and flavor

Preparation:

Preheat your oven to 350°F (175°C) and grease a 9x5 inch loaf pan.

In a large bowl, combine the whole wheat flour, all-purpose flour, slippery elm powder, baking soda, and salt.

In a separate bowl, mix the vegetable or coconut oil, honey or maple syrup, eggs, and buttermilk. Blend these wet ingredients until smooth.

Gradually add the wet mixture to the dry ingredients, stirring until just combined. Avoid overmixing to keep the bread tender.

If using, fold in the nuts or dried fruits at this point.

Pour the batter into the prepared loaf pan and smooth the top with a spatula.

Bake in the preheated oven for 45-55 minutes, or until a toothpick inserted into the center comes out clean.

Let the bread cool in the pan for 10 minutes, then turn it out onto a wire rack to cool completely.

How to Use:

Enjoy slices of Slippery Elm Bread on their own, or serve them with a spread of butter or jam for added flavor. It's also great toasted for breakfast or as a base for sandwiches.

Duration:

Store Slippery Elm Bread in an airtight container at room temperature for up to 3 days or refrigerate for up to a week. For longer storage, wrap well and freeze for up to 3 months.

Slippery Elm Bread provides a nutritious and comforting way to enjoy the benefits of this healing herb, making it an excellent choice for anyone looking to support their digestive health with their diet.

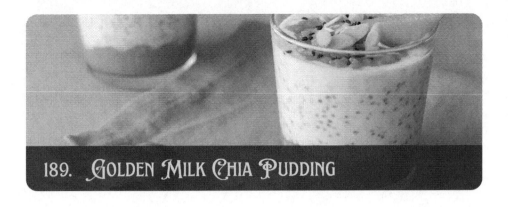

189. GOLDEN MILK CHIA PUDDING

Introduction:

Golden Milk Chia Pudding combines the anti-inflammatory and soothing benefits of golden milk with the nutritious power of chia seeds. This vibrant dessert or breakfast option features turmeric, ginger, and cinnamon for a warm, spicy flavor that's both healing and delicious. Rich in fiber, omega-3 fatty acids, and antioxidants, this pudding is a delightful way to start or end your day with health in mind.

Ingredients and Measurements:

- 1 cup of unsweetened almond milk or coconut milk
- 1 teaspoon of turmeric powder
- 1/2 teaspoon of ground ginger
- 1/4 teaspoon of ground cinnamon
- A pinch of black pepper (to enhance turmeric absorption)
- 2 tablespoons of honey or maple syrup
- 1/2 cup of chia seeds

Preparation:

- In a medium saucepan, gently heat the almond or coconut milk until it is warm but not boiling.
- Stir in the turmeric, ginger, cinnamon, and black pepper, mixing until the spices are fully dissolved.
- Remove the saucepan from the heat and whisk in the honey or maple syrup until it's well incorporated.
- Pour the spiced milk mixture into a bowl and add the chia seeds, stirring thoroughly to ensure the seeds are evenly distributed.
- Let the mixture sit for 5 minutes, then stir again to prevent the chia seeds from clumping.
- Cover the bowl and refrigerate for at least 4 hours or overnight until the pudding has thickened and the chia seeds have absorbed the liquid.

How to Use:

- Serve the Golden Milk Chia Pudding chilled, topped with fresh fruits, a sprinkle of extra cinnamon, or a drizzle of honey for added sweetness.

It makes a perfect breakfast or a soothing, nutritious snack.

Duration:

⏱ Golden Milk Chia Pudding can be stored in the refrigerator in an airtight container for up to 5 days, ensuring you have a ready-to-eat, health-boosting treat whenever you need it.

Golden Milk Chia Pudding offers a fusion of flavors and health benefits, making it a smart choice for anyone looking to enhance their wellness routine with a tasty and nourishing treat.

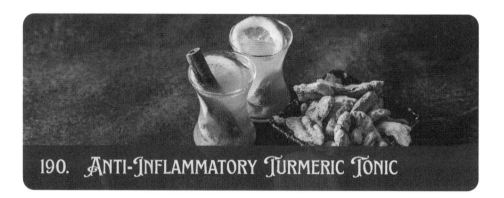

190.   ANTI-INFLAMMATORY TURMERIC TONIC

Introduction:

Anti-Inflammatory Turmeric Tonic is a powerful beverage designed to combat inflammation and boost overall health. Made with turmeric, ginger, and lemon, this tonic is a potent mix of antioxidants and anti-inflammatory compounds that support immune function, enhance digestion, and promote a healthy response to inflammation in the body.

Ingredients and Measurements:

- 4 cups of water
- 2 tablespoons of turmeric powder or freshly grated turmeric root

- 1 tablespoon of freshly grated ginger root
- Juice of 1 lemon
- 2 tablespoons of honey or maple syrup
- A pinch of black pepper (to enhance the absorption of curcumin from turmeric)

Preparation:

🍵 In a saucepan, bring the water to a gentle boil.

🍵 Add the turmeric and ginger to the boiling water and reduce the heat to a simmer. Let it steep for 10-15 minutes, allowing the flavors and nutrients to infuse the water.

- Remove from heat and strain the liquid through a fine-mesh sieve into a pitcher to remove the solids.

- Stir in the lemon juice, honey or maple syrup, and a pinch of black pepper. Mix well until the sweetener is fully dissolved.

- Allow the tonic to cool slightly before serving, or refrigerate to chill.

How to Use:

- Drink a small glass of Anti-Inflammatory Turmeric Tonic daily, preferably in the morning or before meals, to maximize its health benefits. You can enjoy it warm or cold based on your preference.

Duration:

- Store the Anti-Inflammatory Turmeric Tonic in the refrigerator in an airtight container for up to one week. Shake well before each use to redistribute the ingredients.

This tonic provides a simple yet effective way to incorporate the healing powers of turmeric and ginger into your daily routine, ensuring you receive a dose of nature's best anti-inflammatory agents.

PART 09

DETOXIFYING DRINKS AND SMOOTHIES (191-205)

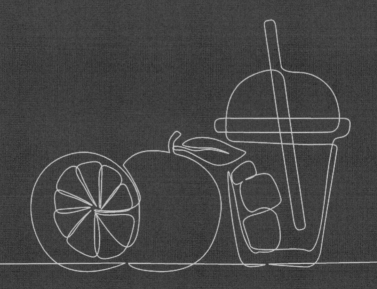

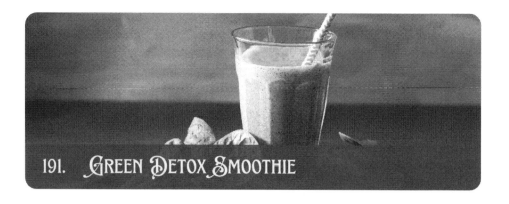

191. GREEN DETOX SMOOTHIE

Introduction:

Green Detox Smoothie is a refreshing and cleansing beverage packed with nutrients to support detoxification and enhance overall health. Combining leafy greens, antioxidant-rich fruits, and purifying ingredients like lemon and ginger, this smoothie helps to flush out toxins while providing a boost of energy and vital nutrients.

Ingredients and Measurements:

- 1 cup of spinach or kale, tightly packed
- 1/2 cucumber, chopped
- 1 apple or pear, cored and chopped
- 1/2 banana, sliced
- 1 tablespoon of fresh ginger, grated
- Juice of 1 lemon
- 1 tablespoon of chia seeds
- 1 cup of coconut water or filtered water

Preparation:

🥄 In a blender, combine the spinach or kale, cucumber, apple or pear, banana, ginger, and lemon juice.

🥄 Add the chia seeds and pour in the coconut water or filtered water for the desired consistency.

🥄 Blend on high until smooth and creamy, ensuring all ingredients are fully incorporated.

🥄 Taste and adjust the sweetness by adding a little more banana or a splash of honey if needed.

How to Use:

🥄 Enjoy the Green Detox Smoothie as a revitalizing breakfast or a mid-day snack to invigorate your body and support detox processes. It's ideal for kick-starting your metabolism and replenishing your system with essential nutrients.

Duration:

🕐 This smoothie is best enjoyed fresh but can be stored in the refrigerator for up to 24 hours. If kept longer, stir or shake well before drinking as separation may occur.

Green Detox Smoothie is an excellent choice for cleansing your system, boosting your nutrient intake, and feeling refreshed and energized throughout the day.

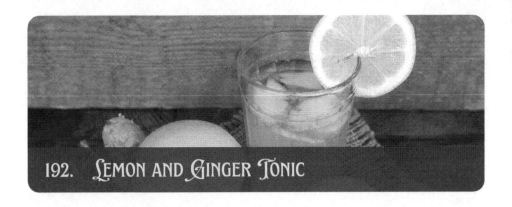

192. LEMON AND GINGER TONIC

Introduction:

Lemon and Ginger Tonic is a vibrant and invigorating drink known for its detoxifying and immune-boosting properties. This tonic combines the cleansing power of lemon with the warming and digestive benefits of ginger, creating a simple yet potent beverage to support overall health and wellness.

Ingredients and Measurements:

- 4 cups of water
- 2 inches of fresh ginger root, peeled and thinly sliced
- Juice of 2 lemons
- 2 tablespoons of honey or maple syrup
- A pinch of cayenne pepper (optional for an extra kick)

Preparation:

- In a saucepan, bring the water to a boil.
- Add the sliced ginger to the boiling water and reduce the heat. Let it simmer for about 15-20 minutes to infuse the water with ginger's spicy flavor.
- Remove from heat and strain the ginger pieces out, pouring the infused water into a heat-resistant pitcher.
- Stir in the lemon juice and honey or maple syrup, mixing until the sweetener is completely dissolved.
- If using, add a pinch of cayenne pepper for added heat and circulation benefits.
- Let the tonic cool to room temperature, then chill in the refrigerator or serve over ice.

How to Use:

- Drink a glass of Lemon and Ginger Tonic in the morning to kickstart your digestion, or enjoy it throughout the day to stay hydrated and flush toxins from your body.

Duration:

- This tonic can be stored in the refrigerator for up to 5 days. Shake or stir well before serving to ensure the flavors are well blended.

Lemon and Ginger Tonic is a straightforward way to incorporate detoxifying elements into your daily routine, offering a delicious and healthful option to enhance your vitality and cleanse your body.

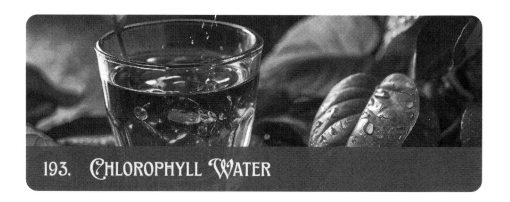

193. CHLOROPHYLL WATER

Introduction:

Chlorophyll Water is a refreshing and detoxifying drink that harnesses the power of chlorophyll, the green pigment in plants responsible for photosynthesis. Known for its ability to purify the body, improve digestion, and boost energy levels, this simple beverage is a great way to hydrate and enrich your body with essential vitamins and minerals.

Ingredients and Measurements:

- 4 cups of filtered water
- 1 tablespoon of liquid chlorophyll
- Juice of 1 lemon
- Optional: a few mint leaves or cucumber slices for added freshness

Preparation:

☕ In a large pitcher, combine the filtered water and liquid chlorophyll, stirring well to ensure it's evenly mixed.

☕ Squeeze in the lemon juice and stir again to blend the flavors.

☕ If desired, add mint leaves or cucumber slices to the pitcher for a hint of extra refreshment.

☕ Refrigerate for at least 30 minutes to allow the flavors to meld and the drink to chill.

How to Use:

🥄 Serve Chlorophyll Water chilled as a daily hydrating beverage to support detoxification and energy levels. It's particularly beneficial first thing in the morning or after workouts to replenish and revitalize your body.

Duration:

○ This drink can be kept in the refrigerator for up to 3 days. Stir or shake well before serving to redistribute the chlorophyll and flavors.

Chlorophyll Water is an effortless and effective way to boost your intake of health-promoting nutrients, promoting a sense of well-being and natural purification with each sip.

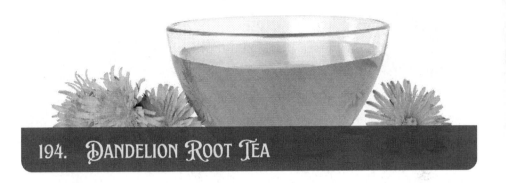

194. DANDELION ROOT TEA

Introduction:

Dandelion Root Tea is a traditional herbal remedy prized for its liver-supportive and detoxifying properties. Made from the roasted roots of the dandelion plant, this tea offers a slightly bitter, earthy flavor that is rich in antioxidants and can help stimulate digestion, reduce inflammation, and cleanse the body of toxins.

Ingredients and Measurements:

- 1 tablespoon of dried, roasted dandelion root
- 4 cups of water
- Optional: honey or lemon to taste

Preparation:

☞ In a medium saucepan, bring the water to a boil.

☞ Add the dried dandelion root to the boiling water and reduce the heat.

☞ Simmer for about 10-15 minutes, allowing the roots to release their full flavor and beneficial compounds.

☞ Strain the tea into a cup or pitcher, removing the dandelion root pieces.

☞ If desired, sweeten with honey or enhance with a squeeze of lemon for added flavor.

How to Use:

↳ Enjoy Dandelion Root Tea warm or chilled as a detoxifying beverage. It can be sipped throughout the day, especially after meals, to aid digestion and support liver health.

Duration:

⊘ This tea can be stored in the refrigerator for up to 3 days. Warm it up or enjoy it cold according to your preference.

Dandelion Root Tea is a natural and effective way to support your body's detox processes and promote overall health, making it a valuable addition to your wellness routine.

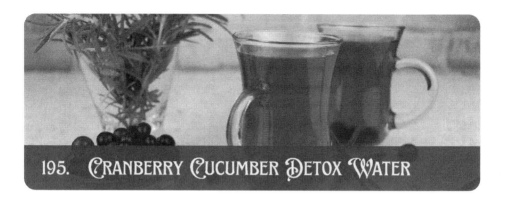

195. CRANBERRY CUCUMBER DETOX WATER

Introduction:

Cranberry Cucumber Detox Water is a hydrating and cleansing beverage that combines the antioxidant properties of cranberries with the refreshing qualities of cucumber. This drink is perfect for flushing toxins from the body, reducing bloat, and enhancing skin health with its mix of vitamins and minerals.

Ingredients and Measurements:

- 4 cups of filtered water
- 1 cup of fresh cranberries
- 1 cucumber, thinly sliced
- Juice of 1 lime
- Optional: a few sprigs of mint for extra freshness

Preparation:

🍶 In a large pitcher, add the cranberries and cucumber slices.

🍶 Pour the filtered water over the cranberries and cucumber, ensuring they are fully submerged.

🍶 Squeeze the lime juice into the pitcher and stir well to combine all the flavors.

🍶 If using, add the mint sprigs to the mixture for an additional layer of flavor.

🍶 Refrigerate the detox water for at least 1 hour or overnight to allow the fruits and herbs to infuse the water fully.

How to Use:

🥄 Serve Cranberry Cucumber Detox Water chilled throughout the day to stay hydrated and support your body's natural detoxification processes. It's particularly beneficial during or after meals to aid digestion and refresh the palate.

Cranberry Cucumber Detox Water is a delightful and effective way to enhance your hydration routine, offering a blend of nutrients that support health and wellness with every sip.

Duration:

⊘ This detox water can be stored in the refrigerator for up to 48 hours. After that, the fruits may begin to break down, but the water will still be flavorful and nutritious.

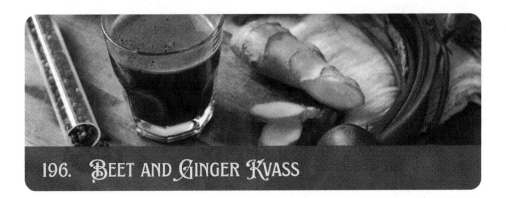

196. BEET AND GINGER KVASS

Introduction:

Beet and Ginger Kvass is a revitalizing fermented beverage that blends the earthy sweetness of beets with the spicy warmth of ginger. This variation on traditional kvass enhances its detoxifying and digestive benefits, making it an excellent choice for supporting liver health and boosting the immune system.

Ingredients and Measurements:

- 2 medium beets, scrubbed and chopped into cubes

- 1 inch of fresh ginger, peeled and sliced
- 1 tablespoon of sea salt
- 4 cups of filtered water
- Optional: a squeeze of lemon for added zest

Preparation:

☞ Place the chopped beets and sliced ginger in a clean, quart-sized glass jar.

☞ Dissolve the sea salt in the filtered water and pour this brine over the beets and ginger, ensuring they are fully submerged. Leave about an inch of space at the top of the jar.

- Cover the jar with a cloth or coffee filter and secure it with a rubber band to allow gases to escape while keeping out contaminants.

- Let the jar sit at room temperature in a cool, dark place for 5-7 days. Check daily to ensure the beets and ginger remain submerged, pressing them down if they rise above the brine.

- Taste the kvass after 5 days; it should have a tangy, slightly sweet flavor with a hint of ginger. If a deeper flavor is desired, allow it to ferment for a couple more days.

- Once fermented to your liking, strain the liquid, discarding the solids, and transfer the kvass to a clean bottle. Refrigerate to slow further fermentation.

How to Use:

- Enjoy a small glass of Beet and Ginger Kvass each morning or before meals to aid digestion and detoxification. You can also use it as a base for salad dressings or to add depth to soups.

Duration:

- Stored in the refrigerator, Beet and Ginger Kvass can last for up to a month. Its flavors will continue to mature, becoming more complex over time.

Beet and Ginger Kvass offers a delicious and healthful way to incorporate the benefits of beets and ginger into your diet, supporting your body's natural cleansing processes and promoting overall well-being.

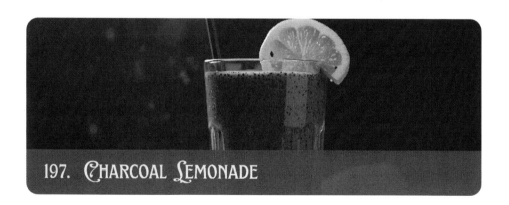

197. CHARCOAL LEMONADE

Introduction:

Charcoal Lemonade is a striking and beneficial detox drink that combines the purifying effects of activated charcoal with the refreshing taste of lemonade. This unique beverage is known for its ability to bind toxins and chemicals, aiding in their removal from the body. Ideal for a cleanse or as a way to reset the digestive system, it offers a crisp, slightly tart flavor with a deep, intriguing color.

Ingredients and Measurements:

- 4 cups of filtered water

- Juice of 3 lemons

- 2 tablespoons of honey or maple syrup

- 1 teaspoon of activated charcoal powder (ensure it's food-grade)

- Optional: a few sprigs of mint or a slice of lemon for garnish

Preparation:

- In a large pitcher, combine the filtered water and lemon juice.

- Stir in the honey or maple syrup until fully dissolved.

- Carefully mix in the activated charcoal powder, ensuring it is evenly distributed without clumps.

- Chill the lemonade in the refrigerator for at least 30 minutes to allow the flavors to meld and the charcoal to fully integrate.

How to Use:

- Serve Charcoal Lemonade chilled, garnished with mint or a lemon slice. It's a great choice for morning detox rituals or as a refreshing drink throughout the day.

Duration:

- This lemonade should be consumed within 24 hours of preparation to maximize the benefits of the activated charcoal. Store it in the refrigerator and stir well before serving, as the charcoal may settle at the bottom.

Charcoal Lemonade is a functional and stylish way to support detoxification, offering a modern twist on traditional lemonade while delivering significant health benefits.

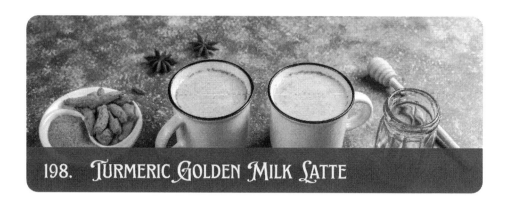

198. TURMERIC GOLDEN MILK LATTE

Introduction:

Turmeric Golden Milk Latte is a warm and comforting drink that combines the anti-inflammatory and antioxidant properties of turmeric with the creamy richness of milk. This soothing beverage is perfect for evenings or as a calming addition to your wellness routine, helping to reduce inflammation, boost immunity, and improve sleep quality.

Ingredients and Measurements:

- 2 cups of almond milk or coconut milk for a dairy-free option
- 1 teaspoon of turmeric powder
- 1/2 teaspoon of ground cinnamon
- 1/4 teaspoon of ground ginger
- A pinch of black pepper (to enhance turmeric absorption)
- 1 tablespoon of honey or maple syrup (adjust to taste)
- Optional: 1 teaspoon of coconut oil or ghee for added creaminess

Preparation:

- In a small saucepan, heat the almond or coconut milk over medium heat until it is warm but not boiling.
- Whisk in the turmeric, cinnamon, ginger, and black pepper until the spices are well integrated and the mixture is smooth.
- Stir in the honey or maple syrup to sweeten and add the coconut oil or ghee if using, whisking until the mixture is frothy and creamy.
- Once the latte is heated through and fully blended, remove it from the heat.

How to Use:

Pour the Turmeric Golden Milk Latte into a mug and enjoy it warm. It's especially beneficial in the evening to unwind before bed or as a soothing start to your day.

Duration:

This latte is best enjoyed fresh but can be stored in the refrigerator for up to 2 days. Reheat gently before serving to preserve the flavors and benefits.

Turmeric Golden Milk Latte is a delightful way to incorporate the healing powers of turmeric into a daily ritual, offering both taste and health benefits in every sip.

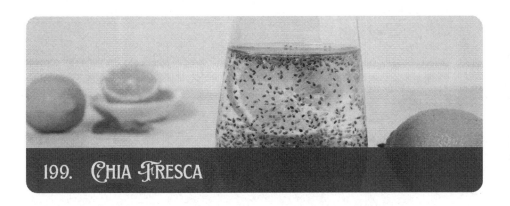

199. CHIA FRESCA

Introduction:

Chia Fresca is a refreshing and hydrating beverage that combines the nutritional power of chia seeds with the invigorating qualities of lemon and water. This simple yet energizing drink is perfect for boosting hydration, providing long-lasting energy, and supporting digestion due to the high fiber content of chia seeds.

Ingredients and Measurements:

- 4 cups of water
- 2 tablespoons of chia seeds
- Juice of 2 lemons
- 2 tablespoons of honey or agave syrup
- Optional: a few slices of cucumber or a sprig of mint for added freshness

Preparation:

🥄 In a large pitcher, add the chia seeds to the water and stir well. Let them sit for about 10 minutes to allow the seeds to swell and form a gel-like consistency.

🥄 Stir again to break up any clumps of seeds, ensuring they are evenly distributed throughout the water.

🥄 Add the lemon juice and honey or agave syrup, mixing until the sweetener is fully dissolved.

🥄 If using, add cucumber slices or mint for extra flavor and let the mixture chill in the refrigerator for at least 30 minutes.

How to Use:

🥄 Serve Chia Fresca chilled as a revitalizing drink throughout the day. It's especially beneficial after workouts or during hot weather to replenish fluids and electrolytes.

Duration:

◎ Chia Fresca can be stored in the refrigerator for up to 24 hours. Stir well before serving, as the chia seeds may settle to the bottom.

Chia Fresca is an excellent choice for anyone looking to enhance their hydration routine with a nutritious and flavorful twist, offering a perfect balance of taste and health benefits.

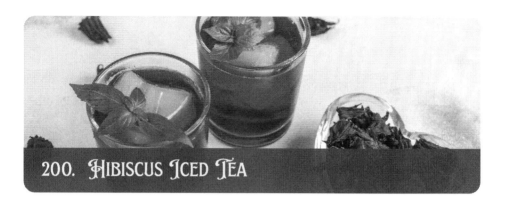

200. Hibiscus Iced Tea

Introduction:

Hibiscus Iced Tea is a vibrant and tangy beverage known for its deep ruby color and refreshing taste. Rich in vitamin C and antioxidants, hibiscus tea helps to lower blood pressure, boost the immune system, and provide a cooling effect on hot days. This drink is not only delicious but also offers numerous health benefits, making it a perfect choice for a revitalizing summer refreshment.

Ingredients and Measurements:

- 4 cups of water
- 1/2 cup of dried hibiscus flowers
- 1/4 cup of honey or sugar (adjust to taste)
- Juice of 1 lime

- Optional: mint leaves or a slice of orange for garnish

Preparation:

☞ In a medium saucepan, bring the water to a boil.

☞ Once boiling, remove from heat and add the dried hibiscus flowers. Cover and let steep for 15-20 minutes, allowing the flowers to infuse the water with their flavor and color.

☞ Strain the tea into a large pitcher, discarding the hibiscus flowers.

☞ While the tea is still warm, stir in the honey or sugar until it dissolves completely.

☞ Add the lime juice and stir to combine.

☞ Refrigerate until chilled, at least 1 hour.

How to Use:

⌕ Serve the Hibiscus Iced Tea over ice, garnished with mint leaves or a slice of orange for an extra touch of elegance and flavor. It's ideal for sipping on warm days or serving at gatherings as a healthy and delightful alternative to sugary drinks.

Duration:

⊘ This iced tea can be kept in the refrigerator for up to 5 days. Ensure it is stored in an airtight container to maintain its freshness and vibrant taste.

Hibiscus Iced Tea is an excellent way to stay hydrated and enjoy the natural benefits of hibiscus, offering a thirst-quenching experience with every sip.

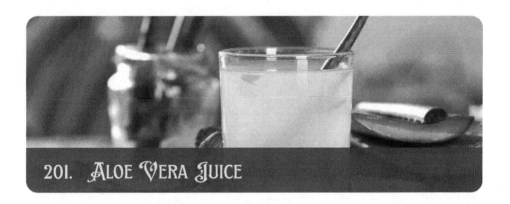

201. ALOE VERA JUICE

Introduction:

Aloe Vera Juice is a soothing and healing beverage known for its extensive health benefits, particularly for the skin and digestive system. Extracted from the flesh of the aloe vera plant, this juice is rich in vitamins, minerals, and antioxidants, making it an excellent choice for enhancing hydration, supporting digestive health, and promoting clear, healthy skin.

Ingredients and Measurements:

- 1 cup of fresh aloe vera gel (from approximately 2 large aloe vera leaves)

- 2 cups of water or coconut water

- Juice of 1 lemon

- 1 tablespoon of honey or agave syrup (optional, for sweetness)

Preparation:

🖙 Carefully slice the aloe vera leaves lengthwise and use a spoon to scoop out the clear gel. Be sure to avoid the yellow latex layer just beneath the skin as it can be irritating.

🖙 In a blender, combine the aloe vera gel, water or coconut water, and lemon juice. Blend until the mixture is smooth.

- Strain the juice through a fine-mesh sieve or cheesecloth to remove any remaining solids.
- Stir in the honey or agave syrup if you prefer a sweeter taste and mix well.
- Chill the juice in the refrigerator or serve immediately over ice for a refreshing drink.

How to Use:

- Drink a small glass of Aloe Vera Juice daily, especially in the morning or before meals, to benefit from its digestive and skin-enhancing properties. It can also be used as a base for smoothies or mixed with other juices for added flavor and nutrients.

Duration:

- Aloe Vera Juice can be stored in the refrigerator in an airtight container for up to 5 days. Shake well before each use to ensure the ingredients are well combined.

Aloe Vera Juice is a versatile and beneficial drink that helps maintain optimal health and vitality, providing a gentle, natural way to support your body's needs.

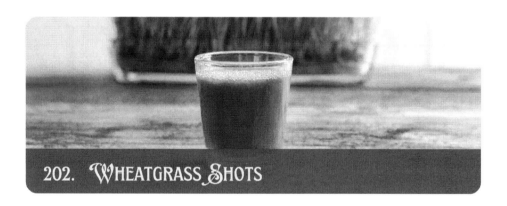

202. WHEATGRASS SHOTS

Introduction:

Wheatgrass Shots are a concentrated source of nutrients, packed with chlorophyll, vitamins, minerals, and enzymes. These powerful little drinks are known for their ability to detoxify the body, boost energy levels, and enhance overall health. Just a small shot can have a significant impact, making it a popular choice for those looking to optimize their wellness routines.

Ingredients and Measurements:

- 1/2 cup of fresh wheatgrass or 1 tablespoon of wheatgrass powder
- 1/2 cup of water (if using wheatgrass powder)

- Optional: a slice of lemon or a small piece of ginger for added flavor

Preparation:

- If using fresh wheatgrass, rinse it thoroughly under cold water. For wheatgrass powder, skip to step 2.

- Using a juicer, juice the fresh wheatgrass. If using wheatgrass powder, mix it with the water until fully dissolved.

- If desired, add a slice of lemon or a small piece of ginger to the juicer to enhance the flavor of the shot.

- Pour the wheatgrass juice into a shot glass or small container.

How to Use:

Take a wheatgrass shot on an empty stomach, preferably in the morning, to maximize its detoxifying and energizing effects. It can be a daily addition to your health regimen or used periodically for a nutrient boost.

Duration:

Fresh wheatgrass juice is best consumed immediately after juicing to preserve its nutritional content. If you must store it, keep it in an airtight container in the refrigerator for no more than 24 hours.

Wheatgrass Shots provide a quick and efficient way to absorb essential nutrients, offering a boost to your health with minimal effort and maximum benefit.

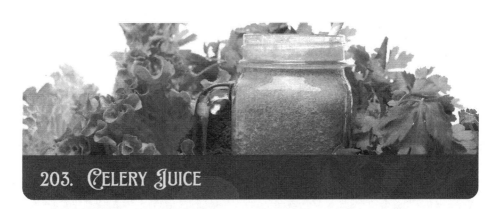

203. CELERY JUICE

Introduction:

Celery Juice has gained popularity for its remarkable health benefits, particularly in supporting digestive health and reducing inflammation. Rich in vitamins, minerals, and electrolytes, this simple green juice helps detoxify the liver, promote hydration, and improve skin health, making it a staple in many wellness routines.

Ingredients and Measurements:

- 1 bunch of fresh celery, approximately 10-12 stalks
- Optional: a squeeze of lemon or lime for added flavor

Preparation:

🍴 Thoroughly wash the celery stalks to remove any dirt or pesticides.

🍴 Chop the celery into manageable pieces that will fit into your juicer.

🍴 Juice the celery in a juicer to extract the liquid. For those without a juicer, blend the chopped celery with a little water in a high-speed blender, then strain through a fine-mesh sieve or nut milk bag to separate the pulp from the juice.

🍴 If desired, enhance the flavor with a squeeze of lemon or lime.

🍴 Pour the celery juice into a glass and serve immediately for the best taste and nutrient content.

How to Use:

🥄 Drink a glass of celery juice first thing in the morning on an empty stomach to maximize its health benefits, especially for digestive support and detoxification.

Duration:

🕐 Celery juice is most beneficial when fresh. However, it can be stored in an airtight container in the refrigerator for up to 24 hours. Shake well before drinking, as separation may occur.

Celery Juice is a simple yet powerful way to support your health, offering a natural boost to various body systems with its hydrating and healing properties.

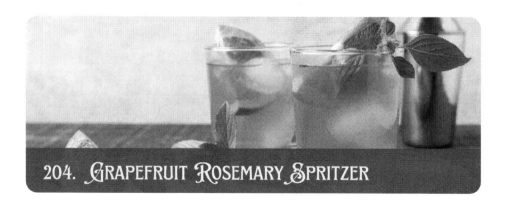

204. GRAPEFRUIT ROSEMARY SPRITZER

Introduction:

Grapefruit Rosemary Spritzer is a refreshing and invigorating beverage that combines the tangy taste of grapefruit with the aromatic essence of rosemary. This drink is not only delicious but also loaded with antioxidants and vitamin C, making it a fantastic choice for boosting immunity, enhancing metabolism, and providing a light, flavorful alternative to sugary sodas.

Ingredients and Measurements:

- 2 cups of fresh grapefruit juice
- 1 cup of sparkling water or club soda
- 2 tablespoons of honey or agave syrup
- A few sprigs of fresh rosemary
- Ice cubes
- Optional: slices of grapefruit or sprigs of rosemary for garnish

Preparation:

☕ In a small saucepan, combine the honey or agave syrup with a sprig of rosemary and heat gently until the sweetener is dissolved and the mixture is infused with rosemary flavor. Remove from heat and let cool.

☕ In a large pitcher, mix the fresh grapefruit juice with the rosemary-infused syrup, stirring well to combine.

☕ Add the sparkling water or club soda and stir gently to maintain the fizz.

☕ Fill glasses with ice cubes and pour the spritzer over the ice.

☕ Garnish with additional slices of grapefruit and a sprig of rosemary for an elegant touch.

How to Use:

🥄 Serve the Grapefruit Rosemary Spritzer chilled as a delightful drink to accompany meals or as a standalone refreshment on warm days or at festive gatherings.

Duration:

🕐 This spritzer is best enjoyed fresh but can be stored in the refrigerator for up to 2 days. Keep it in a sealed container to preserve the carbonation and flavors.

Grapefruit Rosemary Spritzer is a perfect blend of zest and herb, offering a sophisticated twist on traditional refreshments and promoting health with every sip.

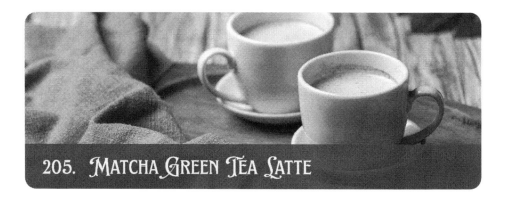

205. Matcha Green Tea Latte

Introduction:

Matcha Green Tea Latte is a creamy and soothing beverage that combines the rich, earthy flavors of matcha with the smooth texture of steamed milk. This drink is packed with antioxidants, particularly EGCG, which boosts metabolism and enhances mood. Its vibrant green color and delicate grassy taste make it a favorite among tea lovers and health enthusiasts alike.

Ingredients and Measurements:

- 1 teaspoon of high-quality matcha powder
- 1/4 cup of hot water (not boiling, about 175°F)
- 3/4 cup of milk (dairy or any plant-based alternative like almond, oat, or soy milk)
- 1 tablespoon of honey or maple syrup (optional, for sweetness)
- Optional: a sprinkle of matcha powder for garnish

Preparation:

- Sift the matcha powder into a bowl or cup to remove any lumps, ensuring a smooth texture.
- Add the hot water to the matcha powder and whisk vigorously in a zigzag motion until the tea is frothy and well mixed.
- Heat the milk in a saucepan or use a milk frother to heat and froth the milk until it's hot and foamy.
- Pour the frothy milk over the matcha mixture, gently stirring to combine.
- Sweeten with honey or maple syrup if desired and stir until dissolved.
- Sprinkle a little matcha powder on top for a decorative touch.

How to Use:

- Enjoy a Matcha Green Tea Latte as a morning beverage or a midday pick-me-up. Its combination of caffeine and L-theanine provides sustained energy without the jitters often associated with coffee.

Duration:

🕐 This latte is best enjoyed immediately after preparation to experience the full flavor and benefits of the matcha. If needed, it can be stored in the refrigerator for a day, but stir well before serving to blend the layers.

Matcha Green Tea Latte is a delightful and healthful choice, offering a unique flavor experience along with numerous wellness benefits.

PART 10

MINDFULNESS AND STRESS MANAGEMENT

(206-220)

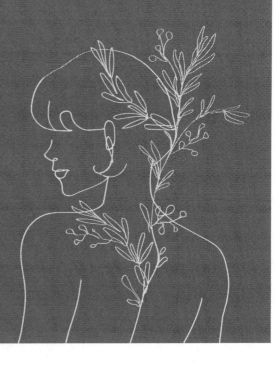

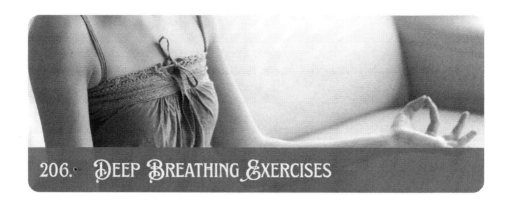

Introduction:

Deep Breathing Exercises are a foundational technique in stress management and mindfulness practices. These exercises involve consciously slowing and deepening your breath to stimulate the body's relaxation response. By focusing on full, deep breaths, you can reduce anxiety, lower blood pressure, and improve overall mental clarity and emotional balance.

Basic Technique and Information:

Deep breathing works by activating the parasympathetic nervous system, which helps counteract the body's stress response. The most common form is diaphragmatic breathing, where you breathe deeply into the lungs, allowing the diaphragm to expand and the abdomen to rise, rather than just filling the upper chest.

Steps to Practice Deep Breathing Exercises:

- **Find a Comfortable Position:** Sit or lie down in a quiet place where you won't be disturbed. Keep your back straight and hands relaxed in your lap or on your thighs.

- **Breathe In Slowly:** Inhale slowly through your nose, counting to four. Feel the air move into your nostrils, down your throat, filling your lungs and expanding your abdomen.

- **Hold Your Breath:** Hold the breath for a count of four. This pause can help increase the absorption of oxygen.

- **Exhale Gradually:** Exhale completely through your mouth or nose, counting to four. As you breathe out, imagine releasing all the stress and tension from your body.

- **Repeat:** Continue this pattern for several minutes, focusing on the rhythm and depth of your breath.

Tips for Enhancing the Practice:

- 💡 Use a quiet and comfortable setting to minimize distractions.
- 💡 Combine with visualization, imagining a peaceful scene or a wave of relaxation flowing over your body as you breathe.
- 💡 Practice regularly, ideally at the same time each day, to cultivate a habit that supports stress reduction and mindfulness.

Benefits:

Regular practice of deep breathing exercises can lead to improved concentration, reduced anxiety, better sleep quality, and a stronger immune response. These exercises are a simple, yet powerful tool to incorporate into daily life for enhancing mental and physical well-being.

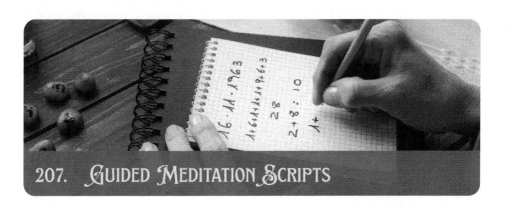

207. GUIDED MEDITATION SCRIPTS

Introduction:

Guided Meditation Scripts are structured narratives or instructions designed to facilitate a focused and calming meditation experience. These scripts guide individuals through a series of mental images or suggestions that enhance relaxation, reduce stress, and promote a sense of peace and well-being. By directing attention and encouraging a deep connection to one's thoughts and feelings, guided meditations help foster a state of mindfulness and presence.

Basic Technique and Information:

Guided meditation often involves a narrator leading the listener through various stages of relaxation and visualization. The process aims to quiet the mind and bring awareness to the present moment, which can be especially helpful for beginners or those struggling with scattered thoughts.

Steps to Practice Using Guided Meditation Scripts:

- **Choose a Quiet Place:** Find a comfortable and quiet space where you won't be interrupted. This could be a seated position on a chair or cushion, or lying down in a relaxed posture.

- **Begin with Deep Breathing:** Start with a few deep breaths to center yourself and prepare your mind and body for meditation.

- **Follow the Script:** Listen to or read the script slowly. If reading, you may want to record yourself in advance or use a pre-recorded audio version.

- **Engage with Visualization:** The script may include visualizing peaceful scenes, focusing on breathing, or noticing sensations in the body. Engage fully with these images or instructions as they are presented.

- **Allow the Experience:** Let go of judgment or expectation. If your mind wanders, gently guide it back to the script's words or your breath.

Example of a Guided Meditation Script:

Imagine you are walking along a quiet beach. The sun is setting, casting a warm, golden glow over the sand and sea. As you walk, notice the feel of the sand beneath your feet and the rhythmic sound of the waves. With each step, breathe in the fresh, salty air, and breathe out any tension or worry. Allow a sense of peace to wash over you, just like the waves on the shore. Continue walking and breathing in this peaceful setting until you feel a deep sense of calm throughout your body and mind.

Tips for Enhancing the Practice:

- Use soothing background music or natural sounds like ocean waves to deepen the relaxation experience.

- Practice regularly, ideally at a set time each day, to establish a routine that strengthens mindfulness and stress management.

- Adjust scripts to fit your needs or mood, focusing on scenarios or themes that resonate with you personally.

Benefits:

Guided meditation scripts can significantly reduce stress, improve focus, lower anxiety levels, and enhance emotional resilience. By guiding the mind through structured narratives or imagery, these meditations help develop a deeper connection to the inner self and a more balanced perspective on life's challenges.

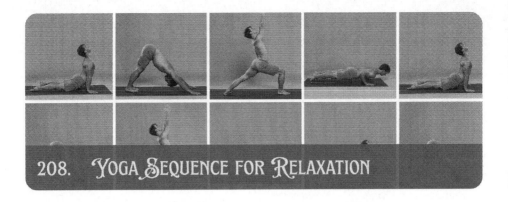

208. Yoga Sequence for Relaxation

Introduction:

A Yoga Sequence for Relaxation is designed to release tension, calm the mind, and bring balance to the body. Through a series of gentle poses and mindful breathing, this sequence helps to alleviate stress, improve flexibility, and foster a deeper sense of peace. Ideal for winding down at the end of the day or as a soothing practice anytime, these poses are accessible to practitioners of all levels.

Basic Technique and Information:

The focus of this yoga sequence is on slow movements, deep breathing, and poses that promote relaxation and reduce muscle tension. The sequence typically includes a mix of seated, lying, and gentle standing poses.

Steps to Practice Yoga Sequence for Relaxation:

- **Child's Pose (Balasana):** Begin on your hands and knees. Sit back on your heels, stretch your arms forward on the mat, and rest your forehead on the ground. Breathe deeply for

1-2 minutes to ground yourself and start the relaxation process.

- **Cat-Cow Pose (Marjaryasana-Bitilasana):** Come to a tabletop position with your wrists under your shoulders and your knees under your hips. Inhale, drop your belly towards the mat, lift your chin and chest, and gaze up (Cow Pose). Exhale, draw your belly to your spine, round your back toward the ceiling, and tuck your chin toward your chest (Cat Pose). Repeat for 5-10 breaths to warm up the spine.

- **Seated Forward Bend (Paschimottanasana):** Sit on the mat with your legs extended in front of you. Inhale and lengthen your spine. As you exhale, hinge at the hips and fold forward over your legs. Hold onto your shins, ankles, or feet, and breathe deeply for 1-2 minutes, releasing tension in your back and hamstrings.

- **Supine Twist (Supta Matsyendrasana):** Lie on your back and bring your knees to your chest. Extend your arms to the sides in a T position. Gently drop your knees to the left, turning your head to the right. Hold for 1-2 minutes, then switch sides. This pose helps relax the spine and improve digestion.

- **Legs-Up-the-Wall Pose (Viparita Karani):** Sit close to a wall and lie back, extending your legs up the wall. Let your arms rest by your sides or on your belly. Stay in this pose for 5-10 minutes, allowing gravity to help with circulation and relaxation.

- **Corpse Pose (Savasana):** Conclude the sequence by lying flat on your back, arms at your sides with palms facing up, and legs slightly apart. Close your eyes and breathe naturally, allowing your body to absorb the benefits of the practice for 5-10 minutes.

Tips for Enhancing the Practice:

- ☀ Use props like cushions, blankets, or yoga blocks for added comfort and support in each pose.

- ☀ Focus on deep, even breaths throughout the sequence to enhance the calming effect.

Benefits:

This yoga sequence for relaxation helps reduce physical and mental stress, promotes better sleep, and improves overall well-being. By integrating gentle movement and mindful breathing, you can achieve a state of deep relaxation and rejuvenation.

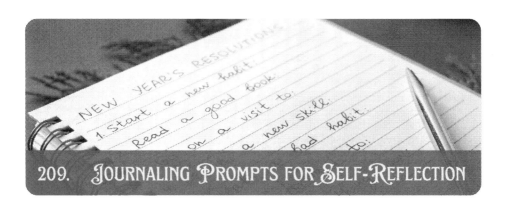

209. JOURNALING PROMPTS FOR SELF-REFLECTION

Introduction:

Journaling for self-reflection is a powerful tool to explore thoughts, emotions, and experiences, leading to deeper self-awareness and personal growth. By responding to targeted prompts, individuals can uncover hidden feelings, clarify their values, and set meaningful goals. This practice encourages introspection and mindfulness, helping to process life's complexities and enhance emotional well-being.

Basic Technique and Information:

To engage in self-reflective journaling, choose a quiet and comfortable space where you can write without interruptions. Use a notebook or digital journal dedicated to this purpose, ensuring privacy and consistency. Begin with a prompt that resonates with you, and write freely without worrying about grammar or structure.

Journaling Prompts to Encourage Self-Reflection:

- What are three things I am grateful for today, and why? Reflecting on gratitude helps shift focus from challenges to blessings, enhancing positivity and resilience.

- What are my biggest strengths, and how did I use them recently? Identifying and appreciating your strengths fosters confidence and encourages their use in daily life.

- What lesson did I learn from a recent challenge or mistake? This prompt helps transform difficulties into opportunities for growth and learning.

- How do I feel right now, and what might be influencing my emotions? Understanding the source of emotions can lead to better emotional regulation and decision-making.

- What are my short-term and long-term goals, and what steps can I take to achieve them? Setting and revisiting goals keeps you focused and motivated.

- In what ways have I changed over the past year, and how do I feel about these changes? Reflecting on personal evolution helps appreciate growth and adapt to ongoing changes.

- When do I feel most at peace, and how can I incorporate more of that into my life? Recognizing sources of peace supports stress management and overall well-being.

- What does success mean to me, and how does my definition align with my current path? Clarifying your vision of success ensures alignment with your actions and values.

- How do I practice self-care, and what new methods can I try? Evaluating and expanding self-care routines boosts mental and physical health.

- What am I avoiding, and what would happen if I faced it? Confronting avoidance can break down barriers to personal growth and happiness.

Tips for Enhancing the Practice:

- Set a regular time for journaling to establish a routine.

- Combine journaling with other mindfulness practices like meditation or deep breathing for enhanced benefits.

- Use your journal as a judgment-free zone where honesty and vulnerability are encouraged.

Benefits:

Journaling for self-reflection promotes clarity, reduces stress, and supports emotional healing. It provides a private space to explore personal narratives, identify patterns, and make conscious changes, leading to increased self-awareness and life satisfaction.

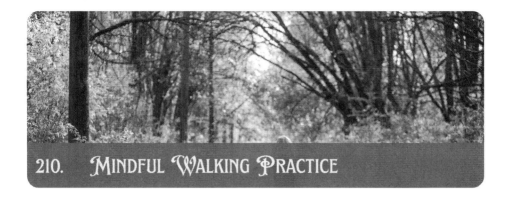

210.   MINDFUL WALKING PRACTICE

Introduction:

Mindful Walking Practice is a form of meditation in motion that combines the physical activity of walking with mindfulness to create a calming, centering experience. This practice helps to ground you in the present moment, reducing stress and enhancing mental clarity by focusing on the sensations of walking and the environment around you.

Basic Technique and Information:

Mindful walking involves paying close attention to the act of walking, noticing each step, the movement of your body, and the sensations you feel as you move. It can be done anywhere, from a quiet path in nature to a busy urban sidewalk, as long as you can maintain a focus on your movements and surroundings.

Steps to Practice Mindful Walking:

- **Start with Intention:** Before you begin walking, take a moment to set an intention for your walk. This could

be to relax, clear your mind, or simply observe the world around you.

- **Focus on Your Breath:** Take a few deep breaths to center yourself. Notice the rhythm of your breathing and let it guide you into a relaxed state.

- **Walk at a Natural Pace:** Begin walking at a comfortable pace. It's not about speed but about being present with each step. Feel your feet touching the ground, the swing of your arms, and the movement of your legs.

- **Engage Your Senses:** As you walk, bring your attention to what you can see, hear, smell, and feel. Notice the colors around you, the sounds of nature or the city, the temperature of the air, and the textures under your feet.

- **Acknowledge Distractions:** When your mind wanders, gently acknowledge the distraction and then bring your focus back to the sensations of walking and your immediate surroundings.

- **Use a Mantra or Count Steps:** To help maintain focus, you might silently repeat a calming word or phrase with each step, or simply count your steps up to ten and then start over.

Tips for Enhancing the Practice:

- 💡 Choose a safe and pleasant route where you can walk without too many interruptions.

- 💡 Practice regularly, ideally at the same time each day, to establish a routine.

- 💡 Combine mindful walking with other mindfulness practices or use it as a warm-up or cool-down for more intense physical activity.

Benefits:

Mindful walking offers a way to integrate mindfulness into daily life, promoting physical health while also reducing anxiety, improving mood, and increasing overall mental well-being. This practice encourages a deeper connection with the environment and a greater appreciation for the simple act of moving through space.

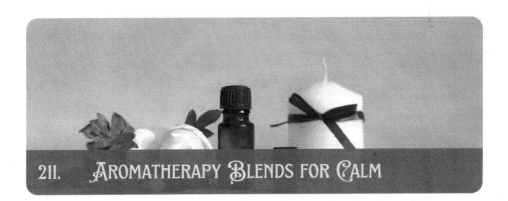

211. AROMATHERAPY BLENDS FOR CALM

Introduction:

Aromatherapy blends for calm utilize essential oils to create a soothing atmosphere that promotes relaxation, reduces stress, and enhances emotional well-being. By combining specific oils known for their calming properties, these blends can be used in diffusers, added to bathwater, or applied topically with a carrier oil to help soothe the mind and body.

Basic Technique and Information:

To create effective aromatherapy blends, it's important to understand the properties of each essential oil and how they work together. For relaxation and stress relief, oils with sedative, antianxiety, and mood-balancing effects are most beneficial. Using these oils in a diffuser or as part of a massage oil can help maximize their calming effects.

Essential Oils and Their Calming Properties:

- **Lavender:** Known for its soothing and sedative properties, lavender oil is a staple in stress reduction and sleep improvement.

- **Chamomile:** With its gentle floral scent, chamomile oil is excellent for easing anxiety and promoting a peaceful state.

- **Bergamot:** A citrus oil that helps reduce stress and anxiety while uplifting mood.

- **Ylang Ylang:** Known for balancing emotions and reducing tension and stress.

- **Frankincense:** Offers deep relaxation and helps alleviate anxiety and chronic stress.

Steps to Create Aromatherapy Blends for Calm:

- **Lavender and Chamomile Blend:** Mix 3 drops of lavender oil with 2 drops of chamomile oil in your diffuser to create a soothing environment, ideal for unwinding before bed or during stressful times.

- **Citrus and Floral Blend:** Combine 2 drops of bergamot oil with 2 drops of ylang ylang and 1 drop of lavender

oil in a diffuser to uplift and soothe the mood simultaneously.

- **Deep Relaxation Blend:** Blend 2 drops of frankincense oil with 2 drops of lavender and 1 drop of chamomile oil for a deeply relaxing and meditative atmosphere.

- **Topical Application:** For a calming massage oil, dilute 5 drops of your chosen blend in 1 ounce of a carrier oil like sweet almond or jojoba. Gently massage onto the neck, shoulders, and temples.

Tips for Enhancing the Practice:

- Always dilute essential oils with a carrier oil before applying them to the skin to avoid irritation.

- Use a diffuser to disperse the oils evenly in your environment for consistent benefits.

- Store essential oils and blends in dark, cool places to preserve their therapeutic properties.

Benefits:

Aromatherapy blends for calm can significantly reduce stress, improve sleep quality, and foster a sense of peace and relaxation. By incorporating these blends into your daily routine, you can create a more balanced and tranquil environment, enhancing both mental and physical well-being.

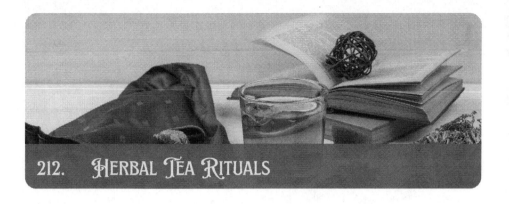

212. Herbal Tea Rituals

Introduction:

Herbal tea rituals are a cherished practice for soothing the mind, nourishing the body, and creating moments of peace in daily life. These rituals involve the preparation and consumption of herbal teas made from plants known for their therapeutic properties. Engaging in this practice can help reduce stress, improve sleep, and foster a deep sense of mindfulness and connection to the natural world.

Basic Technique and Information:

To create a meaningful herbal tea ritual, choose herbs that align with your current needs, whether for relaxation, detoxification, or immune support. The process of brewing the tea and then sitting quietly to enjoy it becomes a meditative practice that encourages slowing down and tuning into your senses.

Herbs Commonly Used in Tea Rituals and Their Benefits:

- **Chamomile:** Promotes relaxation and sleep, and is excellent for calming an upset stomach.

- **Peppermint:** Eases digestive troubles and refreshes the mind, helping to clear mental fog.

- **Lavender:** Known for its stress-relieving properties and its ability to improve sleep quality.

- **Lemon Balm:** Reduces anxiety and improves mood with its calming, lemon-scented leaves.

- **Ginger:** Stimulates digestion, relieves nausea, and boosts immunity with its warming properties.

Steps to Create a Herbal Tea Ritual:

- **Select Your Herbs:** Choose one or a combination of herbs based on your needs. Loose-leaf herbs often provide a richer flavor and more potent benefits than bagged tea.

- **Prepare the Tea:** Boil water and pour it over the herbs, allowing them to steep for 5-10 minutes, depending on the desired strength. Cover the cup or pot to keep the essential oils and flavors intact.

- **Create a Calm Environment:** While the tea steeps, prepare a quiet space where you can sit and enjoy your tea without distractions. This might involve a comfortable chair, soft lighting, and perhaps some soothing music or natural sounds.

- **Mindfully Enjoy the Tea:** Sit with your tea and take a moment to appreciate its aroma before taking the first sip. Notice the taste and feel of the tea as you slowly drink it, allowing its warmth and flavors to soothe you.

- **Reflect and Relax:** Use the time while enjoying your tea to reflect on your day, journal, or simply sit in quiet contemplation. This is a time to connect with yourself and relax deeply.

Tips for Enhancing the Practice:

- Experiment with blending different herbs to create your unique tea blend.

- Use a special cup or teapot reserved for this ritual to make it feel more significant and intentional.

- Incorporate breathing exercises or light stretching before or after your tea time to enhance the calming effect.

Benefits:

Engaging in herbal tea rituals can help reduce stress, support digestion, improve sleep, and elevate your overall sense of well-being. This practice encourages mindfulness and provides a structured way to incorporate self-care into your daily routine, enhancing your connection to nature and your inner self.

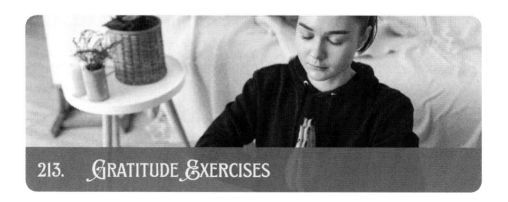

213.   GRATITUDE EXERCISES

Introduction:

Gratitude exercises are transformative practices that focus on appreciating life's blessings, with a special emphasis on expressing thanks to God as the source of all goodness. These exercises foster a deep sense of gratitude for both the significant and the everyday gifts in life, enhancing well-being, deepening faith, and strengthening relationships. By prioritizing thankfulness to God, individuals can cultivate a more profound connection with their spiritual life while experiencing increased overall happiness and reduced stress.

Basic Technique and Information:

Incorporating gratitude to God into these exercises involves consciously acknowledging His role in all aspects of life. This practice can be done through prayer, meditation, journaling, or thoughtful reflection, making it a holistic approach to nurturing one's spiritual and emotional health.

Steps to Practice Gratitude Exercises:

- **Daily Devotion and Prayer:** Start or end your day with prayer, expressing gratitude directly to God for His blessings, guidance, and presence in your life. Focus on specific aspects where you've seen His hand at work, from significant life events to the simple joy of a peaceful moment.

- **Gratitude Journaling:** In a dedicated journal, write down three to five things each day for which you are thankful, beginning with your gratitude towards God. This helps to reinforce the idea that every good thing comes from Him and encourages a deeper appreciation for His continual blessings.

- **Gratitude Walks:** As you walk, mentally or aloud, give thanks to God for the beauty and order of the natural world, the health to walk, and the

senses to enjoy your surroundings. Use this time to connect with God through His creation, acknowledging His creativity and care.

- **Thank You Notes to God:** Write notes or prayers of thanks to God, detailing the ways He has impacted your life. This can be a deeply personal way to reflect on and celebrate the relationship you have with Him.

- **Sharing Gratitude with Others:** Share your gratitude with family and friends, making it clear that your thankfulness begins with God. This not only strengthens your faith but also encourages others to recognize and appreciate God's role in their lives.

Tips for Enhancing the Practice:

- Be specific in your gratitude to deepen the connection and make your thanks more meaningful.

- Combine your gratitude practice with Bible study or other spiritual readings to enrich your understanding and appreciation of God's work in your life.

- Encourage a communal gratitude practice within your family or faith community to build a collective sense of thankfulness and unity.

Benefits:

Regularly practicing gratitude with a focus on God leads to a more resilient spirit, deeper spiritual connections, and a more joyful, contented life. This approach not only improves mental and emotional health but also strengthens one's faith and trust in God, providing a steady anchor in times of uncertainty and change.

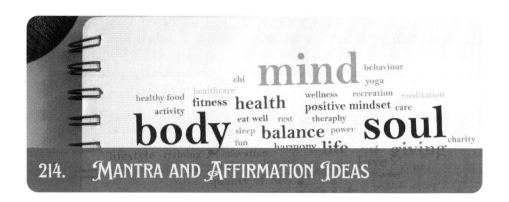

Introduction:

Mantras and affirmations are potent tools designed to reinforce positive thinking, strengthen self-belief, and align thoughts and actions with desired outcomes. These phrases, when repeated regularly, help to shift the mind away from negative self-talk and foster confidence and clarity. By focusing on these positive statements, individuals can improve mental and emotional resilience.

Basic Technique and Information:

Mantras, often seen as sacred sounds or phrases, and affirmations, which are positive statements, are used to support personal growth and emotional well-being. Both are effective in promoting mindfulness and spiritual reflection, guiding individuals towards a balanced and optimistic state of mind.

Steps to Practice Using Mantras and Affirmations:

- **Choose Your Mantras or Affirmations:** Select phrases that

echo your values and the virtues you aim to embody. Ensure they are affirmative, present tense, and clearly reflect your aspirations or areas of personal development.

- **Incorporate Them into Your Routine:** Make time each day to repeat your chosen phrases, whether during quiet reflection, prayer times, or as part of your morning or evening rituals.

- **Use Them Mindfully:** Focus on the meaning behind each mantra or affirmation. Visualize achieving the state or belief it represents, and immerse yourself in the emotions connected to this visualization.

- **Write Them Down:** Maintain a journal or use notes where you write your mantras or affirmations regularly. Seeing them in writing can help solidify their meaning and impact in your life.

Mantra and Affirmation Ideas:

- **For Peace and Calm:** "In the quiet of this moment, I find peace and serenity within myself."

- **For Confidence:** "I am endowed with strength and wisdom to overcome all challenges."

- **For Faith and Trust:** "I trust in the divine plan, knowing all things unfold for my highest good."

- **For Gratitude:** "I am filled with deep gratitude for the blessings that enrich my life each day."

- **For Healing:** "With every breath, divine healing restores my body and soul."

- **For Self-Love:** "I am a creation of great worth, deserving of respect and kindness."

- **For Overcoming Fear:** "I release all fear, embracing courage and clarity guided by faith."

- **For Positivity:** "I choose positivity and light, guided by the wisdom of my heart."

Tips for Enhancing the Practice:

- Pair your mantras or affirmations with deep, mindful breathing or moments of silence to enhance their effects.

- Record these phrases and listen to them during times of reflection or when seeking inner peace.

- Encourage a supportive community or circle where these practices are shared and reinforced.

Benefits:

Using mantras and affirmations regularly transforms your mindset, leading to improved emotional stability, enhanced focus, and a more optimistic life perspective. These practices build resilience, foster personal growth, and help maintain a strong connection to spiritual and ethical values.

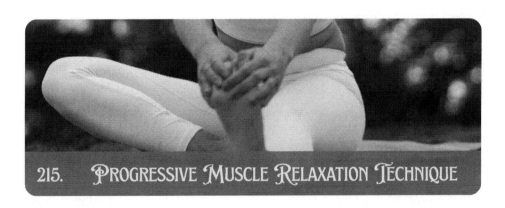

215. PROGRESSIVE MUSCLE RELAXATION TECHNIQUE

Introduction:

Progressive Muscle Relaxation Technique is a systematic method used to alleviate stress and reduce tension in the body. By sequentially tensing and then relaxing different muscle groups, this practice promotes a deep sense of relaxation, helps in managing anxiety, and improves sleep quality. It's a practical approach to mindfulness that encourages bodily awareness and the release of physical stress.

Basic Technique and Information:

This technique involves tightening each muscle group for a short period, then releasing the tension and noticing the contrast between tension and relaxation. This process not only relaxes the muscles but also helps in quieting the mind and easing emotional stress.

Steps to Practice Progressive Muscle Relaxation:

- **Find a Quiet Place:** Choose a comfortable, quiet spot where you can sit or lie down without interruptions. Ensure you won't be disturbed for the duration of the exercise.

- **Start with Deep Breathing:** Take a few deep breaths to initiate a state of relaxation. Inhale slowly through your nose, hold for a few seconds, and then exhale through your mouth.

- **Tense and Relax Muscle Groups:** Begin with your feet and work your way up to your face. For each muscle group, follow these steps:

- Tense the muscles as you inhale for about 5 seconds. Feel the tension but avoid straining.

- Exhale and release the tension in the muscles, noticing the feeling of relaxation. Focus on the difference between tension and relaxation.

- Pause for 10-15 seconds before moving to the next muscle group.

- **Follow a Systematic Order:** Progress through muscle groups in the following order:

- Feet (toes and soles)

- Calves

- Thighs

- Hips and buttocks

- Abdomen

- Chest

- Back (lower and upper)

- Arms (hands, forearms, upper arms)

- Shoulders and neck

- Face (jaw, eyes, forehead)

- **Reflect on the Relaxation:** After completing all muscle groups, take a moment to lie or sit quietly. Breathe deeply and enjoy the sense of relaxation throughout your body.

Tips for Enhancing the Practice:

- Practice regularly, ideally at the same time each day, to establish a routine and enhance the benefits.

- Combine this technique with other relaxation methods like soft background music or natural sounds for a deeper experience.

- Be gentle and listen to your body to avoid over-tensing the muscles, especially if you have any existing injuries or pain.

Benefits:

The Progressive Muscle Relaxation Technique effectively reduces physical tension, lowers stress and anxiety levels, and improves overall mental clarity and emotional balance. Regular practice can lead to better sleep, reduced pain, and a greater sense of calm and well-being.

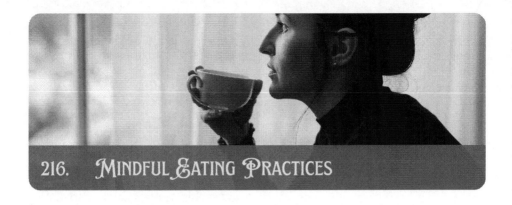

Introduction:

Mindful eating is a technique that encourages being fully attentive to the food and drink you consume, observing how it affects your body and mind at every stage. This practice helps to enhance the dining experience, improve digestion, and promote a healthier relationship with food by slowing down, appreciating the flavors, and recognizing hunger and fullness cues.

Basic Technique and Information:

Mindful eating involves engaging all your senses to fully experience your meal. By focusing on the taste, texture, and aroma of food, you can foster a deeper appreciation for what you eat and make more conscious choices about portions and types of food.

Steps to Practice Mindful Eating:

- **Prepare Your Meal Thoughtfully:** Start by choosing foods that are nourishing and prepared in a way that will satisfy both your body and palate. Consider the source and quality of your ingredients.

- **Set a Calm Environment:** Create a distraction-free dining area. Turn off electronic devices, and ensure the space is clean and inviting. This helps you focus solely on the eating experience.

- **Engage All Senses:** Before eating, take a moment to look at your food and appreciate its colors and presentation. Inhale the aroma and anticipate the flavors. This prepares your mind and body for digestion.

- **Eat Slowly:** Take small bites and chew thoroughly. This not only aids in digestion but also allows you to truly taste and enjoy each bite. Put down your utensils between bites to pace yourself.

- **Notice Your Body's Signals:** Pay attention to hunger and fullness cues. Mindful eating involves recognizing when you are no longer hungry and stopping before you feel overly full.

- **Reflect on Your Experience:** After the meal, take a few moments to reflect on how the food made you feel, the level of satisfaction, and any changes in your physical or emotional state.

Tips for Enhancing the Practice:

- 💡 Use smaller plates to help control portion sizes naturally.
- 💡 Incorporate a variety of textures and flavors to keep your meals interesting and engaging.

- 💡 Practice gratitude before eating, considering the effort and resources that went into preparing your meal.

Benefits:

Mindful eating can transform your relationship with food, leading to improved digestion, reduced overeating, and enhanced satisfaction with meals. It promotes a healthier approach to food that can lead to better weight management and a greater sense of well-being.

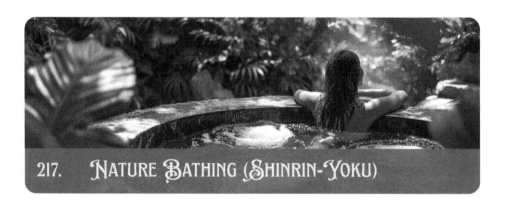

217. NATURE BATHING (SHINRIN-YOKU)

Introduction:

Nature Bathing, also known as Shinrin-Yoku, is a Japanese practice that involves immersing oneself in the natural environment to promote healing and wellness. The term translates to "forest bathing" and focuses on absorbing the atmosphere of the forest or any natural setting through all the senses. This practice is known for reducing stress, enhancing mood, boosting the immune system, and improving overall well-being.

Basic Technique and Information:

Shinrin-Yoku doesn't involve actual bathing; instead, it means taking in the forest atmosphere through mindful walking and observation. The practice encourages a deep connection with nature by engaging sight, smell, hearing, taste, and touch.

Steps to Practice Nature Bathing:

- **Choose a Natural Setting:** Select a forest, park, or natural area that feels safe and inviting. The place should be conducive to walking slowly and comfortably.

- **Leave Distractions Behind:** Turn off your phone or any electronic devices to ensure a fully immersive experience. The goal is to disconnect from daily stresses and reconnect with nature.

- **Engage Your Senses:** As you walk, take the time to observe your surroundings with intention. Notice the colors of the leaves, the patterns of light and shadow, and the texture of the bark. Listen to the sounds of birds, wind, or water. Inhale deeply to take in the scents of the forest, like the fresh, earthy smell of soil or the crisp scent of leaves.

- **Walk Slowly:** Shinrin-Yoku is not about covering distance or exercising; it's about observing and being present. Move at a pace that allows you to absorb the environment without rushing.

- **Touch the Elements:** If comfortable, touch the trees, feel the texture of leaves or the coolness of a stream. Grounding your sense of touch in nature can enhance the therapeutic effects.

- **Sit or Stand in Stillness:** Find a spot to sit or stand quietly and simply be present in the moment. Allow your thoughts to come and go without attachment, focusing instead on the natural world around you.

- **Reflect on Your Experience:** After completing your walk, take a few moments to reflect on how you feel. Notice any changes in your mood, stress level, or physical sensations.

Tips for Enhancing the Practice:

- Practice regularly to cultivate a deeper connection with nature and its healing properties.

- Incorporate mindfulness or meditation techniques during your walk to deepen the relaxation effect.

- If possible, vary your locations to experience different aspects of nature and its seasonal changes.

Benefits:

Nature Bathing (Shinrin-Yoku) offers numerous health benefits, including reduced stress and anxiety, improved concentration, increased energy, and stronger immune function. This practice fosters a profound appreciation for the natural world and its ability to heal and rejuvenate the human spirit.

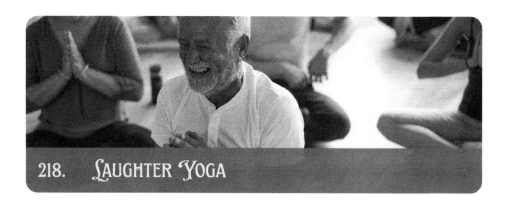

218. ℒAUGHTER ℐOGA

Introduction:

Laughter Yoga is a unique exercise routine that combines laughter with yogic breathing (Pranayama). It's based on the principle that voluntary laughter provides the same physiological and psychological benefits as spontaneous laughter. This practice helps to reduce stress, boost mood, strengthen the immune system, and improve overall health by encouraging deep, playful breathing and the expression of joy through laughter.

Basic Technique and Information:

Laughter Yoga involves a series of laughter exercises that often start with gentle warm-up techniques including stretching, chanting, clapping, and body movement. These exercises aim to cultivate child-like playfulness which leads to genuine and contagious laughter.

Steps to Practice Laughter Yoga:

- Find a Comfortable Space: Choose a quiet and spacious area where you can move freely and laugh without restraint. This could be indoors or outdoors.

- Start with Warm-Up Exercises: Begin with light stretching and deep breathing to relax the body and open the lungs. You can also gently clap and chant to engage the group and create a rhythm.

- Engage in Laughter Exercises: Follow structured exercises that simulate laughter. This can include:

- Greeting Laughter: Mimic greeting someone with a handshake and turn it into laughter.

- Hearty Laughter: Hold your arms up, look up, and laugh heartily from the belly.

- Humming Laughter: Laugh with your mouth closed, feeling the vibration in your body.

- Use Breathing Exercises: Between laughter exercises, use deep yogic breathing to calm the system and prepare for the next round of laughter.

- Incorporate Playfulness: Encourage playfulness by using imaginary scenarios (like laughing at funny hats or slipping on a banana peel) to stimulate laughter.

- End with Relaxation: Conclude the session by lying down, closing your eyes, and relaxing deeply while focusing on the breath. This allows the body to absorb the benefits of the laughter session.

Tips for Enhancing the Practice:

- 💡 Practice regularly to develop a more spontaneous laughter response and deepen the health benefits.
- 💡 Participate in or start a laughter yoga group for communal energy and support.

- 💡 Remain open-minded and refrain from being self-conscious to fully enjoy the benefits of laughter.

Benefits:

Laughter Yoga promotes a joyful and healthy life by reducing stress hormones, increasing the intake of oxygen-rich air, and fostering a positive, optimistic outlook. It enhances emotional resilience, improves interpersonal relationships, and supports overall physical and mental well-being.

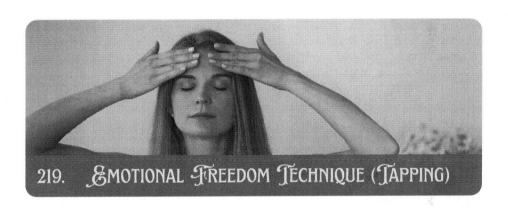

219. EMOTIONAL FREEDOM TECHNIQUE (TAPPING)

Introduction:

The Emotional Freedom Technique (EFT), commonly known as Tapping, is a psychological acupressure technique that combines elements of cognitive therapy with acupressure to relieve stress, anxiety, and emotional distress. By tapping on specific meridian points on the body while focusing on particular negative emotions or physical sensations, EFT helps to balance the

body's energy system and promote healing and well-being.

Basic Technique and Information:

EFT involves tapping with the fingertips on key energy points on the head, face, and upper body while mentally focusing on a specific issue. This process is believed to release blockages within the energy system, thereby reducing emotional stress and physical tension.

Steps to Practice Emotional Freedom Technique (Tapping):

- **Identify the Issue:** Before you begin tapping, pinpoint the specific problem or emotion you want to address. This could be a feeling of anxiety, a painful memory, or a physical symptom like tension or pain.

- **Determine the Intensity:** Assess the intensity of your emotion or pain on a scale from 0 to 10, where 10 is the most intense. This helps to monitor your progress throughout the tapping session.

- **The Setup Statement:** Craft a setup statement that acknowledges the issue and affirms self-acceptance, such as, "Even though I have this [anxiety/fear/pain], I deeply and completely accept myself."

- **Begin Tapping:** Use your fingertips to tap gently but firmly on each of the following points, repeating your setup statement or a reminder phrase at each:

- **Karate Chop (Side of Hand):** Tap with four fingers on the outer edge of the other hand.

- **Eyebrow:** Tap on the point where your eyebrows begin, near the bridge of your nose.

- **Side of the Eye:** Tap on the bone bordering the outside corner of the eye.

- **Under the Eye:** Tap on the bone under an eye, about 1 inch below your pupil.

- **Under the Nose:** Tap in the area between the nose and the upper lip.

- **Chin:** Tap midway between the point of your chin and the bottom of your lower lip.

- **Collarbone:** Tap just below the hard ridge of your collarbone.

- **Under the Arm:** Tap about 4 inches below the armpit.

- **Top of the Head:** Tap on the crown of your head.

- **Reassess the Intensity:** After completing a few rounds of tapping on all points, stop and reassess the intensity level of your problem. Continue tapping until the intensity has significantly decreased or gone.

Tips for Enhancing the Practice:

- Be specific about the issue you are addressing for more effective results.

- Practice regularly, especially during times of stress or when dealing with persistent emotional or physical issues.

- Use gentle but firm pressure – the tapping should be solid but not painful.

Benefits:

EFT (Tapping) is effective in reducing the symptoms of anxiety, depression, PTSD, and physical pain. It helps to improve emotional regulation, enhance mental clarity, and foster a greater sense of peace and well-being. By integrating EFT into a regular self-care routine, individuals can manage stress more effectively and promote lasting emotional and physical health.

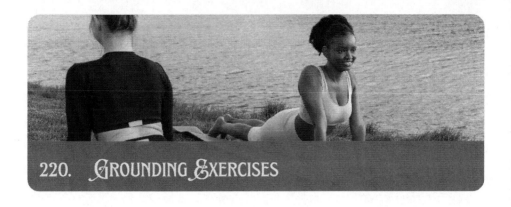

220. GROUNDING EXERCISES

Introduction:

Grounding exercises are techniques used to bring one's focus back to the present moment, particularly during times of stress, anxiety, or emotional overwhelm. These practices help to stabilize the mind by reconnecting with the physical world and the senses, reducing the intensity of distressing thoughts or feelings and promoting a sense of calm and balance.

Basic Technique and Information:

Grounding can be achieved through various sensory engagements and mindfulness practices that encourage a deep connection to the here and now. These methods often involve focusing on physical sensations, environmental details, or simple movements to anchor the mind away from distressing thoughts or feelings.

Steps to Practice Grounding Exercises:

- **5-4-3-2-1 Technique:** This method involves using your senses to list things around you and bring your attention to the present.

- **See:** Identify and name 5 things you can see around you.

- **Touch:** Acknowledge 4 things you can touch or feel (like the texture of your clothing or the surface of your chair).

- **Hear:** Listen and name 3 sounds you can hear in the moment (such as a clock ticking or birds chirping).

- **Smell:** Recognize 2 scents or smells that you can detect, whether nearby or by recalling familiar scents.

- **Taste:** Focus on 1 thing you can taste or imagine tasting a favorite food or drink.

- **Physical Grounding:** Engage your body to help anchor your mind.

- **Breathe Deeply:** Focus on taking slow, deep breaths, feeling the air fill your lungs and then slowly exhale, noticing the rise and fall of your chest or abdomen.

- **Press Your Feet into the Floor:** Stand or sit with both feet firmly on the ground. Press down and feel the solid support beneath you, imagining roots growing from your feet into the ground.

- **Hold or Touch an Object:** Carry a small object like a stone, a piece of jewelry, or a stress ball. Focus on its texture, temperature, and weight in your hand.

- **Mindful Movement:** Simple exercises can help bring you back to the present.

- **Stretching:** Perform gentle stretches, paying attention to the sensations in each muscle group as you move.

- **Walking Mindfully:** Take a slow walk, focusing on each step, how your feet touch and leave the ground, and the rhythm of your movement.

- **Connect with Nature:** Spend time outdoors, feeling the sun, wind, or even rain on your skin. Observing natural elements like trees, water, or sky can profoundly ground and calm the mind.

Tips for Enhancing the Practice:

- Practice regularly, especially in moments of calm, to build familiarity and make these techniques more effective during stressful times.

- Use grounding exercises as a preventive measure in your daily routine to maintain a balanced emotional state.

- Combine grounding with other relaxation techniques like visualization or calming music for a more comprehensive approach to stress management.

Benefits:

Grounding exercises provide immediate relief from acute stress and help manage symptoms of anxiety and PTSD. They promote emotional stability, improve concentration, and foster a sense of safety and control, making them essential tools in personal mental health care.

PART 11

Exercise and Movement (221-235)

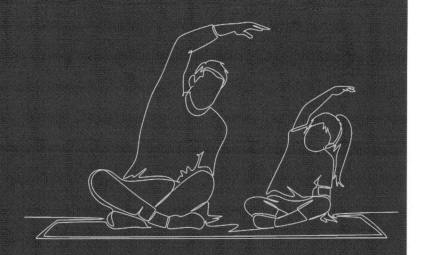

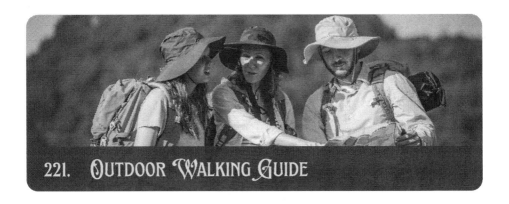

221. OUTDOOR WALKING GUIDE

Introduction:

An Outdoor Walking Guide is designed to help individuals make the most of their walking experiences by exploring various aspects such as routes, pacing, and mindful practices. Walking outdoors not only boosts physical health by improving cardiovascular fitness and strengthening muscles but also enhances mental well-being by connecting with nature and reducing stress.

Basic Technique and Information:

Effective outdoor walking involves choosing the right paths, understanding proper walking form, and being mindful of the environment. It's about finding a balance between physical exertion and relaxation to maximize the benefits of the activity.

Steps to Optimize Outdoor Walking:

- **Choose Your Route:** Select paths that match your fitness level and interest. Consider flat trails for a leisurely walk or hilly terrains for a more challenging workout. Urban parks, nature reserves, and waterfronts are great for variety and scenery.

- **Prepare Appropriately:** Wear comfortable, supportive footwear and weather-appropriate clothing. Bring water to stay hydrated, especially on longer walks, and use sunscreen or wear a hat in sunny conditions.

- **Set Your Pace:** Start at a pace that feels comfortable, gradually increasing intensity as your fitness improves. Aim for a brisk pace where you can talk but not sing to ensure moderate aerobic activity.

- **Incorporate Mindfulness:** Engage your senses to fully experience the environment. Notice the sights, sounds, and smells around you. This can transform a simple walk into a rejuvenating, mindful experience.

- **Use Safety Measures:** Be aware of your surroundings, especially on less familiar or secluded trails. Carry a map or use a GPS app if needed, and let someone know your route and expected return time.

- **Stretch and Cool Down:** After your walk, spend a few minutes stretching to help your muscles recover and prevent stiffness. Focus on areas like your calves, thighs, and lower back.

Tips for Enhancing the Practice:

- 💡 Try different times of the day to experience various aspects of nature, like early morning calm or sunset views.

- 💡 Join walking groups or find a walking buddy for motivation and social interaction.

- 💡 Set goals, such as distance or duration, to track progress and maintain interest.

Benefits:

Regular outdoor walking strengthens the heart, lowers blood pressure, boosts mood and energy levels, and supports weight management. It's an accessible form of exercise that can be adapted to fit any lifestyle, offering a path to improved health and a deeper connection with the natural world.

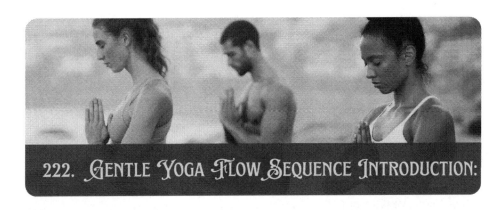

222. GENTLE YOGA FLOW SEQUENCE INTRODUCTION:

Introduction:

A Gentle Yoga Flow Sequence is ideal for those seeking a calming, restorative practice that enhances flexibility, reduces stress, and promotes inner peace. This sequence focuses on slow, fluid movements and deep breathing to gently stretch and strengthen the body while nurturing the mind and spirit.

Basic Technique and Information:

Gentle yoga emphasizes smooth transitions between poses, with an emphasis on mindful breathing and body awareness. It's perfect for beginners, individuals recovering from injuries, or anyone looking for a soothing practice to unwind and relax.

Steps to Practice Gentle Yoga Flow Sequence:

- **Begin with Centering:** Start in a comfortable seated position on your mat, with your hands on your knees and eyes closed. Take a few deep breaths to center yourself and set an intention for your practice.

- **Cat-Cow Stretches (Marjaryasana-Bitilasana):** Move to a tabletop position with hands under shoulders and knees under hips. Inhale as you arch your back downward (Cow Pose), lifting your head and tailbone. Exhale as you round your back upward (Cat Pose), tucking your chin to your chest. Repeat for 5-10 cycles to warm up the spine.

- **Child's Pose (Balasana):** From tabletop, sit back on your heels, stretch your arms forward, and rest your forehead on the mat. Hold for a few breaths to relax and stretch your back.

- **Seated Forward Bend (Paschimottanasana):** Sit with legs extended in front of you. Inhale to lengthen your spine, then exhale and fold forward gently over your legs, reaching for your toes or shins. Hold for several breaths to stretch the hamstrings and calm the mind.

- **Bridge Pose (Setu Bandhasana):** Lie on your back with knees bent and feet flat on the floor, hip-width apart. Press into your feet and lift your hips, creating a straight line from shoulders to knees. Clasp your hands under your back to deepen the stretch or keep your arms flat for support. Hold for a few breaths, then gently lower back down.

- **Supine Twist (Supta Matsyendrasana):** Still lying on your back, bring your knees into your chest and then let them fall to one side while turning your head to the opposite side. Stretch your arms out to form a "T." Hold for a few breaths, then switch sides to balance the stretch.

- **Legs-Up-the-Wall Pose (Viparita Karani):** Sit sideways against a wall, then gently lie back and swing your legs up against the wall. Allow your arms to rest by your sides or on your belly. Stay in this pose for 5-10 minutes to relax deeply and improve circulation.

- **Corpse Pose (Savasana):** End your sequence by lying flat on your back, arms at your sides with palms facing up, and legs slightly apart. Close your eyes and focus on deep, slow breathing. Stay in this pose for 5-10 minutes, allowing your body to absorb the benefits of your practice.

Tips for Enhancing the Practice:

- Use props like cushions, blankets, or yoga blocks to make poses more comfortable and accessible.

- Focus on your breath throughout the sequence to deepen relaxation and enhance the meditative aspect of your practice.

- Listen to your body and modify poses as needed to avoid strain or discomfort.

Benefits:

This gentle yoga flow helps improve flexibility, reduces stress, and promotes relaxation. It's an effective way to unwind after a long day, prepare for sleep, or gently start the day with a focus on well-being and mindfulness.

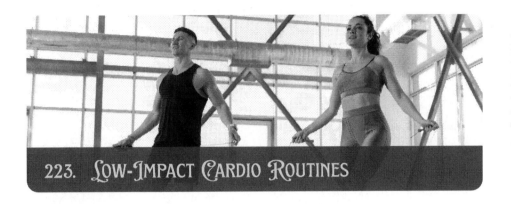

223. Low-Impact Cardio Routines

Introduction:

Low-impact cardio routines are designed to get your heart rate up and improve cardiovascular health without putting excessive stress on the joints. These exercises are ideal for individuals with joint issues, beginners, older adults, or anyone looking for a gentler way to stay active and fit. By focusing on movements that minimize the strain on the body while maximizing health benefits, low-impact cardio can be a sustainable and effective part of a fitness plan.

Basic Technique and Information:

Low-impact cardio involves exercises where at least one foot remains in contact with the ground at all times, reducing the impact on the knees, hips, and back. These routines often include activities like walking, cycling, swimming, and certain types of aerobic workouts.

Steps to Practice Low-Impact Cardio Routines:

- **Warm-Up:** Begin with a 5-10 minute warm-up to prepare your muscles and joints. Gentle stretching and basic movements like arm circles, leg swings, and marching in place can increase blood flow and reduce the risk of injury.

- **Walking or Brisk Walking:** A simple and effective low-impact cardio exercise. Maintain a brisk pace that allows you to talk but makes it hard to sing. Use your arms to increase intensity and engage the upper body.

- **Stationary Cycling:** Use a stationary bike with resistance levels adjusted to your fitness. Cycle for 20-30 minutes at a steady pace, ensuring you're pushing yourself without straining.

- **Elliptical Training:** The elliptical machine provides a fluid motion that mimics running but with reduced impact. Keep a steady pace for 20-30 minutes, varying the resistance and incline for a more challenging workout.

- **Aqua Aerobics or Swimming:** Water provides natural resistance and buoyancy, making it an excellent environment for low-impact cardio. Try aqua aerobics classes or swim laps at a pace that elevates your heart rate.

- **Rowing Machine:** Provides a full-body workout that's low on joint impact. Focus on a smooth, continuous motion, pulling with your arms and legs in a coordinated effort.

- **Cool Down:** Finish your routine with a 5-10 minute cool down, gradually lowering your heart rate with gentle stretching and deep breathing.

Tips for Enhancing the Practice:

- ⚲ Use music to keep your energy and motivation high during your workout.

- ⚲ Incorporate a variety of routines to keep your workouts interesting and work different muscle groups.

- ⚲ Listen to your body and adjust the intensity as needed to avoid overexertion or injury.

Benefits:

Low-impact cardio routines strengthen the heart and lungs, improve endurance, and promote weight management. They also enhance mood and energy levels, making them a key component of a balanced fitness regimen that supports long-term health and mobility.

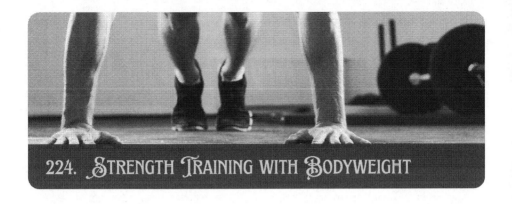

224. STRENGTH TRAINING WITH BODYWEIGHT

Introduction:

Strength Training with Bodyweight is an effective and accessible method to build muscle, improve endurance, and enhance overall fitness without the need for gym equipment. Utilizing your own body's weight as resistance, this approach allows for a variety of exercises that can be done anywhere, making it ideal for those who prefer home workouts or have limited access to fitness facilities.

Basic Technique and Information:

Bodyweight training focuses on using gravity and natural movements to challenge and strengthen different muscle groups. Key principles include maintaining proper form to prevent injury and progressively increasing the intensity or volume of exercises to continue developing strength and stamina.

Steps to Practice Strength Training with Bodyweight:

- **Warm-Up:** Begin with a 5-10 minute warm-up to prepare your muscles and joints for the workout. Include dynamic stretches and light cardio movements like jumping jacks or high knees.

- **Squats:** Stand with feet hip-width apart, arms at your sides or extended in front for balance. Bend your knees and lower your hips as if sitting in a chair, keeping your weight in your heels and your back straight. Push through your heels to return to standing. Aim for 2-3 sets of 10-15 repetitions.

- **Push-Ups:** Start in a plank position with hands slightly wider than shoulder-width apart. Lower your body until your chest nearly touches the floor, elbows bending out to the sides. Press back up to the starting position. Modify by dropping to your knees if needed. Perform 2-3 sets of 8-12 repetitions.

- **Plank:** Lie face down, then lift your body on your toes and forearms, keeping your body in a straight line from head to heels. Engage your core and hold the position for 20-60 seconds, or as long as you can maintain good form.

- **Lunges:** Step forward with one leg, lowering your hips until both knees are bent at about a 90-degree angle. Make sure your front knee is directly above your ankle. Push back to the starting position and repeat with the other leg. Complete 2-3 sets of 10-15 repetitions per leg.

- **Glute Bridges:** Lie on your back with knees bent and feet flat on the floor. Lift your hips off the ground until your knees, hips, and shoulders form a straight line. Squeeze your glutes at the top before slowly lowering back down. Perform 2-3 sets of 15-20 repetitions.

- **Cool Down:** End your session with a cool-down period, including gentle stretching and deep breathing to help your muscles recover and reduce soreness.

Tips for Enhancing the Practice:

- Focus on controlled movements to maximize muscle engagement and effectiveness.

- Gradually increase the number of repetitions or sets as you gain strength.

- Incorporate variations of exercises to challenge different muscle groups and prevent boredom.

Benefits:

Strength Training with Bodyweight enhances muscle tone, boosts metabolic rate, and increases functional strength, aiding in everyday activities. It also supports bone health, improves posture, and contributes to a balanced and healthy physique.

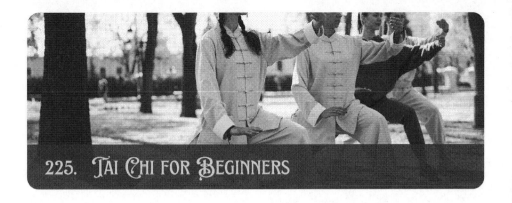

225. Tai Chi for Beginners

Introduction:

Tai Chi is a gentle form of martial arts originating from ancient China, known for its slow, flowing movements and deep breathing. Ideal for beginners and people of all ages, Tai Chi enhances physical health, mental clarity, and emotional balance. It emphasizes mindfulness, coordination, and the cultivation of internal energy, or "chi," making it a holistic practice for improving overall well-being.

Basic Technique and Information:

Tai Chi involves a series of movements, often called "forms," that are performed in a smooth, continuous manner. Each posture flows into the next without pause, ensuring that the body is in constant motion. The focus is on relaxation, controlled breathing, and slow, graceful movements that mirror the rhythms of nature.

Steps to Practice Tai Chi for Beginners:

- **Warm-Up:** Start with a gentle warm-up to loosen your joints and muscles. Simple rotations of the neck, shoulders, wrists, hips, knees, and ankles help prepare your body for the fluid movements of Tai Chi.

- **Basic Stances:** Learn the fundamental Tai Chi stances like "Wu Chi" (an initial, relaxed standing position) and "Horse Stance" (a stable, wide-legged stance). These positions form the foundation for more complex movements.

- **Opening Movement:** Begin with the "Opening of Tai Chi," where you stand with feet together, slowly raise your arms with palms down, and then gently lower them, imagining you are moving through water. This helps you connect with your breath and energy.

- **Single Whip:** From your opening position, step to the side with one foot and extend one arm outward with the hand in a hook position while the other arm sweeps across your body. This movement helps develop balance and coordination.

- **Brush Knee and Push:** Move one hand down past your knee as if brushing it, while the other hand extends forward in a pushing motion. Repeat on both sides to improve flexibility and stimulate energy flow through the body.

- **Parting the Wild Horse's Mane:** This involves stepping forward and extending one arm as if gently pushing a mane away from the face, while the other hand pulls back like drawing a bowstring. This movement enhances balance and grace.

- **Cool Down:** Conclude your practice with slow, meditative breathing and gentle stretching to relax the muscles and integrate the benefits of the session.

Tips for Enhancing the Practice:

- Practice Tai Chi in a calm, quiet environment to enhance concentration and relaxation.

- Focus on your breathing; inhale and exhale deeply with each movement to promote energy flow and relaxation.

- Be patient and consistent. Tai Chi skills and benefits develop over time with regular practice.

Benefits:

Tai Chi for beginners offers numerous health benefits, including improved balance and coordination, reduced stress and anxiety, enhanced flexibility and strength, and a deeper sense of peace and well-being. It's an accessible practice that supports longevity and enhances quality of life by fostering a harmonious connection between body and mind.

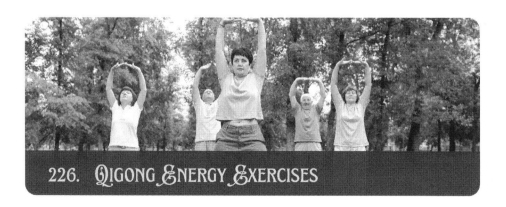

226. QIGONG ENERGY EXERCISES

Introduction:

Qigong is a traditional Chinese exercise system that integrates physical postures, breathing techniques, and focused intention to cultivate and balance the body's life energy, known as "qi." These exercises are designed to enhance vitality, stimulate healing processes, and improve mental clarity. Suitable for all ages and fitness levels, Qigong is a holistic approach to maintaining health and wellness.

Basic Technique and Information:

Qigong involves gentle, rhythmic movements combined with deep, mindful breathing and meditation. The practice aims to open the body's energy pathways, known as meridians, to promote the flow of qi and enhance overall well-being.

Steps to Practice Qigong Energy Exercises:

- **Warm-Up:** Begin with gentle stretching and breathing exercises to loosen the joints and muscles and prepare the body for energy work. Focus on relaxing each part of your body and clearing your mind.

- **Standing Meditation (Zhan Zhuang):** Stand with your feet shoulder-width apart, knees slightly bent, and arms relaxed at your sides. Breathe deeply and visualize your body filling with calming energy with each breath.

- **Opening the Energy Gates:** Start by raising your arms slowly in front of you, palms facing down, as you inhale. Exhale as you lower your arms back to your sides, imagining you are pushing down gently through water. Repeat several times to cultivate awareness of qi.

- **Cloud Hands:** Move your arms side to side in front of your body, with hands following each other in a flowing, wave-like motion. Coordinate this movement with your breath, inhaling as your hands rise and exhaling as they fall, to deepen the sense of energy flow.

- **Golden Ball Exercise:** Visualize holding a ball of energy between your hands. As you breathe in, expand your hands slightly as if the ball is growing; as you breathe out, contract your hands as if compressing the ball. Feel the sensation of energy between your palms.

- **Harvesting Qi:** Gently rotate your waist and let your arms swing loosely, brushing lightly across your body. This movement helps to release tension and distribute qi evenly throughout the body.

- **Cool Down:** Conclude with deep breathing and a final standing meditation, allowing the energy to settle and integrate into your body. Reflect on the sensations experienced during the practice.

Tips for Enhancing the Practice:

- Practice Qigong in a peaceful environment, preferably in nature, to enhance the connection with the earth's energy.

- Focus on the smoothness and fluidity of movements rather than on speed or force.

- Regular practice is key to deepening your sensitivity to qi and reaping the full benefits of Qigong.

Benefits:

Qigong exercises improve physical health by boosting immunity, increasing strength and flexibility, and promoting cardiovascular and respiratory function.

Mentally, it reduces stress, enhances focus, and fosters a greater sense of peace and contentment. Spiritually, it helps in connecting deeply with oneself and the surrounding world, enhancing a sense of harmony and balance.

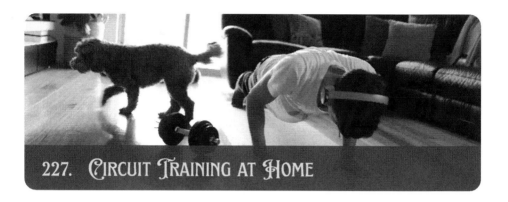

227. Circuit Training at Home

Introduction:

Circuit training at home is an efficient and dynamic way to build strength, improve cardiovascular fitness, and boost overall endurance without needing to go to the gym. This type of workout involves performing a series of exercises in a specific order, targeting different muscle groups with minimal rest between sets. It's perfect for those looking to maximize their workout efficiency and achieve comprehensive fitness results in a short amount of time.

Basic Technique and Information:

Circuit training typically combines strength-building exercises with aerobic components to keep the heart rate up and burn calories. By arranging exercises to alternate between muscle groups, you can keep moving and avoid fatigue, allowing for a continuous, effective workout.

Steps to Practice Circuit Training at Home:

- **Plan Your Circuit:** Decide on 6-10 exercises that cover major muscle groups. Include a mix of upper body, lower body, core, and cardio exercises to ensure a balanced workout. Each exercise should be performed for 30-60 seconds or a specific number of repetitions.

- **Set Up Your Space:** Ensure you have enough room to safely perform all exercises. Gather any equipment you might use, like dumbbells, resistance bands, or a yoga mat, but remember many exercises can be done using just your body weight.

- **Warm-Up:** Start with a 5-10 minute warm-up to get your muscles ready and your heart rate up. This could include jogging in place, dynamic stretches, or light bodyweight movements like squats and arm circles.

- **Perform the Circuit:** Begin your first exercise and complete the set time or repetitions. Move quickly to the next exercise with minimal rest (10-30 seconds). Here's a sample circuit:

- Push-Ups

- Squats

- Jumping Jacks

- Plank

- Lunges

- Burpees

- Bicycle Crunches

- Mountain Climbers

- **Rest and Repeat:** After completing one round of the circuit, rest for 1-2 minutes. Then, start the next round. Aim for 2-4 rounds depending on your fitness level and the intensity of the exercises.

- Cool Down: Finish with a cool-down phase of 5-10 minutes, including stretching and deep breathing to help your muscles recover and prevent soreness.

Tips for Enhancing the Practice:

- Vary your exercises regularly to challenge different muscle groups and prevent boredom.

- Keep track of your progress by timing each circuit or noting the number of repetitions to motivate improvement.

- Listen to your body and modify exercises as needed to suit your fitness level and avoid injury.

Benefits:

Circuit training at home is a versatile and comprehensive workout that improves muscular strength, endurance, flexibility, and cardiovascular health. It's also an excellent way to burn calories and fat, enhancing body composition and boosting metabolic rate. This type of training is adaptable to any fitness level, making it an accessible option for a wide range of individuals looking to improve their health and fitness efficiently.

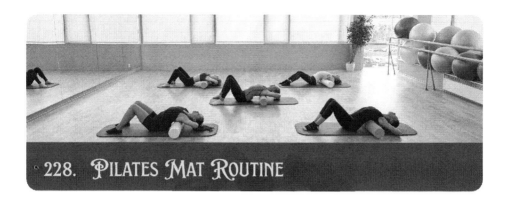

Introduction:

Pilates is a low-impact exercise system designed to strengthen muscles, improve postural alignment, and enhance flexibility. A Pilates mat routine focuses on core strength, balance, and controlled movements, using the body's own resistance. It's ideal for those seeking a harmonious blend of mind and body conditioning, with exercises that can be adapted to all fitness levels.

Basic Technique and Information:

Pilates exercises emphasize precision and control, with a strong focus on the core — the "powerhouse" of your body. The practice involves breathing techniques to support movement and engage deeper abdominal muscles, enhancing the effectiveness of each exercise.

Steps to Practice Pilates Mat Routine:

- **Warm-Up:** Begin with a few minutes of deep breathing and gentle stretches to prepare your body. Focus on elongating the spine and activating your core muscles.

- **The Hundred:** Lie on your back with knees bent into your chest. Lift your head, neck, and shoulders off the mat, and extend your arms by your sides. Pump your arms up and down while breathing in for five counts and out for five counts. Do this for a total of 100 arm pumps.

- **Roll-Up:** Lie flat with your arms extended overhead. Inhale as you lift your arms to the ceiling, then exhale as you roll up into a seated "C" curve, reaching for your toes. Inhale and start rolling back down, vertebra by vertebra, until you're lying flat again. Repeat 5-8 times.

- **Single Leg Circles:** Lie on your back with one leg extended straight up to the ceiling and the other flat on the mat. Circle the raised leg across your body, then down, around, and up, keeping your hips still. Do 5 circles in each direction, then switch legs.

- **Criss-Cross:** Lie on your back with hands behind your head and knees pulled into your chest. Lift your head and shoulders off the mat. Twist your torso, bringing your right elbow to your left knee while extending the right leg.

Switch sides and continue alternating for 10-12 reps on each side.

- **Swan Prep:** Lie face down with hands under shoulders and elbows close to your body. Gently press your hands into the mat to lift your chest up, extending your spine while keeping your abdominal muscles engaged. Lower back down slowly. Repeat 5-6 times.

- **Child's Pose:** After completing the exercises, sit back on your heels with your arms stretched forward on the mat. Relax into Child's Pose to stretch your back and relax your muscles.

Tips for Enhancing the Practice:

- 💡 Focus on the quality of each movement rather than the quantity of repetitions.

- 💡 Use a Pilates or yoga mat for cushioning and support.

- 💡 Breathe deeply and rhythmically to enhance muscle activation and relaxation.

- 💡 Gradually increase the difficulty of exercises as your strength and flexibility improve.

Benefits:

A regular Pilates mat routine enhances core strength, improves posture, increases flexibility, and reduces stress. It's particularly beneficial for stabilizing the spine and building endurance in the deep postural muscles, contributing to overall physical health and well-being.

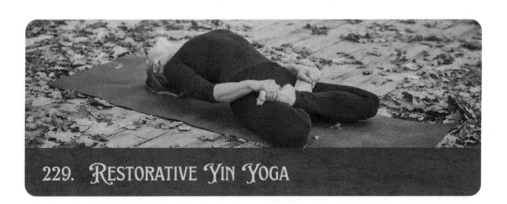

229. RESTORATIVE YIN YOGA

Introduction:

Restorative Yin Yoga is a gentle and meditative practice focused on deep, prolonged stretches and relaxation of the mind and body. By holding poses for several minutes, this form of yoga targets the connective tissues, such as ligaments, bones, and joints, which are often less emphasized in more dynamic styles of yoga. It's ideal for improving flexibility, releasing tension, and fostering a deep sense of calm and mindfulness.

Basic Technique and Information:

Yin Yoga involves passive stretches with little muscular engagement, allowing gravity and time to deepen the stretch and open the body. The practice encourages a softening of the muscles and a focus on breath to support gentle, sustained stretching and mental stillness.

Steps to Practice Restorative Yin Yoga:

- **Prepare Your Space:** Create a calm, comfortable environment with minimal distractions. Use props like yoga blocks, bolsters, and blankets to support your body in the poses.

- **Butterfly Pose (Baddha Konasana):** Sit with the soles of your feet together and knees bent out to the sides. Hold your feet with your hands, and gently fold forward, allowing your back to round and your head to drop toward your feet. Hold for 3-5 minutes, using a pillow or bolster for support if needed.

- **Dragonfly Pose (Upavistha Konasana):** From a seated position, extend your legs wide apart. Inhale to lengthen your spine, then exhale as you fold forward from the hips, bringing your hands or elbows to the floor or onto props. Hold the stretch for 3-5 minutes, relaxing into the pose with each breath.

- **Caterpillar Pose (Paschimottanasana):** Sit with your legs extended straight in front of you. Inhale to lengthen your spine, then exhale as you fold forward, allowing your back to round and

hands to rest wherever comfortable. Use a bolster or folded blanket under your knees if there's strain in your lower back. Hold for 3-5 minutes.

- **Supported Bridge Pose:** Lie on your back with knees bent and feet flat on the floor. Lift your hips and place a yoga block or bolster under your sacrum for support. Allow your arms to rest by your sides, palms facing up. Hold for 4-6 minutes, breathing deeply.

- **Legs-Up-the-Wall Pose (Viparita Karani):** Sit with one hip against the wall, then gently swing your legs up onto the wall as you lie back. Your buttocks can be a few inches from the wall or touching it, based on your comfort. Allow your arms to rest by your sides or on your abdomen. Hold for 5-10 minutes.

- **Savasana with Props:** End your practice by lying flat on your back in Savasana (Corpse Pose), using a bolster under your knees and a blanket over your body for added comfort. Stay in this pose for 5-10 minutes, focusing on deep, relaxing breaths.

Tips for Enhancing the Practice:

- Stay present with your breath throughout each pose to deepen relaxation and mindfulness.

- Adjust the duration in each pose based on your comfort level—longer isn't always better, especially at the beginning.

- Listen to gentle, calming music or nature sounds to enhance the meditative aspect of the practice.

Benefits:

Restorative Yin Yoga is particularly effective for reducing stress and anxiety, enhancing flexibility, and promoting recovery for the body and mind. It helps balance the nervous system, improve joint mobility, and encourage a deep, meditative state that can lead to profound inner peace and rejuvenation.

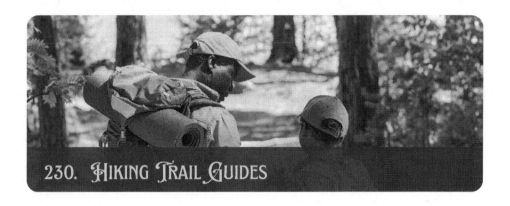

230. HIKING TRAIL GUIDES

Introduction:

Hiking Trail Guides are essential tools for navigating and enjoying the natural world through hiking. These guides provide detailed information about trails, including their length, difficulty, terrain type, and points of interest. Whether you're a novice hiker or an experienced adventurer, a well-structured guide can enhance your experience by ensuring safety, promoting environmental awareness, and enriching the journey with historical and ecological insights.

Basic Technique and Information:

Effective hiking involves preparation and awareness. A good hiking trail guide helps you prepare by offering maps, descriptions of the trail conditions, and advice on what to expect regarding weather, wildlife, and necessary gear.

Steps to Use Hiking Trail Guides Effectively:

- **Choose the Right Trail:** Based on your fitness level and hiking experience, select a trail that matches your abilities. Look for guides that categorize trails by length, elevation gain, and technical difficulty.

- **Prepare Your Gear:** Based on the guide's recommendations, pack essential items such as water, snacks, a first aid kit, appropriate clothing, and navigation tools like a compass or a GPS device.

- **Understand the Route:** Study the trail guide to familiarize yourself with key waypoints, water sources, camping spots, and potential hazards. Knowing these can help you pace your hike and make informed decisions on the trail.

- **Respect the Environment:** Follow the principles of Leave No Trace to minimize your impact. This includes staying on marked trails, packing out all trash, and being respectful of wildlife and other hikers.

- **Stay Safe:** Use the guide to learn about local wildlife, weather patterns, and any specific safety advice for the area. Always let someone know your hiking plan and expected return time.

- **Take Breaks and Stay Hydrated:** Use the guide to identify good spots for rest and hydration, especially on longer or more challenging trails. Regular breaks can prevent fatigue and injury.

- **Document Your Experience:** Take notes or photographs to remember your hike and provide feedback or updates to the guide if you encounter new conditions or obstacles.

Tips for Enhancing the Practice:

- Combine the hiking guide with a digital app for real-time navigation and updates.

- Join a hiking group or find a hiking buddy to share the experience and ensure additional safety.

- Take time to learn about the natural history and cultural background of the area to deepen your appreciation and connection to the landscape.

Benefits:

Using hiking trail guides enhances your outdoor experience by ensuring you are well-prepared and informed, leading to safer and more enjoyable hikes. It fosters a connection to nature, improves physical health, and provides a refreshing escape from the daily routine, contributing to mental well-being and personal growth.

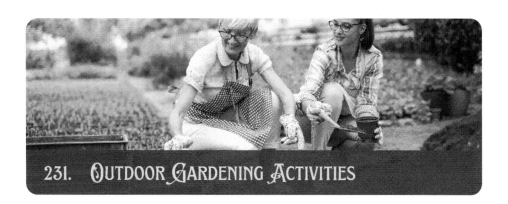

231. OUTDOOR GARDENING ACTIVITIES

Introduction:

Outdoor gardening is a rewarding and enriching activity that connects individuals with nature while enhancing their living environment. Whether you're growing vegetables, cultivating flowers, or maintaining a landscape, gardening offers therapeutic benefits, physical exercise, and the satisfaction of nurturing life from the earth. It's a versatile hobby suitable for all ages and skill levels, providing endless opportunities for creativity and discovery.

Basic Technique and Information:

Successful gardening requires a basic understanding of plant types, soil preparation, planting techniques, and ongoing care. Engaging in a variety of gardening activities can maximize the health and aesthetic benefits of your garden while offering a fulfilling, hands-on experience.

Steps to Engage in Outdoor Gardening Activities:

- **Plan Your Garden:** Decide on the type of garden you want, whether it's a vegetable plot, a flower bed, or a mixed-use area. Consider the climate, soil type, and sunlight exposure of your space to choose suitable plants.

- **Prepare the Soil:** Start with soil testing to understand its nutrient content and pH level. Amend the soil with compost, manure, or other organic matter to enhance fertility and drainage.

- **Choose Your Plants:** Select plants based on their compatibility with your garden's conditions and your personal preferences. Include a mix of perennials, annuals, and bulbs for year-round interest.

- **Planting:** Follow the best practices for planting each type of plant. This includes digging appropriate-sized holes, spacing plants correctly, and

watering them after planting to help establish roots.

- **Maintenance:** Regularly water, weed, and prune your garden to promote healthy growth. Monitor for pests and diseases and apply natural or recommended treatments to protect your plants.

- **Harvesting and Enjoying:** For vegetable gardens, harvest your produce at peak ripeness for the best flavor and nutritional value. Enjoy the blooms from your flower garden by creating bouquets or simply appreciating the beauty and wildlife they attract.

- **Seasonal Activities:** Engage in seasonal gardening tasks such as mulching in winter, planting spring bulbs, summer pruning, and fall cleanup to keep your garden thriving year-round.

Tips for Enhancing the Practice:

- Use gardening as an opportunity to learn about different plant species and gardening techniques through books, workshops, or community groups.

- Involve family and friends in gardening activities to share the benefits and make it a communal endeavor.

- Experiment with container gardening, vertical gardening, or raised beds if space or soil conditions are limited.

Benefits:

Outdoor gardening improves physical health by providing exercise and promoting time spent outdoors. It reduces stress, enhances mood, and can lead to improved diet quality when growing your own fruits and vegetables. Additionally, it contributes to biodiversity and supports local wildlife, making it a sustainable practice that benefits both personal well-being and the environment.

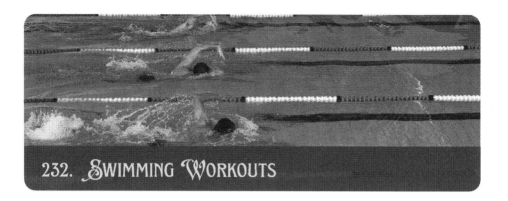

232. SWIMMING WORKOUTS

Introduction:

Swimming workouts are a highly effective form of exercise that provides a full-body workout while being gentle on the joints. Ideal for all ages and fitness levels, swimming improves cardiovascular health, builds strength, enhances flexibility, and reduces stress. The buoyancy of water offers natural resistance, making swimming an excellent choice for both conditioning and rehabilitation.

Basic Technique and Information:

Effective swimming workouts combine various strokes, intensities, and drills to challenge different muscle groups and improve overall fitness. Understanding the basics of each stroke and incorporating interval training can maximize the benefits of your time in the pool.

Steps to Engage in Swimming Workouts:

- **Warm-Up:** Begin with a light swim or water-based stretching to prepare your muscles and joints for the workout. This could involve swimming a few easy laps using a comfortable stroke, like the freestyle or breaststroke.

- **Drills and Techniques:** Focus on specific techniques to improve your stroke efficiency. This can include drills like catch-up freestyle to enhance arm movement, single-arm drills for balance, or kicking drills to strengthen the legs.

- **Interval Training:** Mix periods of high-intensity swimming with periods of rest or light swimming. For instance, swim one lap at a fast pace, then one lap at a slower pace to recover. This approach boosts cardiovascular fitness and burns more calories.

- **Stroke Variety:** Incorporate different strokes into your workout to engage various muscle groups. A mix of freestyle, backstroke, breaststroke, and butterfly can help develop balanced muscle strength and prevent boredom.

- **Endurance Building:** Gradually increase the distance or duration of continuous swimming. This could involve swimming for a set time, like 20-30 minutes, without stopping, or completing a specific number of laps without a break.

- **Cool Down:** Finish your workout with a slow swim or gentle floating to allow your heart rate to return to normal and to stretch your muscles. This helps prevent muscle soreness and aids recovery.

Tips for Enhancing the Practice:

- 💡 Use pool equipment like kickboards, pull buoys, or fins to target specific muscles and add variety to your workouts.

- 💡 Pay attention to your breathing technique, aiming for rhythmic and controlled breaths to maintain endurance and stability in the water.

- 💡 Consider swimming lessons or joining a swim club to get professional guidance and structured workouts.

Benefits:

Swimming workouts offer comprehensive health benefits, including enhanced lung capacity, improved cardiovascular endurance, increased muscle tone, and better joint mobility. Additionally, swimming is a relaxing and meditative exercise that can help reduce anxiety and promote a sense of well-being.

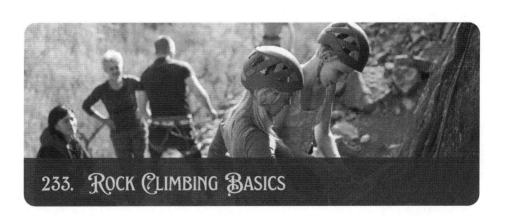

233. ROCK CLIMBING BASICS

Introduction:

Rock climbing is an exhilarating sport that combines physical strength, mental focus, and technical skill to ascend natural or artificial rock formations. Suitable for adventurous spirits of all ages and skill levels, it offers a unique way to connect with nature, challenge oneself, and build confidence through overcoming obstacles.

Basic Technique and Information:

Whether you're bouldering, sport climbing, or traditional climbing, understanding the fundamentals of grip, footwork, and body positioning is essential. Safety is paramount in climbing, so familiarizing yourself with equipment, techniques, and communication is crucial for a successful experience.

Steps to Engage in Rock Climbing:

- **Choose the Right Gear:** Essential equipment includes climbing shoes for better grip, a harness for roped climbing, a helmet for protection, and chalk to improve hand grip. For outdoor climbing, additional gear like ropes, carabiners, and belay devices is necessary.

Learn Basic Techniques:

- **Grip:** Use your fingers, not your whole hand, to hold onto rocks. This conserves energy and provides more control.

- **Footwork:** Focus on placing your feet precisely and using the edges of your climbing shoes to stand on small footholds.

- **Body Positioning:** Keep your body close to the wall to maintain balance. Use your legs to push upwards rather than pulling with your arms.

- **Start with Bouldering:** Bouldering involves climbing short routes (called "problems") without ropes over crash pads. It's a great way to practice techniques and build strength without the complexities of roped climbing.

- **Practice Indoor Climbing:** Many cities have indoor climbing gyms where you can safely learn and practice under the guidance of experienced instructors. This environment is ideal for beginners to build skills and confidence.

- **Understand Belaying:** Learn the basics of belaying — a technique to manage the rope and ensure the safety of the climber. Always practice this with a knowledgeable partner and under professional supervision when starting.

- **Climb with a Partner:** Rock climbing is often a two-person sport, with one climbing and the other belaying. Communication is key, so develop clear signals and dialogue with your partner.

- **Join a Climbing Community:** Engage with local climbing clubs or groups to learn from more experienced climbers, share tips, and enjoy group outings.

Tips for Enhancing the Practice:

- Start with easier routes and gradually progress to more challenging climbs as your skills improve.

- Take rest days to let your muscles recover and prevent injuries.

- Attend workshops or courses to learn advanced techniques and safety protocols.

Benefits:

Rock climbing offers a full-body workout that strengthens muscles, improves flexibility, and enhances cardiovascular fitness. Beyond the physical benefits, it sharpens problem-solving skills, boosts mental resilience, and fosters a sense of achievement and camaraderie among climbers.

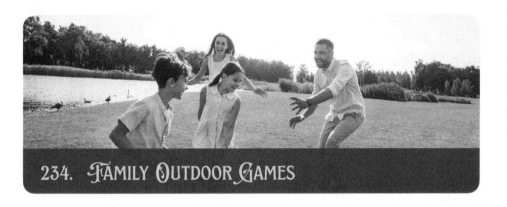

234. FAMILY OUTDOOR GAMES

Introduction:

Family outdoor games are a fantastic way to encourage physical activity, strengthen family bonds, and create lasting memories. These games are suitable for participants of all ages and can be played in backyards, parks, or any spacious outdoor setting. Engaging in these activities promotes teamwork, improves coordination, and offers a fun, interactive way to enjoy the outdoors together.

Basic Technique and Information:

Selecting games that are inclusive, easy to understand, and safe for all participants is important. The key is to choose activities that encourage movement, laughter, and healthy competition without requiring specialized skills or equipment.

Steps to Engage in Family Outdoor Games:

- **Choose Appropriate Games:** Select games that fit the age range and physical abilities of all family members. Consider classics like tag, hide and seek, or new favorites that encourage movement and teamwork.

- **Prepare the Play Area:** Ensure the space is safe, removing any obstacles or hazards. Mark boundaries clearly if needed, using cones, ropes, or natural landmarks.

- **Explain the Rules:** Before starting, clearly explain the rules to everyone. Keep instructions simple and concise to maintain interest and ensure fair play.

- **Rotate Games:** To keep the excitement high and cater to different interests, rotate between several games during your outdoor time.

This variety helps engage all family members and prevents boredom.

- **Encourage Fair Play and Teamwork:** Emphasize the importance of fair play, sportsmanship, and teamwork. Make sure everyone feels included and valued, regardless of the game's outcome.

- **Stay Hydrated and Protected:** Provide plenty of water and encourage regular breaks, especially on hot days. Apply sunscreen and wear hats to protect against the sun.

Popular Family Outdoor Games:

- **Tag:** A simple game where one person is "it" and tries to tag others to make them "it."

- **Hide and Seek:** One person counts while others hide; the seeker then tries to find everyone.

- **Frisbee or Catch:** Toss a frisbee or ball back and forth, adjusting the difficulty based on age and skill.

- **Relay Races:** Set up a course and divide the family into teams for a series of relay challenges.

- **Obstacle Course:** Create a course with stations like jumping, crawling, and balancing tasks.

- **Sack Races:** Use burlap sacks or pillowcases for a hopping race from start to finish.

Benefits:

Family outdoor games enhance physical fitness, improve motor skills, and foster positive emotional and social development. These activities offer a break from screens and technology, encouraging creativity and active play while building a foundation for a healthy lifestyle.

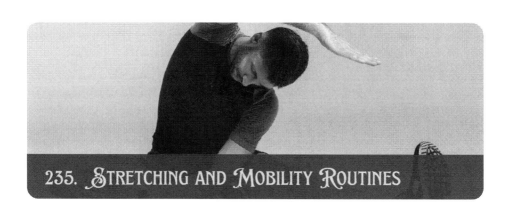

235. STRETCHING AND MOBILITY ROUTINES

Introduction:

Stretching and mobility routines are essential components of a comprehensive fitness plan, designed to enhance flexibility, reduce the risk of injury, and improve overall movement quality. These routines are beneficial for people of all ages and fitness levels, helping to maintain muscle health, alleviate stiffness, and promote better posture and balance.

Basic Technique and Information:

Effective stretching involves both static and dynamic movements. Static stretches involve holding a position for a period to lengthen the muscle, while dynamic stretches involve moving parts of the body gradually to increase range of motion and warm up the muscles.

Steps to Engage in Stretching and Mobility Routines:

- **Warm-Up:** Begin with a light warm-up to raise your body temperature and prepare your muscles for stretching. This could include walking, light jogging, or dynamic movements like arm circles and leg swings.

- **Focus on Major Muscle Groups:** Include stretches that target key areas such as the neck, shoulders, back, hips, legs, and ankles. Ensure each major muscle group is addressed to maintain balance and flexibility.

- **Hold Static Stretches:** For static stretches, hold each position for 15-30 seconds, feeling a gentle but not painful stretch in the muscle. Breathe deeply to help relax the muscles further.

- **Perform Dynamic Stretches:** Dynamic stretches should be controlled and gradual. Move

through the full range of motion of each joint, repeating each movement 8-10 times.

- **Incorporate Mobility Drills:** Include exercises like hip circles, shoulder rolls, and ankle rotations to improve joint mobility and function.

- Cool Down: End your routine with a series of slower, deeper stretches to cool down the body and further improve flexibility. This is also a good time for deep breathing and relaxation.

Tips for Enhancing the Practice:

- Be consistent with your routines to see progressive improvements in flexibility and mobility.

- Listen to your body and avoid pushing into pain. Stretching should feel challenging but not painful.

- Use props like yoga straps, blocks, or foam rollers to help deepen stretches and work on tight areas more effectively.

Benefits:

Regular stretching and mobility routines can lead to improved range of motion, decreased muscle soreness, enhanced performance in physical activities, and better overall health. These practices also contribute to mental relaxation and stress reduction, offering a holistic approach to wellness.

PART 12

Sustainable Living Practices

(236-250)

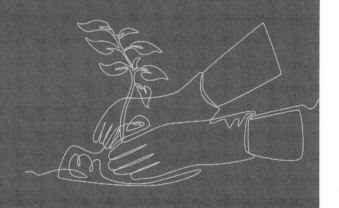

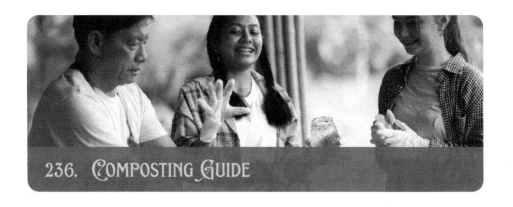

Introduction:

Composting is a key sustainable living practice that transforms organic waste into nutrient-rich soil, reducing landfill use and enhancing garden health. This natural process involves the breakdown of organic materials like food scraps and yard waste by microorganisms, resulting in compost that enriches the soil and supports plant growth.

Basic Technique and Information:

Composting requires a balance of green (nitrogen-rich) and brown (carbon-rich) materials, proper moisture, and air circulation to facilitate the decomposition process. By managing these elements, you can turn kitchen and garden waste into valuable compost.

Steps to Engage in Composting:

- **Choose a Composting Method:** Decide between a compost bin, tumbler, or an open pile. Bins and tumblers are more contained and can speed up the process, while open piles are simpler but require more space and manual turning.

Gather Your Materials:

- Green materials include fruit and vegetable scraps, coffee grounds, fresh grass clippings, and plant trimmings.

- Brown materials consist of dried leaves, straw, sawdust, paper, and cardboard.

- Balance these materials in roughly equal parts to ensure efficient decomposition.

- **Set Up Your Compost Area:** Choose a convenient, shaded spot in your yard. If using a bin or tumbler, ensure it has adequate drainage and ventilation.

- **Layer Your Materials:** Start with a layer of coarse brown materials at the bottom for drainage. Then alternate layers of green and brown materials, adding a little soil or finished compost between layers to introduce microorganisms.

- **Maintain Moisture and Aeration:** Keep the compost moist like a wrung-out sponge. Turn the pile regularly (about once a week) to introduce air, which speeds up the decomposition process.

- **Monitor the Compost:** Check for signs of progress like a decrease in volume and a dark, crumbly texture with an earthy smell. Adjust moisture and aeration as needed.

- **Harvest Your Compost:** Depending on conditions, your compost should be ready in 3-6 months. Finished compost will be dark, crumbly, and free of the original material's odor or appearance.

Tips for Enhancing the Practice:

- ☼ Avoid adding meat, dairy, or oily foods to prevent odors and pests.
- ☼ Cut or shred larger items to speed up the decomposition process.
- ☼ Use a compost thermometer to monitor the pile's temperature and ensure optimal conditions.

Benefits:

Composting reduces waste sent to landfills, decreases greenhouse gas emissions, and enriches the soil, promoting healthier plant growth. It's a simple yet impactful way to contribute to a more sustainable ecosystem and enhance the fertility of your garden.

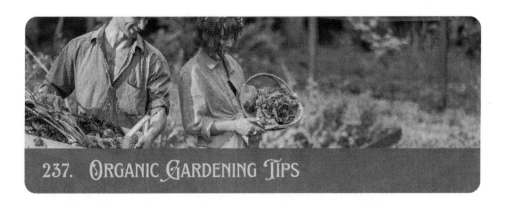

237. ORGANIC GARDENING TIPS

Introduction:

Organic gardening is an environmentally friendly approach to cultivating plants without synthetic chemicals or genetically modified organisms. This method focuses on building healthy soil, using natural pest management, and supporting biodiversity to grow robust, nutritious plants. It's ideal for anyone looking to create a sustainable, toxin-free garden that benefits both the environment and the people who enjoy its produce.

Basic Technique and Information:

Successful organic gardening involves nurturing the ecosystem as a whole, emphasizing soil health, plant diversity, and natural cycles. It requires patience, observation, and a willingness to work with nature rather than trying to control it.

Steps to Engage in Organic Gardening:

- **Build Healthy Soil:** Start with a soil test to understand its nutrient content and pH level. Amend the soil with organic matter like compost, aged manure, or green manure crops to enhance fertility and structure.

- **Choose the Right Plants:** Select plant varieties that are well-suited to your climate, soil type, and sunlight availability. Opt for native plants or heirloom varieties that are naturally more resilient to pests and diseases.

- **Natural Pest Control:** Avoid synthetic pesticides by using integrated pest management (IPM) techniques. Encourage beneficial insects, use barriers or traps, and apply natural remedies like neem oil or insecticidal soap only when necessary.

- **Water Wisely:** Use drip irrigation or soaker hoses to deliver water directly to the roots, minimizing waste and reducing the likelihood of fungal diseases. Water in the early morning to give plants time to dry out during the day.

- **Crop Rotation and Companion Planting:** Rotate crops annually to prevent soil nutrient depletion and break pest and disease cycles. Use companion planting to naturally repel pests and enhance plant growth. For example, plant marigolds near tomatoes to deter nematodes.

- **Mulching:** Apply organic mulch like straw, leaves, or wood chips around your plants to conserve moisture, suppress weeds, and add nutrients to the soil as it decomposes.

- **Regular Observation and Maintenance:** Regularly inspect your garden for signs of pests or diseases. Promptly remove affected plant parts or use organic treatments to manage issues.

Tips for Enhancing the Practice:

- Keep a garden journal to track what works and what doesn't, helping you plan and improve each season.

- Incorporate permaculture principles for a more holistic approach to sustainability.

- Engage with local organic gardening groups or workshops to learn from others and share your experiences.

Benefits:

Organic gardening enhances the health of the soil and the biodiversity of your garden, leading to stronger, more resilient plants. It reduces your exposure to harmful chemicals, ensures healthier food, and contributes to a healthier environment by supporting pollinators and wildlife.

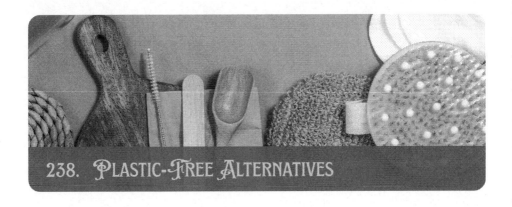

238. PLASTIC-FREE ALTERNATIVES

Introduction:

Reducing plastic usage is crucial for environmental conservation and health. Plastic pollution is a significant global issue affecting wildlife, ecosystems, and human health due to its long-lasting impact and toxicity. By choosing plastic-free alternatives, individuals can contribute to reducing waste, conserving resources, and promoting a sustainable lifestyle.

Basic Technique and Information:

Switching to plastic-free alternatives involves identifying areas in daily life where plastic is commonly used and replacing those items with sustainable, reusable, or biodegradable options. This transition not only minimizes waste but also supports a circular economy.

Steps to Engage in Using Plastic-Free Alternatives:

- **Assess Your Plastic Use:** Identify the most common plastic items in your household, such as bags, bottles, packaging, and personal care products. Note which items you can easily replace with sustainable alternatives.

- **Choose Reusable Bags and Containers:** Replace plastic shopping bags with cloth or canvas bags. Use glass or stainless steel containers for food storage instead of plastic containers or wrap.

- **Opt for Bulk and Unpackaged Goods:** Shop for food and household items in bulk to avoid single-use plastic packaging. Bring your own containers and bags to bulk stores, farmers' markets, and even some supermarkets.

- **Switch to Sustainable Personal Care:** Replace plastic toothbrushes with bamboo ones, use bar soaps instead of bottled, and opt for reusable or biodegradable personal care items like cotton swabs and menstrual products.

- **Refuse Single-Use Plastics:** Avoid disposable plastic items like straws, cutlery, and plates. Carry your own reusable versions, or choose products made from bamboo, wood, or stainless steel.

- **Support Plastic-Free Brands:** Purchase from companies that prioritize plastic-free packaging and sustainable practices. This encourages more businesses to adopt environmentally friendly methods.

- **Educate and Advocate:** Share your knowledge and experiences with family and friends. Support local and global initiatives that aim to reduce plastic pollution and promote sustainable living.

Tips for Enhancing the Practice:

- Start gradually to make the transition manageable and sustainable.

- Repair and repurpose items when possible instead of buying new.

- Stay informed about new sustainable products and technologies that can further reduce plastic use.

Benefits:

Choosing plastic-free alternatives significantly reduces waste and environmental impact, conserving resources and protecting wildlife. It also reduces exposure to harmful chemicals found in plastics, contributing to better health and a cleaner environment for future generations.

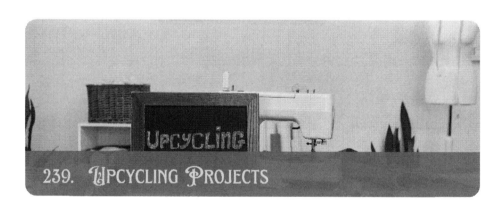

239. UPCYCLING PROJECTS

Introduction:

Upcycling is the creative process of transforming by-products, waste materials, or unwanted items into new materials or products of higher quality or value. This practice not only reduces waste and conserves resources but also encourages creativity and innovation. Upcycling can turn everyday objects into functional, artistic, or decorative items, adding unique character and sustainability to your environment.

Basic Technique and Information:

To successfully engage in upcycling, start by identifying materials that are commonly discarded and envisioning new uses for them. This involves assessing the potential of items before throwing them away and considering how they can be repurposed or enhanced.

Steps to Engage in Upcycling Projects:

- **Identify Potential Items:** Look around your home for items that are no longer used or are destined for the trash. Common candidates include old furniture, clothing, containers, and construction materials.

- **Gather Materials and Tools:** Depending on the project, you may need basic hand tools, paint, glue, or other crafting supplies. Make sure you have everything you need before starting your project.

- **Plan Your Project:** Sketch out your ideas or create a mood board. Determine the steps needed to transform the item and any additional materials or alterations required.

- **Clean and Prepare the Item:** Ensure the item is clean and free of any debris or residue. Sand, prime, or treat surfaces as needed to prepare them for transformation.

- **Execute the Transformation:** Follow your plan to alter, decorate, or rebuild the item. This could involve painting, sewing, cutting, assembling, or other crafting techniques.

- **Add Finishing Touches:** Once the main work is done, add any final details like varnish, decorative elements, or protective coatings to ensure the item's durability and enhance its appearance.

- **Use and Display Your Upcycled Item:** Place or use the upcycled item in its intended new role. This could be as home decor, a functional piece of furniture, clothing, or even as a gift.

Tips for Enhancing the Practice:

- Stay inspired by following upcycling blogs, social media accounts, or joining community groups.

- Experiment with different materials and techniques to continually develop your skills.

- Teach others about upcycling by hosting workshops or sharing your projects online.

Benefits:

Upcycling promotes environmental sustainability by reducing waste and the need for new materials. It fosters creativity and can lead to personalized and meaningful items that reflect individual style and values. Additionally, upcycling can be a cost-effective way to refresh your living space and wardrobe without the environmental impact of purchasing new items.

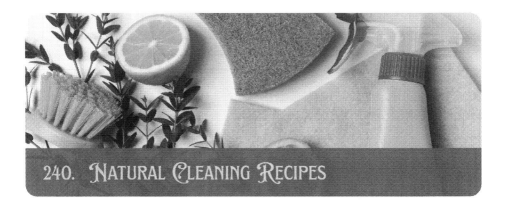

Introduction:

Natural cleaning recipes offer an eco-friendly and health-conscious alternative to commercial cleaning products, which often contain harsh chemicals. By using simple, natural ingredients, you can create effective cleaning solutions that are safe for your family, pets, and the environment. These recipes are not only gentle but also cost-effective and easy to make with common household items.

Basic Technique and Information:

The foundation of natural cleaning involves a few key ingredients like vinegar, baking soda, lemon, and essential oils. These ingredients have natural antibacterial, antifungal, and deodorizing properties, making them powerful allies in maintaining a clean and healthy home.

Steps to Engage in Making Natural Cleaning Recipes:

All-Purpose Cleaner:

- **Ingredients:** 1 part white vinegar, 1 part water, a few drops of essential oil (like lemon, tea tree, or lavender for scent and additional antibacterial properties).

- **Preparation:** Mix ingredients in a spray bottle. Shake well before each use. This cleaner is excellent for countertops, appliances, and most surfaces but should be avoided on marble and granite as vinegar can etch natural stone.

Glass Cleaner:

- **Ingredients:** ¼ cup white vinegar, ¼ cup rubbing alcohol, 1 tablespoon cornstarch, 2 cups water, and a few drops of essential oil for scent.

- **Preparation:** Combine all ingredients in a spray bottle and shake well to dissolve the cornstarch. Use this solution with a microfiber cloth for streak-free windows and mirrors.

Scrubbing Paste for Tough Grime:

- **Ingredients:** ½ cup baking soda, a few tablespoons of water to make a paste, and 10 drops of essential oil (optional).

- **Preparation:** Mix baking soda with water until it forms a paste. Use a sponge or brush to scrub sinks, tubs, and tiles. Rinse well with water.

Carpet Deodorizer:

- **Ingredients:** 1 cup baking soda, 10-20 drops of essential oil (like lavender or eucalyptus).
- **Preparation:** Mix the baking soda and essential oils. Sprinkle on carpets, let sit for at least 15 minutes or overnight, then vacuum up. This helps refresh and deodorize the carpets.

Wood Polish:

- **Ingredients:** ¼ cup olive oil, ¼ cup white vinegar, and 10 drops of lemon essential oil.
- **Preparation:** Mix the ingredients in a jar or bottle. Apply with a soft cloth to wood surfaces, then buff with a clean, dry cloth for a natural shine.

Tips for Enhancing the Practice:

- ⚲ Label your homemade cleaners clearly and store them safely, especially away from children and pets.
- ⚲ Test any new cleaner on a small, inconspicuous area first to ensure it does not damage the surface.
- ⚲ Reuse old cleaning product bottles or invest in durable glass spray bottles for long-term use.

Benefits:

Using natural cleaning recipes reduces exposure to toxic chemicals, minimizes environmental impact, and can alleviate allergies or sensitivities triggered by commercial cleaners. These homemade solutions are effective, sustainable, and contribute to a healthier living environment.

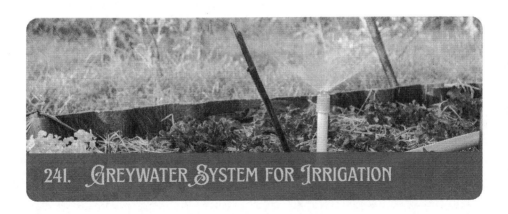

241. GREYWATER SYSTEM FOR IRRIGATION

Introduction:

A greywater system for irrigation is an eco-friendly approach to water management that reuses water from household sources like sinks, showers, and washing machines to irrigate gardens and landscapes. This method conserves water, reduces wastewater treatment demand, and provides a sustainable source of irrigation that is rich in nutrients beneficial for plant growth.

Basic Technique and Information:

Greywater systems vary in complexity from simple bucketing to advanced plumbing systems. The key is to use greywater safely and effectively without introducing harmful chemicals into your garden. It's essential to ensure that the water used doesn't contain harsh detergents, bleach, or other substances harmful to plants and soil life.

Steps to Engage in Using a Greywater System for Irrigation:

- **Identify Suitable Greywater Sources:** Common sources include bath, shower, sink, and laundry water. Ensure that the detergents and soaps used are biodegradable and free from harmful chemicals.

- **Design Your System:** Decide between a direct use system, where greywater is used immediately, or a storage system. Simple systems can involve a hose leading from a washing machine to the garden. More complex systems may include filters, pumps, and storage tanks.

- **Install Necessary Components:** For a basic system, adapt the plumbing to divert greywater from the source to the garden. For more complex systems, install a three-way valve to switch between the sewer and the greywater system, filters to remove lint and debris, and a pump if elevation changes require it.

- **Use Appropriate Irrigation Methods:** Drip irrigation or subsurface irrigation are the best methods to use with greywater, as they reduce the risk of human contact and prevent the spread of pathogens.

- **Monitor Soil and Plant Health:** Regularly check soil moisture and nutrient levels to avoid over-irrigation and nutrient imbalances. Adjust your greywater usage based on the needs of your plants and the condition of your soil.

- **Maintain the System:** Clean filters, check pipes and hoses for clogs, and ensure all parts are functioning correctly to prevent backups and leaks.

Tips for Enhancing the Practice:

- Educate yourself on local regulations regarding greywater use, as some areas have specific guidelines or restrictions.

- Use low-phosphate, salt-free, and biodegradable cleaning products to protect your plants and soil.

- Regularly rotate the areas irrigated with greywater to prevent salt and nutrient buildup in the soil.

Benefits:

Using a greywater system for irrigation conserves potable water, reduces the burden on municipal water treatment facilities, and lowers water bills. It also recycles nutrients back into the garden, supporting plant health and promoting a sustainable gardening practice that aligns with ecological principles.

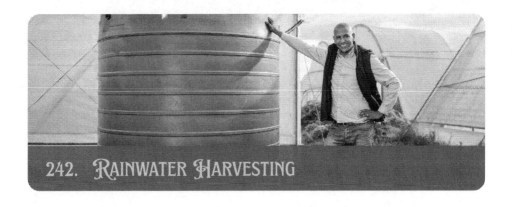

Introduction:

Rainwater harvesting is a sustainable practice of collecting and storing rainwater from rooftops, land surfaces, or rock catchments for later use. This approach helps conserve water, reduce dependence on municipal water systems, and mitigate flooding and erosion. It's particularly beneficial in areas with water scarcity or for anyone looking to reduce their environmental footprint and water bills.

Basic Technique and Information:

The process of rainwater harvesting involves capturing rainwater, filtering it to remove debris, and storing it in tanks or barrels. The stored water can be used for irrigation, washing, flushing toilets, and with proper treatment, even for drinking.

Steps to Engage in Rainwater Harvesting:

- **Assess Your Needs and Local Regulations:** Determine how much water you need and can realistically collect based on your roof area and local rainfall patterns. Also, check local regulations regarding rainwater harvesting, as some areas have specific guidelines or restrictions.

- **Choose a Catchment Area:** Typically, the roof is used as the catchment area. Ensure it's made of suitable materials that don't leach harmful chemicals into the water.

- **Install Gutters and Downspouts:** Ensure your roofing system has gutters and downspouts in good condition to direct rainwater efficiently. Fit these with mesh guards to keep out leaves and debris.

- **Set Up a Filtration System:** Before storing, filter the water to remove particles and debris. Simple systems use a first-flush diverter that discards the initial water which carries most of the debris.

- **Choose Appropriate Storage:** Use barrels or tanks to store the harvested water. These should be made of food-grade material if the water is intended for consumption. Dark, opaque containers help prevent algae growth.

- **Connect to a Usage System:** Depending on your use, connect the storage system to your irrigation system, toilets, or washing machines. For garden use, a simple spigot or hose connection at the bottom of the barrel may suffice.

- **Maintain the System:** Regularly clean gutters, inspect and clean filters, and check storage containers for leaks or contamination. Ensure the system is winterized if necessary to prevent freezing damage.

Tips for Enhancing the Practice:

- Consider a larger system with underground tanks for long-term storage and a broader range of uses.

- Use gravity to your advantage by placing tanks higher than the point of use to reduce the need for pumping.

- Engage in community or group initiatives to learn from others and share experiences in rainwater harvesting.

Benefits:

Rainwater harvesting reduces the demand on municipal water supplies, lowers water bills, and provides a source of soft, low-sodium water ideal for gardens and some household uses. It helps mitigate flooding and erosion around buildings and contributes to sustainable water management in the community.

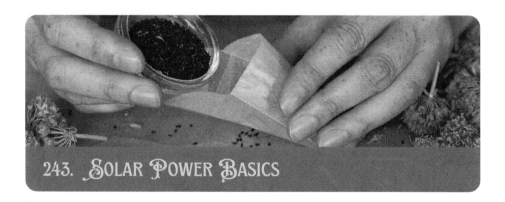

243. Solar Power Basics

Introduction:

Solar power harnesses the sun's energy to generate electricity, providing a clean, renewable source that reduces reliance on fossil fuels and decreases greenhouse gas emissions. It's an increasingly popular choice for homeowners and businesses looking to reduce their energy costs and environmental impact.

Basic Technique and Information:

Solar power systems convert sunlight into electricity using photovoltaic (PV) panels or mirrors that concentrate solar radiation. These systems can be installed on rooftops or in large-scale solar farms and can include battery storage to provide power during non-sunny periods.

Steps to Engage in Solar Power Use:

- **Assess Your Energy Needs:** Calculate your average electricity usage to determine how many solar panels you need. Look at your utility bills to get a sense of your monthly and annual consumption.

- **Evaluate Your Site:** Check the orientation and tilt of your roof or available land. South-facing roofs with little to no shade are ideal for maximizing solar energy production in the Northern Hemisphere.

- **Choose the Right Solar Panels:** There are various types of solar panels available, including monocrystalline, polycrystalline, and thin-film. Each has different efficiencies and costs, so choose based on your budget and space constraints.

- **Consider Inverters:** Solar panels produce direct current (DC), but homes use alternating current (AC). Inverters convert DC into AC. Choose between string inverters, which connect a series of panels, or microinverters, which are attached to each panel for individual optimization.

- **Installation:** Engage a professional installer certified in solar panel installation. The process includes mounting the panels, connecting the

electrical systems, and integrating with the grid if applicable.

- **Apply for Incentives:** Many regions offer tax incentives, rebates, or grants for installing solar power systems. Research local programs to reduce initial costs and improve your return on investment.

- **Maintenance and Monitoring:** Solar panels require minimal maintenance, mainly keeping them clean and free of debris. Monitoring systems can track energy production and help detect any issues.

Tips for Enhancing the Practice:

- Consider adding battery storage to use your solar power during nighttime or cloudy days.

- Regularly clean your panels to maintain their efficiency, especially after dust storms or snow.

- Stay informed about technological advances in solar energy to potentially upgrade components in the future.

Benefits:

Using solar power significantly reduces electricity bills and provides a stable energy price over time. It increases the value of your property and contributes to a sustainable future by reducing carbon emissions and promoting energy independence.

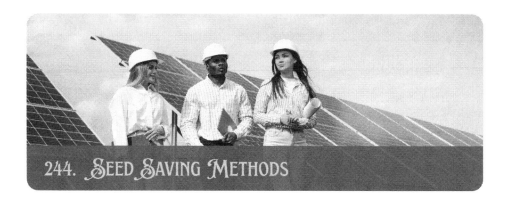

Introduction:

Seed saving is the practice of collecting and preserving seeds from plants for future planting. This age-old tradition helps maintain biodiversity, saves money, and ensures the continuation of plant varieties that have adapted to local conditions. It's an essential part of sustainable gardening, allowing gardeners to become more self-reliant and fostering a deeper connection with the life cycle of plants.

Basic Technique and Information:

Effective seed saving involves selecting healthy plants, proper timing, and appropriate methods for drying and storing seeds. Different plants require different approaches, but the basic principles are the same: ensure the seeds are mature, dry them carefully, and store them in conditions that preserve their viability.

Steps to Engage in Seed Saving:

- **Select the Right Plants:** Choose healthy, vigorous plants that show desirable traits, such as disease resistance, productivity, or excellent flavor. It's best to save seeds from open-pollinated or heirloom varieties as they produce true-to-type plants, unlike hybrid varieties.

- **Harvest Seeds at the Right Time:** Wait until the seeds are fully mature before harvesting. For many vegetables and flowers, this means allowing pods, fruits, or heads to dry on the plant until they brown or the seeds rattle inside.

- **Dry the Seeds:** Carefully remove the seeds from the plant and spread them out on a clean, dry surface out of direct sunlight. Allow them to dry completely, which can take several days to a few weeks depending on the seed size and humidity.

- **Clean the Seeds:** Once dry, separate the seeds from any chaff, husks, or other plant materials. For larger seeds, you can use a sieve or gently blow to remove debris. For smaller seeds, careful hand-picking might be necessary.

- **Test for Viability:** To ensure the seeds are worth saving, you can perform a simple germination test by placing a few seeds between moist paper towels in a warm area. Check for germination after a few days to a week.

- **Label and Store:** Place the dried seeds in labeled envelopes, jars, or containers. Include the plant type, variety, and date of harvest. Store them in a cool, dark, and dry place. A refrigerator is often ideal, especially if you're saving seeds for more than one season.

Tips for Enhancing the Practice:

💡 Participate in seed swaps or local gardening clubs to share seeds and experiences.

💡 Keep a garden journal to record details about the plants you save seeds from, including their performance and any specific care they required.

💡 Use silica gel packets in storage containers to help maintain dryness and prolong seed viability.

Benefits:

Seed saving encourages genetic diversity, reduces dependency on commercial seed suppliers, and allows gardeners to develop plant varieties uniquely suited to their local environment. It's an economical way to garden, reduces waste, and can be a rewarding educational activity for all ages.

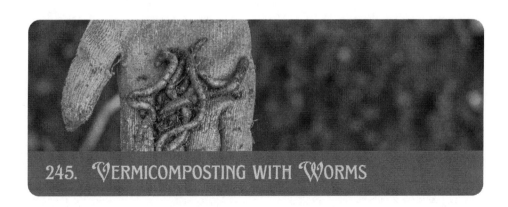

245. VERMICOMPOSTING WITH WORMS

Introduction:

Vermicomposting is the process of using worms, primarily red wigglers, to convert organic waste into nutrient-rich compost. This method is an efficient, environmentally friendly way to recycle kitchen scraps, paper waste, and other biodegradable materials into valuable soil amendment known as worm castings.

Ideal for both indoor and outdoor settings, vermicomposting accelerates the composting process while minimizing odor and space requirements.

Basic Technique and Information:

To start vermicomposting, you need a suitable bin, bedding, and the right type of worms. The process relies on the natural activity of worms to break down organic matter, turning it into compost rich in nutrients that are easily absorbed by plants.

Steps to Engage in Vermicomposting:

- **Set Up Your Worm Bin:** Choose or build a worm bin that is shallow and wide, as worms are surface feeders. The bin should have good ventilation and drainage to prevent excess moisture and odors.

- **Prepare the Bedding:** Use shredded newspaper, cardboard, coir, or aged compost as bedding. Moisten the bedding so it's damp but not soggy, providing a comfortable environment for the worms.

- **Add the Worms:** Red wigglers (Eisenia fetida) are the most common worms used for vermicomposting. Introduce a sufficient quantity to your bin based on its size — typically, a pound of worms (about 1,000 worms) for each square foot of surface area.

- **Feed Your Worms:** Start by adding small amounts of kitchen scraps like fruit and vegetable peelings, coffee grounds, and eggshells. Avoid

meat, dairy, and oily foods, which can attract pests and cause odors. Burry the food under the bedding to prevent fruit flies and other insects.

- **Maintain the Bin:** Keep the bedding damp and the bin at a moderate temperature (between 55-77°F or 13-25°C). Turn or fluff the bedding occasionally to prevent compaction and to ensure oxygen flow.

- **Harvest the Castings:** After 3-6 months, the worms will have converted much of the bedding and food waste into castings. To harvest, move all the contents to one side of the bin and add fresh bedding and food to the other side. Over a few weeks, the worms will migrate to the fresh food, allowing you to collect the castings from the other side.

- **Use the Worm Castings:** Mix the castings into your garden soil or use them as top dressing for houseplants. Worm castings are an excellent, balanced fertilizer that can significantly enhance plant health.

Tips for Enhancing the Practice:

- Keep the worm bin out of direct sunlight and protect it from extreme temperatures to keep the worms healthy.

- Chop food waste into small pieces to speed up the decomposition process.

- Regularly check for and manage moisture levels in the bin to prevent overly wet or dry conditions, which can stress the worms.

Vermicomposting reduces household waste, lowers your carbon footprint, and produces high-quality compost full of beneficial microorganisms and nutrients. It's a simple, cost-effective way to improve soil health and support sustainable gardening practices.

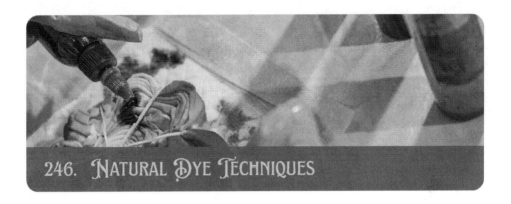

246. NATURAL DYE TECHNIQUES

Introduction:

Natural dye techniques involve using plants, minerals, and other natural sources to color fabric, yarn, and other materials. This ancient art offers a sustainable alternative to synthetic dyes, reducing harmful environmental impacts and providing a unique, organic aesthetic. Natural dyes produce vibrant, rich colors that are deeply connected to the local environment and cultural traditions.

Basic Technique and Information:

To achieve successful natural dyeing, you need to understand the properties of different natural materials, proper mordant use to fix the color, and the techniques for applying dye to fabric or yarn. The process can vary based on the material being dyed and the desired color outcome.

Steps to Engage in Natural Dye Techniques:

- **Choose Your Dye Material:** Common natural dye sources include onion skins, berries, leaves, bark, roots, and flowers. Each material yields different colors, and the season and location can affect the intensity.

- **Prepare the Fabric or Yarn:** Before dyeing, clean the material to remove any oils, dirt, or chemicals that could affect dye uptake. Known as scouring, this process ensures that the fabric or yarn is ready to absorb the dye evenly.

- **Use a Mordant:** A mordant is a substance that fixes dye to the fabric, ensuring colorfastness. Common mordants include alum, iron, and vinegar. Choose your mordant based on the fabric type and the desired color strength.

- **Extract the Dye:** Place the dye material in a large pot of water and slowly bring it to a simmer. The length of time will vary depending on the material, but generally, an hour of simmering will release the dye. Strain the plant material from the liquid to obtain the dye bath.

- **Dye the Material:** Wet the fabric or yarn and immerse it in the dye bath. Heat gently and maintain a simmer, allowing the material to absorb the color. This can take from 30 minutes to several hours, depending on the desired depth of color.

- **Rinse and Dry:** Once the desired color is achieved, remove the material and rinse it in cool water until the water runs clear. Hang the dyed fabric or yarn to dry away from direct sunlight to prevent fading.

Tips for Enhancing the Practice:

- Experiment with different mordants and dye materials to discover unique color combinations and effects.

- Overdyeing (dyeing the material multiple times with different colors) can create complex, layered colors.

- Document your process, including the materials and ratios used, to replicate successful recipes or tweak future projects.

Benefits:

Natural dyeing is environmentally friendly and often hypoallergenic, making it suitable for sensitive skin. It connects crafters with nature and tradition, offering a creative outlet that is both artistic and ecological. The practice fosters a deeper appreciation for the natural world and the subtle beauty of its colors.

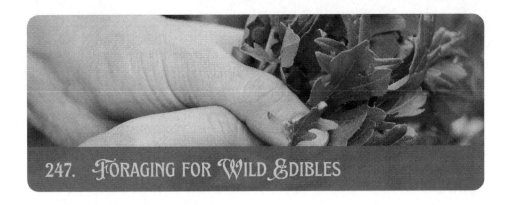

247. FORAGING FOR WILD EDIBLES

Introduction:

Foraging for wild edibles is a practice that involves searching for and harvesting food resources like plants, mushrooms, berries, and nuts from their natural, often wild, habitats. This activity connects individuals with nature, providing a sustainable way to source fresh, nutritious, and often unique flavors while encouraging a deeper understanding of local ecosystems.

Basic Technique and Information:

Successful foraging requires knowledge of plant identification, understanding the best seasons for harvesting, and awareness of local laws and guidelines. Safety is paramount to avoid poisonous species and ensure sustainable harvesting practices.

Steps to Engage in Foraging for Wild Edibles:

- **Learn About Local Flora:** Before foraging, educate yourself about the edible plants and mushrooms in your area. Use field guides, apps, or join local foraging tours or workshops led by experts to accurately identify safe and edible species.

- **Understand the Laws and Ethics:** Check local regulations regarding foraging in public lands, parks, and other areas. Practice ethical foraging by taking only what you need, leaving enough for wildlife and other foragers, and never uprooting plants.

- **Prepare for the Field:** Bring essentials like a good field guide, a knife or scissors for harvesting, bags or baskets for collecting, gloves, and appropriate clothing for protection against the elements and insects.

- **Harvest Responsibly:** When you find an edible plant or mushroom, verify its identity using multiple sources. Harvest in a way that allows the plant to continue growing, such as by cutting leaves or stems rather than pulling up roots unless the entire plant is edible and abundant.

- **Process and Store Properly:** Clean and process your foraged items as soon as possible. Some items may require cooking or other preparation to be safe to eat. Learn the best ways to preserve or cook each type of wild edible for maximum flavor and safety.

- **Cook with Wild Edibles:** Incorporate foraged foods into your meals thoughtfully. Wild herbs, greens, berries, and mushrooms can enhance a variety of dishes, adding unique flavors and nutrients.

Tips for Enhancing the Practice:

☞ Start with easily recognizable and common edibles to build confidence and knowledge.

☞ Keep a foraging journal to record locations, dates, and experiences with different plants and mushrooms.

☞ Share your foraging adventures with others to foster community learning and appreciation for local ecosystems.

Benefits:

Foraging promotes physical activity and outdoor time, contributing to overall health and wellness. It offers an opportunity to learn about and contribute to local biodiversity while enjoying fresh, seasonal, and organic foods. Foraging also fosters a sense of self-sufficiency and deepens one's connection to the environment.

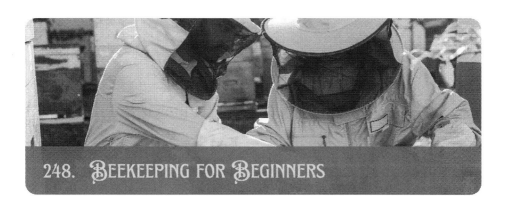

248. BEEKEEPING FOR BEGINNERS

Introduction:

Beekeeping, or apiculture, is the practice of managing honeybee colonies, typically in man-made hives, to produce honey, beeswax, and other products, as well as to pollinate crops and support the health of the local ecosystem. For beginners, beekeeping offers a fascinating insight into the natural world, providing both environmental benefits and the joy of producing your own honey.

Basic Technique and Information:

Successful beekeeping requires understanding bee behavior, hive management, and the seasonal needs of bees. Beginners should start with the basics of hive setup, bee biology, and routine maintenance to ensure the health and productivity of their colonies.

Steps to Engage in Beekeeping for Beginners:

- **Educate Yourself:** Before starting, learn about bee behavior, life cycles, and beekeeping practices. Attend workshops, read books, or join a local beekeeping club to gain knowledge and support.

- **Choose the Right Equipment:** Basic beekeeping equipment includes a hive (such as Langstroth or top-bar), a bee suit with gloves and veil, a smoker, and hive tools. Start with at least one hive to learn the ropes.

- **Obtain Your Bees:** Purchase bees from a reputable supplier. You can start with a nucleus colony (a small, established colony) or a package of bees (a queen and workers without comb). Spring is the best time to establish a new hive.

- **Set Up Your Hive:** Choose a suitable location for your hive — a sunny spot with some shade, protection from strong winds, and easy access for maintenance. Ensure it's away from high traffic areas and secure against predators.

- **Install the Bees:** Carefully introduce the bees to the hive. If using a package, place the queen in her cage first, then gently shake the worker bees into the hive. If using a nucleus, transfer the frames directly into your hive.

- **Monitor and Maintain the Hive:** Regularly inspect the hive every 7-10 days during active seasons to check for the health of the queen, signs of disease, and sufficient space for honey and brood. Use the smoker to calm the bees before inspections.

- **Manage Pests and Diseases:** Learn to identify and treat common bee pests and diseases, such as varroa mites and American foulbrood. Use integrated pest management strategies to minimize chemical use.

- **Harvest Honey Responsibly:** Once your bees have filled the combs and capped the cells with wax, you can harvest honey. Use an extractor or crush and strain methods, ensuring you leave enough honey for the bees to survive winter.

Tips for Enhancing the Practice:

- Keep detailed records of your beekeeping activities to track the health and productivity of your hive.

- Engage with the beekeeping community for advice and to stay updated on best practices.

- Plant a bee-friendly garden with a variety of flowers that bloom throughout the seasons to support your bees.

Benefits:

Beekeeping promotes biodiversity, supports pollination for gardens and local agriculture, and yields natural products like honey and beeswax. It's also a rewarding hobby that fosters a deeper connection with nature and provides educational opportunities for all ages.

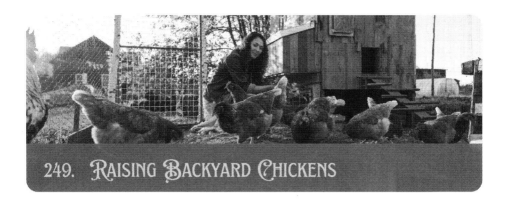

249. RAISING BACKYARD CHICKENS

Introduction:

Raising backyard chickens has become a popular practice for many, offering a sustainable source of fresh eggs, natural pest control, and the joy of caring for these lively creatures. It's an engaging way to connect with food sources, teach responsibility, and enjoy the companionship of chickens in a suburban or rural setting.

Basic Technique and Information:

Successful chicken keeping requires understanding the needs of chickens, including shelter, food, water, and protection from predators. Ensuring the health and happiness of your flock involves regular care, attention, and some basic knowledge of poultry management.

Steps to Engage in Raising Backyard Chickens:

- **Check Local Regulations:** Before getting chickens, ensure your local zoning laws permit them. Some areas have restrictions on the number of chickens you can keep or prohibit roosters due to noise concerns.

- **Choose Your Chickens:** Decide on breeds based on your climate, the egg production you desire, and temperament. Popular breeds for beginners include Buff Orpingtons, Rhode Island Reds, and Plymouth Rocks due to their hardiness and friendly nature.

- **Prepare the Coop:** Your chickens need a secure coop to protect them from weather and predators. The coop should have nesting boxes for laying eggs, perches for sleeping, and enough space for each chicken to move comfortably (typically 3-4 square feet per chicken inside the coop).

- **Set Up an Outdoor Run:** Provide a fenced outdoor area where chickens can forage, dust bathe, and exercise. Ensure the run is secure from predators, with a wire mesh buried around the perimeter to prevent digging.

- **Provide Proper Nutrition:** Feed your chickens a balanced diet of commercial poultry feed supplemented with grains, greens, and occasional treats like fruits or mealworms. Ensure they have continuous access to fresh water.

- **Regular Health Checks and Care:** Monitor your chickens for signs of illness or distress, such as changes in eating habits, abnormal droppings, or lethargy. Keep the coop clean to prevent disease and parasites.

- **Collect Eggs Regularly:** Chickens can start laying eggs as early as 5-6 months old. Collect eggs daily to ensure freshness and encourage continued laying.

- **Learn About Chicken Behavior:** Understanding the social dynamics of your flock will help in managing them better. Chickens establish a "pecking order," and occasional squabbles are normal, but ensure there is no persistent bullying.

Tips for Enhancing the Practice:

- Engage with local chicken-keeping communities or online forums for support and advice.

- Plant a chicken-friendly garden with herbs and plants that chickens enjoy and that can boost their health.

- Consider rotational grazing if you have space, to allow chickens to access fresh grass and naturally fertilize different areas.

Benefits:

Raising backyard chickens reduces reliance on store-bought eggs, provides an opportunity to teach children about animal care and food sources, and contributes to a sustainable household ecosystem. Chickens also help with pest control and provide rich manure that can be composted and used in gardens.

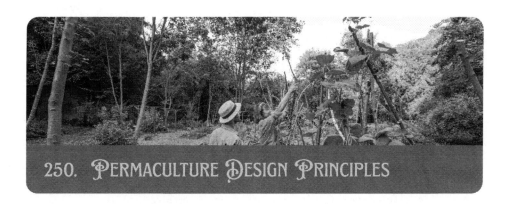

250. PERMACULTURE DESIGN PRINCIPLES

Introduction:

Permaculture is a holistic approach to designing sustainable and self-sufficient agricultural systems that mimic the patterns and relationships found in natural ecosystems. It integrates land, resources, people, and the environment through mutually beneficial synergies, emphasizing sustainability, resilience, and the harmonious integration of human activities with the natural world.

Basic Technique and Information:

Permaculture design is guided by ethical principles — care for the earth, care for people, and fair share — and utilizes a set of design principles derived from the observation of natural systems. These principles help create landscapes that are both productive and sustainable, reducing waste, conserving resources, and supporting a diversity of life.

Steps to Engage in Permaculture Design:

- **Observe and Interact:** Spend time observing the land and its patterns throughout the seasons. Understand the flow of water, sunlight, wind, and how local wildlife interacts with the area. This helps inform your design decisions to work with nature rather than against it.

- **Catch and Store Energy:** Use resources when they are abundant to meet needs during scarcity. This can be done by collecting rainwater, storing solar energy, or creating biomass through composting and mulching.

- **Obtain a Yield:** Ensure that your design produces useful and valuable outputs, like food, fiber, or energy, to provide for the needs of people and wildlife. Diversify your crops and

livestock to create resilience and reduce risk.

- **Apply Self-Regulation and Accept Feedback:** Regularly assess and adapt your system based on its performance. Learn from both successes and failures to evolve and improve the design over time.

- **Use and Value Renewable Resources:** Maximize the use of renewable resources to reduce dependency on non-renewable inputs. This includes growing food, using natural building materials, and utilizing renewable energy sources.

- **Produce No Waste:** Design systems that recycle waste back into the system, turning outputs from one element into inputs for another. Compost organic waste, reuse greywater, and recycle nutrients within the system.

- **Design from Patterns to Details:** Start with broad landscape patterns (such as water flow, wind patterns, and sunlight exposure) and then move to specific details (like plant selection and placement). This ensures coherence and synergy in the overall design.

- **Integrate Rather than Segregate:** Place elements in the design so they can work together and support each other. For example, plant nitrogen-fixing legumes near nutrient-hungry crops, or use chickens to help manage pests and fertilize the soil.

- **Use Small and Slow Solutions:** Start with small-scale, manageable interventions that can grow and evolve over time. This allows for better adaptation and reduces the risk of large-scale failures.

- **Use and Value Diversity:** Include a variety of species and elements in your design to create a resilient ecosystem. Diversity in plants, animals, and microorganisms helps stabilize the system and adapt to changing conditions.

- **Use Edges and Value the Marginal:** The interface between different elements, like the edge of a forest and a field, often holds the most diversity and productivity. Design to maximize these edge spaces in your landscape.

- **Creatively Use and Respond to Change:** View change as an opportunity, not a threat. Be flexible in your approach and ready to adapt your design to evolving conditions and new knowledge.

Benefits:

Permaculture design reduces ecological footprints by creating sustainable and productive landscapes. It enhances biodiversity, improves soil health, and creates a more resilient local ecosystem. By fostering a deeper connection with the environment, permaculture also contributes to community well-being and a more sustainable future.

PART 13

Glossary of 25 Common Herbs And Their Uses

(251-275)

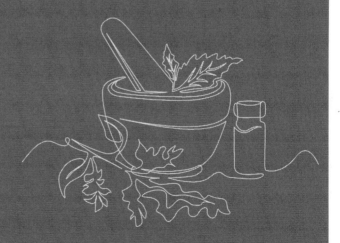

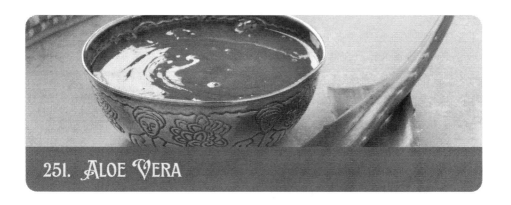

251. ALOE VERA

Introduction:

Aloe Vera is a succulent plant known for its thick, fleshy leaves filled with a clear gel. This plant has been used for thousands of years for its medicinal properties, particularly in skincare, wound healing, and as a dietary supplement. Its soothing, moisturizing, and healing attributes make it a staple in many traditional and modern health and beauty routines.

Basic Uses and Information:

The gel inside Aloe Vera leaves is rich in vitamins, minerals, enzymes, and amino acids, which contribute to its many health benefits. It is commonly applied topically to soothe burns, cuts, and other skin irritations and can also be consumed in juice form for digestive and immune system support.

Detailed Uses of Aloe Vera:

Skin Care:

- **Burn Relief:** Aloe Vera gel is well-known for its ability to soothe and heal sunburns and minor burns. Its anti-inflammatory and cooling properties provide immediate relief.

- **Moisturizing:** The gel is an excellent moisturizer for the skin, especially for dry or sensitive skin types. It helps to lock in moisture without leaving a greasy residue.

- **Acne Treatment:** Due to its antimicrobial and anti-inflammatory properties, Aloe Vera is effective in treating acne. It can reduce redness and inflammation and promote faster healing of acne scars.

Wound Healing:

- The gel accelerates the healing process of cuts and scrapes by boosting collagen production and fighting bacteria.

Digestive Health:

- When taken orally, Aloe Vera juice can help soothe the lining of the stomach and intestines, aiding in the relief of digestive disorders like irritable bowel syndrome (IBS) and acid reflux.

Immune Support:

- Aloe Vera contains immune-boosting polysaccharides that help the body to ward off infections.

Hair Care:

- Aloe Vera can be used as a scalp conditioner, reducing dandruff and promoting a healthy scalp. It can also add shine and strength to hair when used as a hair mask.

Tips for Enhancing the Use of Aloe Vera:

🖤 Harvest Aloe Vera gel from the freshest leaves of the plant for the best quality. Cut a leaf from the base, slice it open, and scoop out the gel.

🖤 Mix Aloe Vera gel with other natural ingredients like honey or turmeric for added skin care benefits.

🖤 For digestive health, ensure that Aloe Vera juice is decolorized and purified to remove aloin, which can be harmful in large quantities.

Benefits:

Aloe Vera's versatile range of uses and benefits makes it a valuable plant for health and wellness. Its ability to heal, soothe, and nourish the body, both inside and out, contributes to its longstanding popularity in natural medicine and cosmetics.

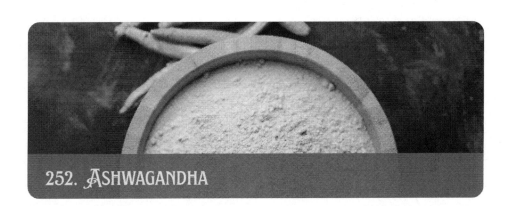

252. ASHWAGANDHA

Introduction:

Ashwagandha, also known as Withania somnifera or Indian ginseng, is a prominent herb in Ayurvedic medicine renowned for its adaptogenic properties. This ancient herb is celebrated for its ability to combat stress and anxiety, enhance stamina, and improve overall well-being.

Basic Uses and Information:

Ashwagandha contains various bioactive compounds, including withanolides, which are thought to contribute to its therapeutic effects. It's traditionally used to strengthen the immune system, stabilize mood, and support mental and physical health.

Detailed Uses of Ashwagandha:

Stress and Anxiety Reduction:

- Ashwagandha is well-known for its ability to lower cortisol levels, the body's stress hormone. Regular consumption can lead to significant reductions in stress and anxiety symptoms.

- The herb enhances resistance to stress by modulating the body's stress response systems, promoting a sense of calm and well-being.

Cognitive Function and Memory:

- Ashwagandha supports brain health by protecting nerve cells from harmful free radicals. Studies suggest it can improve cognitive functions, including memory, attention, and processing speed.

Sleep Improvement:

- The herb has been shown to improve sleep quality and help treat insomnia, primarily due to its calming effects on the nervous system.

Physical Performance and Recovery:

Ashwagandha can boost muscle strength, increase endurance, and speed up recovery in athletes and those engaged in physical activities by enhancing oxygen use during exercise.

Balancing Hormones and Fertility:

- In men, Ashwagandha can improve testosterone levels and reproductive health. In women, it helps in regulating hormonal balance and may alleviate symptoms of stress-related conditions like polycystic ovary syndrome (PCOS).

Tips for Enhancing the Use of Ashwagandha:

- Start with a low dose to assess tolerance and gradually increase as needed. Standard dosages can range from 300-500 mg of a root extract taken twice daily.

- Pair Ashwagandha with a healthy lifestyle, including a balanced diet and regular exercise, to maximize its benefits.

- Consult with a healthcare provider before starting Ashwagandha, especially if you are pregnant, nursing, or on medication, as it can interact with other drugs.

Benefits:

Ashwagandha's adaptogenic properties make it a powerful tool for managing stress and enhancing overall health. By improving mental and physical performance and supporting hormonal balance, this herb offers a holistic approach to well-being that harmonizes body and mind.

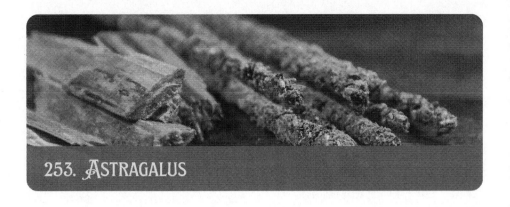

253. ASTRAGALUS

Introduction:

Astragalus is a perennial plant whose roots are used in traditional Chinese medicine to enhance the immune system, promote healing, and support overall vitality. Known scientifically as Astragalus membranaceus, this herb has been used for centuries to prevent illness and stimulate the body's natural defenses.

Basic Uses and Information:

Astragalus contains several compounds, including polysaccharides, saponins, and flavonoids, which contribute to its health-promoting properties. It is primarily recognized for its ability to strengthen immunity, but it also offers benefits for cardiovascular health and stress management.

Detailed Uses of Astragalus:

Immune System Enhancement:

- Astragalus is renowned for its ability to boost the immune system. It stimulates the production and activity of white blood cells, particularly T-cells and macrophages, which are essential for immune response.

- The herb increases the production of antibodies, enhancing the body's ability to fight off viral and bacterial infections.

Cardiovascular Health:

- Astragalus supports heart health by improving blood flow and lowering blood pressure. It has been shown to help prevent plaque buildup in arteries and reduce the risk of heart disease.

Anti-Aging and Longevity:

- The antioxidant properties of Astragalus help combat oxidative stress and reduce inflammation, contributing to its reputation as an anti-aging remedy.

- It is believed to protect the telomeres, parts of the chromosomes linked to aging, thereby promoting longer cell life.

Support for Energy and Stamina:

- Astragalus can increase energy levels and reduce fatigue by enhancing the body's metabolic efficiency and encouraging better oxygen utilization.

Healing and Recovery:

- The herb is used to speed up wound healing and improve recovery from injuries or surgeries due to its ability to stimulate tissue regeneration.

Tips for Enhancing the Use of Astragalus:

- ☀ Astragalus can be taken in various forms, including capsules, tinctures, and teas. Ensure you use a high-quality source to maximize its health benefits.

- ☀ Combine Astragalus with other immune-boosting herbs like echinacea or elderberry for a more comprehensive approach to immune health.

- ☀ While generally safe, consult with a healthcare provider before starting Astragalus, especially if you have autoimmune diseases or are on immunosuppressive medications.

Benefits:

Astragalus is a versatile herb that strengthens the immune system, supports cardiovascular health, and promotes healing and vitality. Its broad range of benefits makes it a valuable addition to a preventive health care regimen, especially for those looking to naturally enhance their body's resilience and longevity.

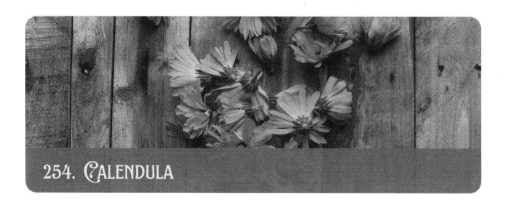

254. CALENDULA

Introduction:

Calendula, often known as pot marigold, is a vibrant herb renowned for its bright yellow and orange flowers. It has been used for centuries in traditional medicine for its healing properties. The active compounds in calendula, including flavonoids and triterpenoids, contribute to its antiseptic and anti-inflammatory effects, making it an excellent choice for skin care and wound healing.

Basic Uses and Information:

Calendula is primarily used topically in creams, salves, and oils to soothe and heal the skin. It can also be used in teas and tinctures for internal benefits, particularly for gastrointestinal and immune health.

Detailed Uses of Calendula:

Skin Care and Healing:

- **Wound Healing:** Calendula accelerates the healing of cuts, scrapes, and other wounds by promoting new tissue growth and reducing inflammation.

- **Soothing Skin Conditions:** It is effective in treating eczema, psoriasis, and dermatitis due to its anti-inflammatory and moisturizing properties.

- **Burns and Sunburns:** The herb provides relief from burns and sunburns by reducing pain, swelling, and redness.

Oral Health:

- **Mouth and Gum Health:** Calendula's antiseptic properties make it beneficial for reducing oral infections, soothing inflamed gums, and healing mouth ulcers when used as a mouthwash.

Digestive Health:

- **Gastrointestinal Relief:** Calendula tea can help soothe the digestive tract, alleviate cramps, and treat ulcers due to its anti-inflammatory and healing effects.

Immune Support:

Lymphatic Health: Calendula supports the lymphatic system, which is crucial for detoxification and immune function.

Antifungal and Antimicrobial:

- **Fungal Infections:** Calendula is effective against common fungal skin infections, including athlete's foot and ringworm.

Tips for Enhancing the Use of Calendula:

- For skin applications, infuse calendula flowers in a carrier oil like olive or almond oil for several weeks to make a potent healing oil.

- To prepare a calendula tea, steep dried calendula flowers in boiling water for about 10 minutes and strain before drinking.

- Combine calendula with other healing herbs like chamomile or lavender for enhanced skin-soothing effects.

Benefits:

Calendula's multifaceted benefits make it a staple in natural health and beauty routines. It enhances skin health, supports digestive and immune systems, and provides antifungal and antimicrobial protection. This versatility, combined with its gentle nature, makes calendula an invaluable herb for holistic wellness.

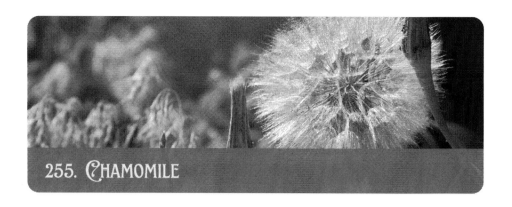

255. CHAMOMILE

Introduction:

Chamomile is a daisy-like plant known for its gentle, soothing properties, widely recognized in herbal medicine for its ability to aid digestion and promote relaxation and sleep. There are two main types: German chamomile (Matricaria recutita) and Roman chamomile (Chamaemelum nobile), both used for their calming effects and pleasant, mildly sweet aroma.

Basic Uses and Information:

Chamomile is most commonly consumed as tea, but it is also available in extracts, tinctures, and topical applications such as creams and ointments. Its active compounds, including flavonoids and apigenin, contribute to its anti-inflammatory, antispasmodic, and sedative effects.

Detailed Uses of Chamomile:

Digestive Health:

- **Soothing Stomach Ailments:** Chamomile tea is effective in soothing an upset stomach, reducing gas and bloating, and alleviating abdominal cramps due to its antispasmodic properties.

- **Improving Digestion:** Regular consumption can help improve overall digestion and alleviate symptoms of conditions like irritable bowel syndrome (IBS).

Sleep and Relaxation:

- **Promotes Restful Sleep:** Chamomile tea is a popular nighttime beverage because it contains apigenin, an antioxidant that binds to certain receptors in the brain to promote sleepiness and reduce insomnia.

- **Reduces Anxiety and Stress:** Its mild sedative effect helps to calm nerves and reduce anxiety, making it a useful aid in managing stress.

Skin Care:

- **Anti-inflammatory and Healing:** Chamomile is applied topically to reduce inflammation, soothe skin irritations like eczema and psoriasis, and accelerate the healing of minor wounds and burns.

- **Natural Beauty Enhancer:** Chamomile infusions are used in facial steams and baths to brighten the complexion and soothe sensitive skin.

Immune Support:

- **Cold and Flu Relief:** Drinking chamomile tea can provide comfort during colds and flu by relieving sore throat, congestion, and reducing fever.

Tips for Enhancing the Use of Chamomile:

- ☀ Brew chamomile tea by steeping dried flowers in hot water for 5-10 minutes to fully release its beneficial compounds.

- ☀ For skin applications, create a chamomile compress by soaking a cloth in cooled chamomile tea and applying it to affected areas.

- ☀ Combine chamomile with other calming herbs like lavender or mint for enhanced flavor and relaxation benefits.

Benefits:

Chamomile offers a holistic approach to health, providing natural relief for digestive issues, promoting restful sleep, soothing skin conditions, and supporting the immune system. Its gentle nature makes it suitable for all ages, contributing to its longstanding popularity in herbal remedies.

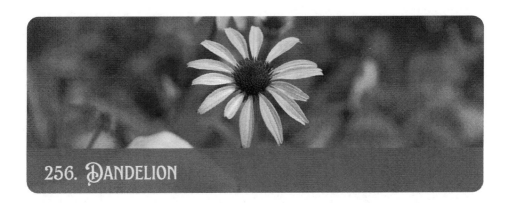

256. DANDELION

Introduction:

Dandelion, often seen as a common weed, is a powerhouse of nutrition and has been used in herbal medicine for centuries. With its bright yellow flowers and deeply rooted leaves, every part of the dandelion plant, from root to flower, is edible and packed with vitamins and minerals. Dandelion is especially known for its ability to support liver health and act as a natural diuretic.

Basic Uses and Information:

Rich in vitamins A, C, K, and E, along with minerals like iron, calcium, magnesium, and potassium, dandelion offers a range of health benefits. Its bitter compounds stimulate digestion and detoxification, particularly in the liver, and its diuretic properties help reduce water retention.

Detailed Uses of Dandelion:

Liver Detoxification:

- **Stimulates Liver Function:** Dandelion root is used in herbal medicine to cleanse and detoxify the liver, promoting improved liver function and bile flow.

- **Supports Overall Detox:** The compounds in dandelion aid in removing toxins from the bloodstream and improving digestive health.

Natural Diuretic:

- **Reduces Water Retention:** Dandelion leaves are effective as a natural diuretic, helping to eliminate excess water from the body without depleting potassium, unlike many synthetic diuretics.

- **Supports Kidney Health:** By increasing urine production, dandelion helps in flushing out waste, salt, and excess water through the kidneys, aiding in kidney function and health.

Digestive Health:

- **Promotes Digestive Enzymes:** The bitter qualities of dandelion stimulate the appetite and help in the secretion of digestive enzymes, improving digestion and alleviating issues like bloating and constipation.

Nutritional Supplement:

- **Rich Source of Nutrients:** Dandelion greens can be eaten raw in salads, cooked like spinach, or brewed into a tea, providing a significant boost of vitamins and minerals.

- **Anti-inflammatory Properties:** The high antioxidant content helps reduce inflammation throughout the body, contributing to overall health and well-being.

Tips for Enhancing the Use of Dandelion:

- Harvest dandelion from clean, pesticide-free areas to ensure they are safe for consumption.

- Use dandelion roots roasted and ground as a caffeine-free coffee substitute or steep them as a tea.

- Combine dandelion leaves with other greens in smoothies or salads to balance their bitter taste with sweeter flavors.

Benefits:

Dandelion's comprehensive health benefits make it a valuable addition to a balanced diet and holistic health routine. By supporting liver function, aiding in fluid balance, and providing a nutritional boost, dandelion enhances overall health and promotes natural body detoxification.

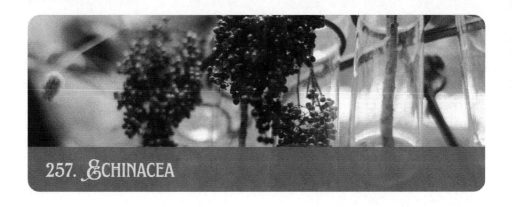

257. ECHINACEA

Introduction:

Echinacea, often referred to as the purple coneflower, is a native North American plant that has long been celebrated for its medicinal properties. It's especially renowned for its ability to enhance the immune system and combat infections, particularly the common cold and other respiratory ailments.

Basic Uses and Information:

Echinacea is available in various forms, including capsules, tinctures, teas, and topical creams. Its active compounds, such as alkamides, polyphenols, and glycoproteins, contribute to its immune-boosting and anti-inflammatory effects.

Detailed Uses of Echinacea:

Immune System Support:

- **Boosts Immune Response:** Echinacea stimulates the production and activity of immune cells like macrophages and T-cells, enhancing the body's ability to fight off infections.

- **Reduces Cold and Flu Symptoms:** Regular use of echinacea at the onset of cold or flu symptoms can reduce the duration and severity of these illnesses.

Anti-Inflammatory Properties:

- **Soothes Inflammation:** Echinacea's anti-inflammatory properties make it beneficial in reducing inflammation associated with various conditions, including skin disorders and inflammatory diseases.

- **Aids in Wound Healing:** Applied topically, echinacea can accelerate the healing process of cuts, burns, and other skin injuries by promoting tissue regeneration and reducing inflammation.

Respiratory Health:

- **Relieves Upper Respiratory Issues:** Echinacea is effective in treating symptoms of upper respiratory infections, such as sore throats, coughs, and sinus congestion.

- **Supports Lung Health:** By enhancing immune function, echinacea helps the body combat and recover from respiratory ailments.

Pain Relief:

- **Natural Analgesic:** The compounds in echinacea can provide relief from pain, especially in conditions like headaches, toothaches, and pains related to inflammatory responses.

Tips for Enhancing the Use of Echinacea:

- Start taking echinacea at the first sign of illness to maximize its effectiveness in reducing symptoms.

- For immune support during cold and flu season, use echinacea in cycles to avoid diminishing its effectiveness—three weeks on, one week off is a common approach.

- Combine echinacea with other immune-supportive herbs like elderberry or vitamin C for a more comprehensive approach to preventing illness.

Benefits:

Echinacea's role in supporting the immune system and reducing inflammation makes it a valuable herb in both preventive health and the treatment of acute conditions. By enhancing the body's natural defenses, echinacea contributes to overall health resilience and recovery from a range of infections.

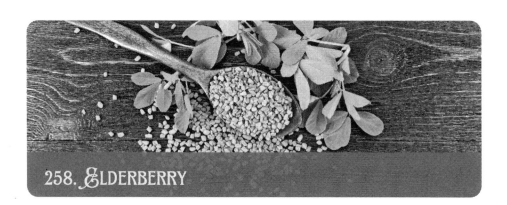

258. ELDERBERRY

Introduction:

Elderberry is recognized for its deep purple berries and fragrant flowers, both of which have been used for centuries in traditional medicine across various cultures. Most notably, the berries are lauded for their antiviral properties and ability to enhance the immune system, making them a popular remedy for colds, flu, and other viral infections.

Basic Uses and Information:

Elderberries are rich in vitamins A, B, and C, as well as antioxidants like anthocyanins, which give the berries their characteristic dark color. These nutrients contribute to the berries' health benefits, particularly their capacity to fight infections and boost immunity.

Detailed Uses of Elderberry:

Cold and Flu Prevention and Treatment:

- **Reduces Severity and Duration:** Consuming elderberry syrup at the onset of flu symptoms has been shown to significantly reduce the duration and severity of the illness, thanks to its antiviral properties.

- **Preventative Measures:** Regular intake of elderberry extract can help strengthen the immune system against respiratory viruses.

Antioxidant Support:

- **Fights Oxidative Stress:** The high levels of antioxidants in elderberries help protect cells from damage caused by free radicals, supporting overall health and reducing the risk of chronic diseases.

- **Promotes Healthy Aging:** These antioxidants also contribute to skin health and are believed to help prevent signs of aging.

Heart Health:

- **Improves Circulation and Lowers Blood Pressure:** Elderberry can help improve heart health by reducing blood pressure and improving blood vessel function, thanks to its high flavonoid content.

- **Lowers Cholesterol:** Regular consumption of elderberry can contribute to lowering LDL cholesterol levels, further protecting cardiovascular health.

Anti-Inflammatory Effects:

- Alleviates Pain and Swelling: Elderberry's anti-inflammatory properties make it effective in reducing pain and inflammation, particularly in joint disorders like arthritis.

Tips for Enhancing the Use of Elderberry:

- Elderberries must be cooked before consumption, as the raw berries contain compounds that can be toxic.

- Elderberry syrup or extract is a convenient way to consume the berries. You can make your own syrup by simmering the berries with water and sweetening with honey or sugar.

- Combine elderberry with other immune-boosting ingredients like ginger, honey, or lemon for added benefits and improved flavor.

Benefits:

Elderberry's antiviral and immune-enhancing properties make it a potent natural remedy for preventing and treating viral infections, particularly those affecting the respiratory system. Its rich antioxidant content also supports overall health and helps combat inflammation, contributing to a robust and resilient immune system.

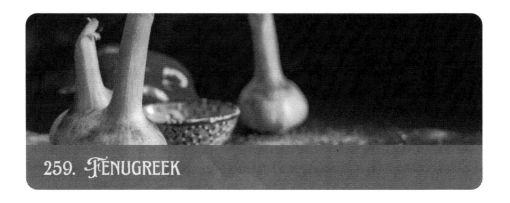

259. FENUGREEK

Introduction:

Fenugreek is a versatile herb known for its distinct aromatic seeds and leaves, widely used in culinary and medicinal applications. One of its most notable health benefits is its ability to increase milk supply in breastfeeding mothers, a property attributed to its phytoestrogen content.

Basic Uses and Information:

Fenugreek seeds contain a range of beneficial nutrients, including dietary fiber, protein, B vitamins, iron, and several phytochemicals. These compounds are believed to stimulate milk production and enhance overall lactation.

Detailed Uses of Fenugreek:

Lactation Support:

- **Stimulates Milk Production:** Fenugreek is commonly recommended to nursing mothers to enhance milk supply. It works by possibly increasing the production of hormones responsible for breast milk flow.

- **Improves Milk Quality:** The nutrients in fenugreek can contribute to the nutritional quality of breast milk, benefiting the infant's health.

Digestive Health:

- **Soothes Digestive Issues:** Fenugreek seeds are rich in soluble fiber, which can help relieve constipation, reduce inflammation in the digestive tract, and improve overall digestive health.

- **Regulates Blood Sugar Levels:** The herb has been shown to improve glucose tolerance and reduce blood sugar levels, making it beneficial for people with diabetes.

Menstrual and Reproductive Health:

- **Eases Menstrual Discomfort:** Fenugreek has antispasmodic and anti-inflammatory properties that can help alleviate menstrual cramps and discomfort.

- **Balances Hormones:** It may also help in balancing hormones and reducing symptoms of menopause due to its phytoestrogenic effects.

Respiratory Health:

- **Relieves Congestion and Coughs:** Fenugreek acts as an expectorant, helping to clear mucus from the lungs and soothe irritated throat tissues.

Tips for Enhancing the Use of Fenugreek:

- To increase milk supply, nursing mothers can take fenugreek in capsule form, as tea, or by incorporating the ground seeds into their diet.

- Start with a lower dose to gauge your body's response and gradually increase as needed, typically between 500 mg to 1000 mg three times a day.

- Ensure adequate hydration, as fenugreek can increase perspiration and urine production due to its diuretic properties.

Benefits:

Fenugreek's multifaceted health benefits extend beyond lactation support, including digestive health improvement, blood sugar regulation, menstrual pain relief, and respiratory system support. Its nutritional profile and phytochemicals make it a valuable addition to a balanced diet and holistic health regimen.

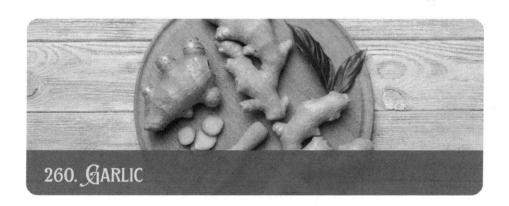

260. GARLIC

Introduction:

Garlic, a member of the Allium family alongside onions and leeks, is celebrated for its pungent flavor and numerous health benefits. It has been used for millennia in cooking and medicine for its potent antimicrobial properties and its ability to lower cholesterol and improve heart health.

Basic Uses and Information:

The key compounds in garlic, particularly allicin, are responsible for its health benefits. Allicin is produced when garlic is chopped, crushed, or chewed, releasing its characteristic strong aroma and flavor. This compound is a powerful antioxidant and contributes to garlic's antiviral, antibacterial, and antifungal effects.

Detailed Uses of Garlic:

Antimicrobial Effects:

- **Fights Infections:** Garlic is effective against a wide range of pathogens, including bacteria, viruses, and fungi. It can help prevent and treat common colds, flu, and other infections.

- **Topical Use for Skin Health:** Applied topically, garlic can treat fungal infections like athlete's foot and ringworm due to its antifungal properties.

Cardiovascular Health:

- **Lowers Cholesterol:** Regular consumption of garlic has been shown to reduce levels of LDL (bad) cholesterol while mildly increasing HDL (good) cholesterol, contributing to overall heart health.

- **Reduces Blood Pressure:** Garlic acts as a natural blood thinner, helping to lower high blood pressure and reduce the risk of heart disease and stroke.

Antioxidant Properties:

- **Protects Against Oxidative Stress:** The antioxidants in garlic help combat free radicals, reducing oxidative stress and preventing chronic diseases, including certain cancers.

- **Enhances Immune Function:** By boosting the immune system, garlic helps the body fight off illnesses more effectively.

Detoxification:

- **Supports Liver Function:** Garlic assists in detoxifying the body by enhancing liver function and aiding in the elimination of toxins.

Tips for Enhancing the Use of Garlic:

- For maximum health benefits, consume garlic raw or let crushed or chopped garlic sit for a few minutes before cooking to maximize allicin production.

- Combine garlic with other heart-healthy foods like olive oil and leafy greens to create nutrient-rich, protective meals.

- If concerned about garlic breath, consume parsley or mint after eating, or opt for aged garlic supplements which have similar benefits without the strong odor.

Benefits:

Garlic's comprehensive health-promoting properties make it a powerful food for enhancing overall wellness. Its ability to improve cardiovascular health, fight infections, and boost the immune system, alongside its use in a myriad of culinary dishes, secures its place as a staple in both the kitchen and natural medicine cabinet.

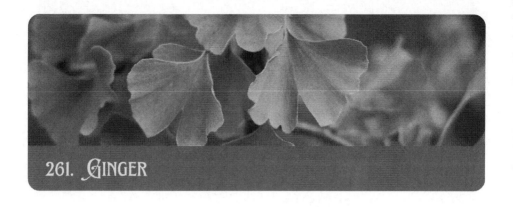

261. GINGER

Introduction:

Ginger is a root known for its zesty flavor and medicinal properties. Cultivated for thousands of years, ginger is used globally in cooking and herbal medicine. It's particularly valued for its anti-inflammatory effects and ability to relieve nausea, making it a favored remedy for a variety of digestive issues.

Basic Uses and Information:

The active compounds in ginger, particularly gingerol, give it potent anti-inflammatory and antioxidant properties. These compounds are responsible for ginger's distinctive spicy flavor and its health benefits, including soothing upset stomachs, reducing pain, and promoting overall well-being.

Detailed Uses of Ginger:

Digestive Health:

- **Relieves Nausea and Vomiting:** Ginger is effective in reducing symptoms of nausea related to motion sickness, pregnancy, and chemotherapy. It can also alleviate morning sickness in pregnant women.

- **Improves Digestion:** By stimulating saliva, bile, and gastric enzymes, ginger enhances the digestion process and helps relieve indigestion, bloating, and gas.

Anti-inflammatory and Pain Relief:

- **Reduces Inflammation:** Ginger's anti-inflammatory properties make it beneficial for treating conditions like arthritis, reducing swelling and pain in joints.

- **Soothes Muscle Pain:** It can help alleviate muscle soreness and pain following exercise or physical activity due to its natural analgesic properties.

Cardiovascular Health:

- **Lowers Blood Pressure:** Ginger can help improve circulation and lower blood pressure by relaxing the muscles surrounding blood vessels.

- **Reduces Blood Sugar Levels:** Regular consumption of ginger can help stabilize blood sugar levels, beneficial for people with diabetes.

Immune System Support:

- **Boosts Immunity:** The antioxidant properties of ginger help strengthen the immune system, making it more capable of fighting off infections and illnesses.

Tips for Enhancing the Use of Ginger:

- For nausea relief, consume ginger in the form of tea, capsules, or chew fresh ginger slices. Ginger tea can be made by steeping fresh ginger root in hot water for several minutes.

- Add fresh ginger to smoothies, soups, or stir-fries to incorporate its health benefits into your daily diet.

- If using ginger to reduce inflammation or pain, consider combining it with other anti-inflammatory herbs or foods, such as turmeric or honey, for synergistic effects.

Benefits:

Ginger's versatile therapeutic properties make it a powerful natural remedy for a range of ailments, from digestive issues to inflammatory conditions. Its ease of use in various forms, from fresh root to powders and supplements, ensures that ginger can be conveniently included in daily health routines for significant benefits.

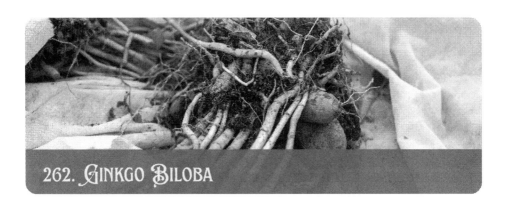

262. GINKGO BILOBA

Introduction:

Ginkgo biloba, one of the oldest living tree species, is renowned for its distinctive fan-shaped leaves and its long history of medicinal use, particularly in traditional Chinese medicine. It is most acclaimed for its ability to enhance cognitive function and improve circulation, making it a popular supplement for memory support and overall brain health.

Basic Uses and Information:

The active compounds in ginkgo leaves include flavonoids and terpenoids, which are known for their potent antioxidant and vasodilatory properties.

These compounds help protect the nervous system, improve blood flow, and combat oxidative stress, contributing to improved cognitive function and vascular health.

Detailed Uses of Ginkgo Biloba:

Cognitive Enhancement:

- **Boosts Memory and Concentration:** Ginkgo biloba is often taken to improve memory, particularly in older adults experiencing mild memory impairment or those looking to enhance cognitive performance.

- **Supports Brain Health:** Its antioxidant properties help protect the brain from damage caused by free radicals, potentially slowing the progression of age-related cognitive decline.

Circulatory Health:

- **Improves Blood Flow:** Ginkgo's ability to dilate blood vessels enhances circulation, particularly to the brain and extremities, which can alleviate symptoms of claudication and support overall vascular health.

- **Reduces Risk of Stroke:** By improving blood flow and reducing blood viscosity, ginkgo may lower the risk of ischemic strokes and other circulatory issues.

Eye Health:

- **Protects Against Age-Related Eye Diseases:** The antioxidants in ginkgo can help protect the eyes from oxidative damage and age-related conditions like macular degeneration.

Mental Health Support:

- **Reduces Anxiety and Depression:** Some studies suggest that ginkgo can help alleviate symptoms of anxiety and depression by improving brain function and reducing stress.

Tips for Enhancing the Use of Ginkgo Biloba:

- To ensure consistent results, use standardized extracts of ginkgo biloba, typically containing 24% flavonoid glycosides and 6% terpene lactones.

- Start with a lower dose to assess your body's response and gradually increase as needed, usually around 120-240 mg per day.

- Consult with a healthcare provider before starting ginkgo, especially if you are taking blood thinners or other medications, as ginkgo can interact with several drugs.

Benefits:

Ginkgo biloba's impact on cognitive function, circulation, and overall well-being makes it a valuable supplement for those seeking to maintain or enhance brain health and improve quality of life. Its long history of use and current research support its role as a beneficial herb in promoting mental clarity and vascular health.

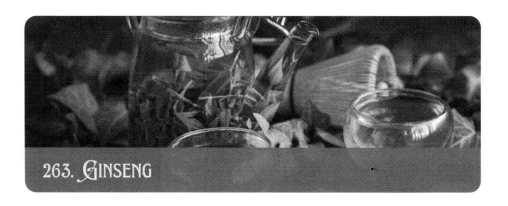

263. GINSENG

Introduction:

Ginseng is a revered herb in traditional medicine, especially within Asian and North American cultures, known for its root that possesses significant health-promoting properties. It comes in various forms, such as American ginseng (Panax quinquefolius) and Asian ginseng (Panax ginseng), each with unique benefits. Ginseng is celebrated for its ability to enhance energy, increase stamina, and support overall well-being.

Basic Uses and Information:

Ginseng contains active compounds called ginsenosides, which are believed to be responsible for its health benefits. These compounds help modulate the body's response to stress, improve cognitive function, and support physical endurance.

Detailed Uses of Ginseng:

Energy and Stamina:

- **Boosts Physical Performance:** Ginseng is often used by athletes

and those seeking natural ways to enhance physical performance and recover more quickly from exercise-induced fatigue.

- **Reduces Fatigue:** It helps combat general lethargy and chronic fatigue by enhancing cellular energy production and improving oxygen uptake in tissues.

Cognitive Function:

- **Improves Mental Performance:** Regular consumption of ginseng can lead to improvements in cognitive abilities like memory, concentration, and mental clarity.

- **Neuroprotective Effects:** Ginsenosides in ginseng have been shown to protect the brain against oxidative stress and may reduce the risk of neurodegenerative diseases.

Immune System Support:

- **Strengthens Immunity:** Ginseng's immunomodulatory properties help strengthen the immune system, making the body more resilient against infections and illnesses.

- **Accelerates Recovery:** By boosting the immune response, ginseng can help shorten the duration of colds and respiratory infections.

Mood and Stress Management:

- **Reduces Stress and Anxiety:** Ginseng has adaptogenic properties that help the body cope with stress, reduce anxiety levels, and promote a sense of calm.

Tips for Enhancing the Use of Ginseng:

- Start with a moderate dose of ginseng, typically around 200-400 mg of standardized extract, and adjust based on your response and health goals.

- For sustained energy and cognitive benefits, take ginseng regularly for several weeks, followed by a break to prevent tolerance build-up.

- Pair ginseng with a balanced diet and regular exercise for comprehensive health benefits.

Benefits:

Ginseng's multifaceted effects on energy, cognitive function, immune health, and stress resilience make it a powerful supplement for those looking to enhance their physical and mental capacities. Its adaptogenic qualities support the body in maintaining balance and efficiency, contributing to overall health and well-being.

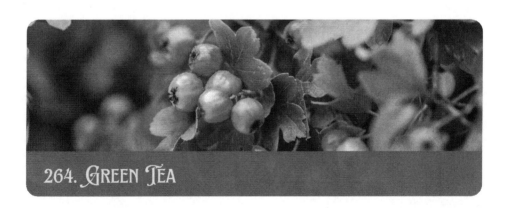

264. GREEN TEA

Introduction:

Green tea, derived from the leaves of the Camellia sinensis plant, is one of the healthiest beverages available, celebrated for its abundance of antioxidants and numerous health benefits. Unlike black tea, green tea is processed in a way that preserves its natural antioxidants, particularly catechins like epigallocatechin gallate (EGCG), which are responsible for many of its health-promoting properties.

Basic Uses and Information:

Green tea is enjoyed worldwide for its refreshing taste and health benefits. It can be consumed hot or cold and is often used in supplements, extracts, and even topical applications for its antioxidant properties.

Detailed Uses of Green Tea:

Antioxidant Protection:

- **Combats Oxidative Stress:** The high levels of antioxidants in green tea help protect cells from damage caused by free radicals, reducing the risk of chronic diseases, including certain cancers.

- **Enhances Skin Health:** Topical application or oral consumption of green tea can improve skin health by reducing inflammation and protecting against sun damage.

Weight Management:

- **Boosts Metabolism:** The combination of caffeine and catechins in green tea can enhance metabolic rate and increase fat burning, supporting weight loss and management.

- **Reduces Appetite:** Some studies suggest that green tea can help regulate hunger signals, aiding in weight control.

Cardiovascular Health:

- **Lowers Cholesterol and Blood Pressure:** Regular consumption of green tea has been shown to reduce levels of LDL (bad) cholesterol and improve arterial function, lowering the risk of heart disease and stroke.

- **Improves Blood Flow:** The antioxidants in green tea help improve blood vessel function, enhancing circulation and overall heart health.

Cognitive Health:

- **Enhances Brain Function:** Caffeine and L-theanine in green tea work synergistically to improve cognitive function, including better attention, alertness, and memory.

- **Neuroprotective Effects:** EGCG and other catechins have potential protective effects against neurodegenerative diseases like Alzheimer's and Parkinson's.

Tips for Enhancing the Use of Green Tea:

- Brew green tea at lower temperatures (around 175-185°F or 80-85°C) to prevent bitterness and preserve antioxidants.

- Combine green tea with a healthy diet rich in fruits, vegetables, and whole grains for a holistic approach to wellness.

- For those sensitive to caffeine, consider decaffeinated green tea or consume it earlier in the day to avoid sleep disturbances.

Benefits:

Green tea's rich antioxidant profile makes it a powerful beverage for enhancing overall health, offering benefits from improved metabolic health and weight management to reduced risk of chronic diseases. Its gentle stimulant effect also makes it a preferred choice for those seeking a healthier alternative to coffee or sugary drinks.

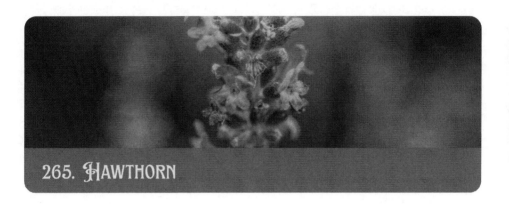

265. HAWTHORN

Introduction:

Hawthorn is a shrub or small tree with berries, flowers, and leaves that have been used in traditional medicine for centuries, primarily as a heart tonic. The plant's active compounds, including flavonoids and oligomeric procyanidins, contribute to its beneficial effects on cardiovascular health.

Basic Uses and Information:

Hawthorn is available in various forms, including teas, tinctures, capsules, and extracts. It's particularly valued for its ability to strengthen the heart muscle, enhance blood flow, and regulate blood pressure and cholesterol levels.

Detailed Uses of Hawthorn:

Cardiovascular Health:

- **Improves Heart Function:** Hawthorn enhances cardiac output by increasing the force of heartbeats and the flow of blood through arteries and veins. This support is particularly beneficial for those with heart failure or weakened heart muscles.

- **Regulates Blood Pressure:** The herb helps dilate blood vessels, which can lower high blood pressure and improve overall circulatory health.

Cholesterol Management:

- **Lowers Cholesterol Levels:** Hawthorn can aid in reducing levels of LDL (bad) cholesterol and triglycerides, while potentially raising HDL (good) cholesterol, contributing to better heart health.

Angina Relief:

- **Reduces Chest Pain:** By improving blood flow to the heart, hawthorn can help alleviate angina pectoris, or chest pain, which occurs when the heart muscle doesn't receive enough oxygen.

Antioxidant Protection:

- **Combats Oxidative Stress:** The flavonoids in hawthorn provide potent antioxidant protection, reducing damage to heart tissue and supporting overall cardiovascular function.

Tips for Enhancing the Use of Hawthorn:

- ☼ Start with a lower dose of hawthorn and gradually increase as needed, typically under the guidance of a healthcare provider, especially if you are already taking heart medications.

- ☼ Consistency is key with hawthorn; benefits are usually observed after several weeks or months of regular use.

- ☼ Combine hawthorn with lifestyle changes like a balanced diet, regular exercise, and stress management techniques for comprehensive cardiovascular health.

Benefits:

Hawthorn's role as a heart tonic makes it a significant herb for enhancing cardiovascular function and preventing heart-related conditions. Its ability to improve blood flow, regulate heart rhythm, and protect against oxidative stress ensures that it supports not only physical but also overall well-being.

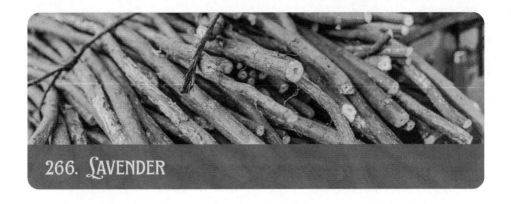

266. LAVENDER

Introduction:

Lavender is celebrated for its fragrant purple flowers and soothing properties, making it a staple in aromatherapy, skincare, and herbal medicine. Known scientifically as Lavandula angustifolia, lavender's calming effects are attributed to its essential oils, which are rich in compounds like linalool and linalyl acetate.

Basic Uses and Information:

Lavender is versatile, used in essential oils, teas, extracts, and even culinary applications. Its most noted for its ability to reduce anxiety, promote relaxation, and enhance sleep quality.

Detailed Uses of Lavender:

Stress and Anxiety Reduction:

- **Calms the Nervous System:** The aroma of lavender essential oil is known to lower levels of stress hormones in the brain, helping to alleviate anxiety and create a sense of calm.

- **Aids in Relaxation:** Using lavender in aromatherapy or in a warm bath can help soothe tension and promote a peaceful state of mind.

Sleep Enhancement:

- **Improves Sleep Quality:** Placing lavender sachets near the pillow or using lavender essential oil in a diffuser can help improve sleep onset, duration, and quality by inducing a more relaxed state.

- **Treats Insomnia:** Regular use of lavender can help those with insomnia by decreasing wakefulness and increasing restful sleep.

Skin Care:

- **Soothes Skin Irritations:** Lavender's anti-inflammatory and antiseptic properties make it effective in treating skin conditions like eczema, psoriasis, and acne.

- **Promotes Wound Healing:** Applying diluted lavender oil or lotions can accelerate the healing of cuts, burns, and insect bites by promoting tissue regeneration.

Pain Relief:

- **Alleviates Headaches and Migraines:** Inhaling lavender oil or applying it to the temples can help reduce the severity of headaches and migraines.

- **Reduces Muscle and Joint Pain:** Massaging with lavender-infused oils can relieve muscle stiffness, soreness, and joint pain.

Tips for Enhancing the Use of Lavender:

- For maximum therapeutic benefits, choose high-quality, pure lavender essential oil for aromatherapy and topical applications.

- Combine lavender with other calming herbs like chamomile or valerian for enhanced sleep and relaxation effects.

- When using lavender topically, dilute it with a carrier oil to prevent skin irritation, especially for those with sensitive skin.

Benefits:

Lavender's broad range of uses, from enhancing sleep and reducing stress to improving skin health and providing pain relief, makes it an invaluable herb in natural wellness practices. Its pleasant fragrance and gentle effects ensure it remains a favorite for promoting relaxation and well-being.

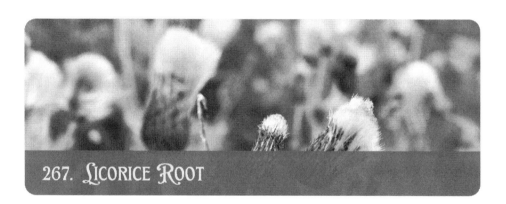

267. ℒICORICE ℛOOT

Introduction:

Licorice root, derived from the Glycyrrhiza glabra plant, has been used for thousands of years in various cultures for its medicinal properties. It's particularly valued for its ability to soothe sore throats and support respiratory health, thanks to its natural sweetness and soothing compounds.

Basic Uses and Information:

Licorice root contains glycyrrhizin, a compound up to 50 times sweeter than sugar, which is responsible for much of its healing properties. This compound has anti-inflammatory and immune-boosting effects, making licorice root an effective remedy for various ailments, especially those involving the throat and digestive system.

Detailed Uses of Licorice Root:

Respiratory Health:

- **Soothes Sore Throats:** Licorice root is a common ingredient in throat lozenges and teas because it helps coat and soothe the throat, reducing irritation and easing pain.

- **Relieves Cough and Bronchial Issues:** Its expectorant properties help loosen and expel phlegm, making it beneficial for treating bronchitis and other respiratory conditions.

Digestive System Support:

- **Treats Ulcers and Heartburn:** Licorice root has a protective effect on the stomach lining, which can prevent and heal ulcers and reduce the symptoms of heartburn and acid reflux.

- **Aids in Digestion:** Its anti-inflammatory properties help soothe inflammation in the gastrointestinal tract, aiding in the treatment of conditions like gastritis and irritable bowel syndrome (IBS).

Adrenal Support:

- **Supports Adrenal Function:** Licorice root can help modulate cortisol levels, providing support for the adrenal glands, especially in times of chronic stress.

Anti-inflammatory and Antiviral Effects:

- **Reduces Inflammation:** The glycyrrhizin and flavonoids in licorice root help reduce inflammation throughout the body.

- **Fights Viral Infections:** Licorice root has been shown to have antiviral properties, effective against viruses like herpes simplex and influenza.

Tips for Enhancing the Use of Licorice Root:

- For sore throat relief, drink licorice root tea or chew on a small piece of the root to release its soothing properties.

- Be mindful of dosage and duration of use, as excessive consumption of licorice root can lead to side effects like hypertension and low potassium levels due to its glycyrrhizin content.

- Consider using deglycyrrhizinated licorice (DGL) for long-term use, especially for digestive health, as it has the glycyrrhizin removed to minimize side effects while maintaining beneficial properties.

Benefits:

Licorice root's diverse therapeutic effects make it a versatile natural remedy for enhancing respiratory and digestive health, reducing inflammation, and supporting the body's response to stress. Its sweet flavor and soothing properties make it a pleasant and effective treatment for a variety of conditions.

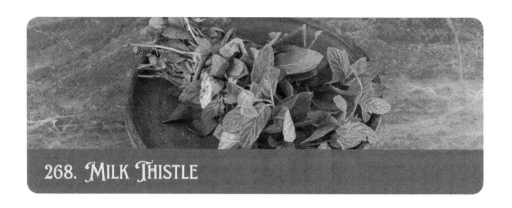

268. Milk Thistle

Introduction:

Milk thistle is a flowering herb related to the daisy and ragweed family, renowned for its benefits to liver health. The active ingredient in milk thistle, silymarin, is a complex of flavonolignans which has potent antioxidant and anti-inflammatory properties that protect liver cells and promote liver regeneration.

Basic Uses and Information:

Milk thistle is commonly used to treat liver disorders such as cirrhosis, jaundice, hepatitis, and gallbladder disorders. It is available in various forms, including capsules, tablets, teas, and extracts, making it accessible for different therapeutic needs.

Detailed Uses of Milk Thistle:

Liver Protection and Detoxification:

- **Supports Liver Function:** Milk thistle helps protect the liver from toxins, including drugs like acetaminophen, which can cause liver damage in high doses. It promotes the repair of liver cells and reduces inflammation.

- **Enhances Detoxification Processes:** The silymarin in milk thistle supports the liver's role in filtering harmful substances from the blood and aids in detoxifying the body from environmental toxins and alcohol.

Liver Disease Management:

- **Reduces Liver Enzyme Levels:** Regular use of milk thistle can help lower elevated liver enzyme levels, indicating improved liver health.

- **Slows Progression of Liver Diseases:** It is used to slow the progression of chronic liver diseases like fatty liver disease, hepatitis, and even liver cancer by protecting liver cells and promoting regeneration.

Antioxidant Effects:

Scavenges Free Radicals: Milk thistle's antioxidant action helps combat oxidative stress and cell damage, contributing to overall health and prevention of various diseases.

Digestive Health Support:

- **Improves Gallbladder Function:** By stimulating bile production, milk thistle can improve digestion and prevent or treat gallstones.

Tips for Enhancing the Use of Milk Thistle:

- ⚘ To maximize benefits, choose standardized milk thistle extracts containing 70% to 80% silymarin.

- ⚘ Combine milk thistle with a healthy diet rich in fruits, vegetables, and lean proteins to support overall liver health.

- ⚘ Consult with a healthcare provider before starting milk thistle, especially if you have existing liver disease or are taking medications, as it can interact with some drugs.

Benefits:

Milk thistle's protective and regenerative effects on the liver make it a valuable supplement for maintaining liver health and supporting the body's natural detoxification processes. Its use can contribute to improved liver function, better digestion, and enhanced resilience against liver-related diseases.

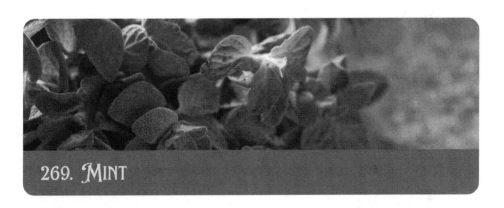

269. MINT

Introduction:

Mint, known for its refreshing aroma and cooling sensation, is a popular herb in culinary and medicinal applications. Belonging to the Mentha genus, mint varieties like peppermint and spearmint are widely used for their digestive benefits and as natural breath fresheners. These plants contain menthol, which provides their characteristic cooling effect and aids in various health benefits.

Basic Uses and Information:

Mint is versatile, used fresh or dried in teas, cooking, and topical applications. Its active compounds, including menthol, have antispasmodic, anti-inflammatory, and antimicrobial properties, making mint effective for soothing digestive issues and freshening breath.

Detailed Uses of Mint:

Digestive Health:

- Soothes Digestive Disorders: Mint helps relax the muscles of the digestive tract, relieving symptoms of irritable bowel syndrome (IBS), bloating, and gas. Peppermint tea is a common remedy for settling the stomach and aiding digestion.

- Alleviates Nausea: The aroma and soothing properties of mint can help reduce nausea and motion sickness.

Breath Freshener:

- **Neutralizes Bad Odor:** Mint's strong, pleasant scent and antimicrobial properties make it effective in combating bad breath, often used in toothpaste, mouthwash, and chewing gum.

- **Improves Oral Health:** The antibacterial qualities of mint help prevent dental plaque and contribute to healthier gums and teeth.

Respiratory Relief:

- **Clears Congestion:** Menthol in mint acts as a natural decongestant, helping to clear sinuses and relieve symptoms of colds and allergies.

- **Soothes Sore Throats:** Mint can alleviate throat irritation and coughing due to its cooling and anti-inflammatory effects.

Skin Care:

- **Cools and Soothes Skin:** Applied topically, mint can relieve itching and reduce redness in conditions like insect bites, sunburns, and minor rashes.

- **Natural Insect Repellent:** The strong scent of mint can help repel insects, making it a useful addition to natural repellent formulations.

Tips for Enhancing the Use of Mint:

- For digestive relief, drink mint tea after meals or chew fresh mint leaves to promote digestion and freshen breath.

- Incorporate mint into salads, beverages, and desserts for a refreshing flavor and health benefits.

- When using mint topically, mix it with a carrier oil or lotion to avoid skin irritation, especially for sensitive skin.

Benefits:

Mint's combination of digestive aid, oral health improvement, respiratory relief, and skin soothing properties make it a multifaceted herb for both culinary and medicinal uses. Its refreshing flavor and scent enhance a variety of dishes and products, making it a favorite worldwide.

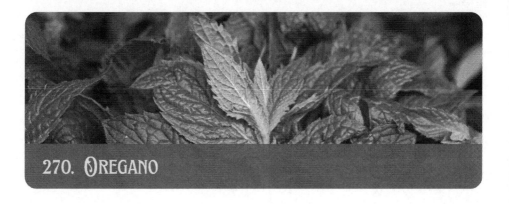

270. ❂REGANO

Introduction:

Oregano is a robust herb known for its potent flavor and medicinal properties, widely used in Italian, Greek, and Mexican cuisines. Beyond its culinary use, oregano is celebrated for its natural antibiotic properties, primarily due to its high content of phenolic compounds such as carvacrol and thymol.

Basic Uses and Information:

Oregano can be used fresh or dried and is available in various forms, including oil, capsules, and tinctures. These forms harness oregano's antimicrobial and antioxidant properties, making it effective against bacteria, fungi, and certain viruses.

Detailed Uses of Oregano:

Antimicrobial Properties:

- **Fights Bacterial Infections:** Oregano oil is particularly effective against a wide range of bacteria, including strains resistant to traditional antibiotics, like E. coli and Staphylococcus aureus.

- **Combats Fungal Infections:** The antifungal action of oregano helps treat conditions like athlete's foot, candidiasis, and other fungal infections.

Immune System Support:

- **Boosts Immune Health:** Regular use of oregano, especially in its oil form, can strengthen the immune system, helping the body ward off infections.

- **Reduces Inflammation:** The anti-inflammatory properties of oregano contribute to its effectiveness in reducing symptoms of inflammatory conditions.

Respiratory Health:

- **Eases Respiratory Conditions:** Oregano can help relieve congestion, coughs, and symptoms of respiratory tract infections due to its expectorant properties.

- **Soothes Sore Throats:** Gargling with oregano tea or using oregano oil diluted in water can alleviate sore throat discomfort.

Digestive Health:

- **Improves Digestion:** Oregano stimulates bile flow and aids in the efficient digestion and absorption of nutrients.

- **Relieves Digestive Discomfort:** Its antispasmodic effects help soothe upset stomachs, reduce bloating, and ease cramps.

Tips for Enhancing the Use of Oregano:

- For internal health benefits, especially for fighting infections, consider taking oregano oil capsules or adding a few drops of oregano oil to a glass of water.

- Incorporate fresh or dried oregano in cooking to benefit from its antimicrobial properties and enhance the flavor of dishes.

- If using oregano oil topically, always dilute it with a carrier oil to prevent skin irritation, as it is highly concentrated and potent.

Benefits:

Oregano's natural antibiotic, anti-inflammatory, and immune-supportive properties make it a valuable herb for maintaining health and treating a range of conditions. Its versatility in both culinary and medicinal applications underscores its importance as a staple in natural health practices.

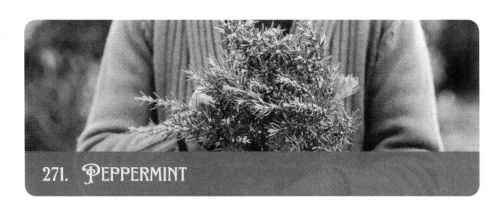

271. PEPPERMINT

Introduction:

Peppermint is a popular aromatic herb in the mint family, known for its cooling sensation and refreshing flavor. It is valued not only for its culinary use but also for its medicinal properties, particularly its effectiveness in relieving nausea and muscle spasms.

Basic Uses and Information:

Peppermint is available in various forms, including fresh leaves, dried leaves for tea, essential oil, capsules, and extracts. Its active compound, menthol, is responsible for the herb's cooling effect and many of its therapeutic benefits.

Detailed Uses of Peppermint:

Digestive Health:

- **Relieves Nausea:** Peppermint is often recommended for its ability to soothe nausea and prevent vomiting, especially related to motion sickness, pregnancy, and post-operative conditions.

- **Improves Digestion:** The herb helps relax the muscles of the digestive tract, reducing symptoms of indigestion, bloating, and gas. It also stimulates bile flow, aiding in the digestion of fats.

Muscle and Nerve Pain:

- **Eases Muscle Spasms:** Peppermint's antispasmodic properties make it effective in relaxing smooth muscle in the intestines, relieving cramps and spasms.

- **Soothes Headaches and Migraines:** Applied topically as an essential oil, peppermint can alleviate tension headaches and migraines by relaxing muscles and improving circulation.

Respiratory Relief:

- **Clears Congestion:** The menthol in peppermint acts as a natural decongestant, helping to clear nasal passages and relieve symptoms of colds and allergies.

- **Soothes Sore Throats:** Peppermint can alleviate throat irritation and coughing due to its cooling and anti-inflammatory properties.

Skin Care:

- **Cools and Soothes Skin:** Applied topically, peppermint provides relief from itching, sunburns, and skin irritations due to its cooling effect.

- **Antimicrobial Action:** The natural antibacterial properties help treat acne and prevent infections in minor cuts and scrapes.

Tips for Enhancing the Use of Peppermint:

- Brew peppermint tea from fresh or dried leaves to enjoy its digestive and nausea-relieving benefits. Let the tea steep for 5-10 minutes for full effect.

- For headaches, dilute peppermint essential oil with a carrier oil and apply it to the temples and forehead for quick relief.

- Incorporate peppermint into aromatherapy practices or use in a diffuser to benefit from its respiratory and mood-enhancing effects.

Benefits:

Peppermint's wide array of health benefits, from aiding digestion and relieving nausea to soothing muscle and nerve pain, makes it a versatile and essential herb in natural health remedies. Its pleasant taste and aroma also make it a favorite for both culinary and therapeutic uses.

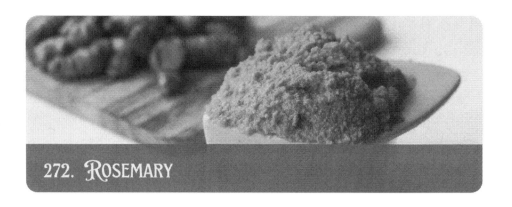

272. ROSEMARY

Introduction:

Rosemary is an aromatic evergreen herb in the mint family, prized for its needle-like leaves and distinctive fragrance. Known for its culinary uses, rosemary also offers significant health benefits, including enhancing circulation and supporting memory and cognitive function.

Basic Uses and Information:

Rosemary contains a variety of active compounds, such as rosmarinic acid, carnosic acid, and essential oils like cineole. These contribute to its antioxidant, anti-inflammatory, and neuroprotective properties, making it a valuable herb for both physical and mental health.

Detailed Uses of Rosemary:

Circulatory System:

- **Enhances Blood Flow:** Rosemary stimulates blood circulation, which can help improve the delivery of oxygen and nutrients to tissues, enhancing overall vitality and energy.

- **Supports Cardiovascular Health:** The herb's ability to improve circulation also contributes to better heart health, potentially reducing the risk of circulatory disorders.

Cognitive Function and Memory:

- **Boosts Memory and Concentration:** The aroma of rosemary has been shown to enhance memory, attention, and concentration. Studies suggest that inhaling rosemary essential oil can improve cognitive performance in tasks requiring speed and accuracy.

- **Neuroprotective Effects:** Compounds in rosemary may protect brain cells from damage and support brain health, potentially lowering the risk of neurodegenerative diseases like Alzheimer's.

Digestive Health:

- **Relieves Digestive Discomfort:** Rosemary aids in digestion by stimulating the production of digestive enzymes and bile, helping to alleviate indigestion, bloating, and cramps.

- **Antimicrobial Properties:** The herb can help combat gastrointestinal pathogens, contributing to a healthier gut environment.

Respiratory Health:

- **Clears Respiratory Tract:** Rosemary's cineole content helps decongest the respiratory tract, easing symptoms of colds, sinusitis, and asthma.

- **Soothes Coughs and Sore Throats:** Its anti-inflammatory and antispasmodic properties can relieve coughs and soothe sore throats.

Tips for Enhancing the Use of Rosemary:

- Use fresh or dried rosemary in cooking to impart flavor and gain its health benefits. Rosemary pairs well with meats, vegetables, and bread.

- For cognitive and circulatory benefits, try inhaling rosemary essential oil or using a diffuser to spread its aroma throughout your space.

- Steep rosemary leaves in hot water to make a tea that supports digestion and provides antioxidant benefits.

Benefits:

Rosemary's ability to improve circulation, enhance memory, and support digestive and respiratory health makes it a versatile and essential herb in both the kitchen and the natural medicine cabinet. Its aromatic and flavorful profile further ensures its popularity and frequent use in a variety of dishes and health remedies.

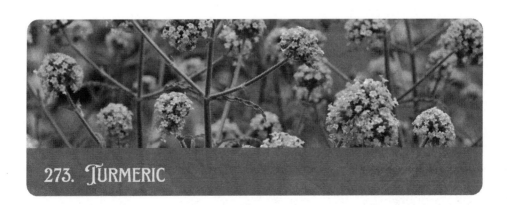

273. TURMERIC

Introduction:

Turmeric is a vibrant yellow-orange spice known for its potent anti-inflammatory properties and significant role in traditional medicine, particularly in Ayurveda and Chinese healing practices. Derived from the root of the Curcuma longa plant, turmeric contains curcumin, a compound that gives the spice its distinctive color and is responsible for many of its health benefits.

Basic Uses and Information:

Turmeric is commonly used in powdered form in cooking, especially in curries and other Asian dishes. It is also available as capsules, extracts, teas, and topical ointments. The bioactive compounds in turmeric, especially curcumin, have powerful antioxidant, anti-inflammatory, and antimicrobial properties.

Detailed Uses of Turmeric:

Anti-Inflammatory and Pain Relief:

- **Reduces Inflammation:** Curcumin in turmeric is highly effective in reducing inflammation throughout the body, making it a natural treatment for inflammatory conditions such as arthritis, inflammatory bowel disease, and psoriasis.

- **Alleviates Pain:** Due to its anti-inflammatory properties, turmeric can help relieve pain associated with arthritis and other chronic pain conditions.

Cognitive Health:

- **Supports Brain Function:** Curcumin has been shown to improve memory and cognitive function by reducing inflammation and oxidative damage in the brain. It may also lower the risk of neurodegenerative diseases like Alzheimer's.

- **Boosts Mood:** Turmeric can enhance mood and may be beneficial in treating depression, partly due to its anti-inflammatory effects.

Cardiovascular Health:

- **Improves Heart Health:** Turmeric helps improve cardiovascular health by reducing inflammation and oxidation, which can contribute to heart disease. It also helps regulate blood pressure and prevent blood clotting.

- **Lowers Cholesterol:** Regular consumption of turmeric can help reduce levels of LDL (bad) cholesterol and triglycerides, enhancing overall heart health.

Digestive Health:

- **Soothes Digestive System:** Turmeric aids in digestion and can help relieve symptoms of indigestion and bloating. It's also used to treat ulcerative colitis and other inflammatory bowel conditions.

- **Detoxifies the Liver:** Turmeric supports liver function and helps detoxify the body by enhancing the liver's ability to process and eliminate toxins.

Tips for Enhancing the Use of Turmeric:

- To increase the bioavailability of curcumin, combine turmeric with black pepper, which contains piperine, a compound that enhances absorption by up to 2000%.

- Incorporate turmeric into your diet by adding it to soups, stews, smoothies, and teas, or use it as a spice in various dishes.

- For topical use, create a paste of turmeric powder and water or oil and apply it to the skin to reduce inflammation and treat skin conditions.

Benefits:

Turmeric's broad range of health benefits, from potent anti-inflammatory and antioxidant effects to cognitive and cardiovascular support, makes it a cornerstone in natural health practices. Its vibrant color and earthy flavor also make it a popular culinary spice, enriching dishes with both flavor and a boost of health.

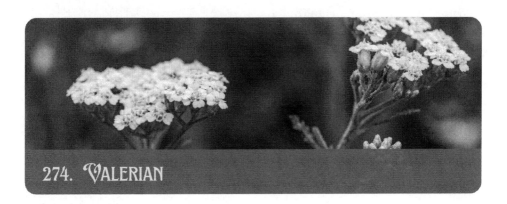

274. VALERIAN

Introduction:

Valerian is a perennial flowering plant native to Europe and Asia, renowned for its sedative and calming properties. The root of the valerian plant is most commonly used in herbal medicine to promote relaxation and improve sleep quality. It is one of the most widely recognized natural sleep aids available today.

Basic Uses and Information:

Valerian root contains a number of compounds, including valerenic acid, isovaleric acid, and a variety of antioxidants that contribute to its sedative effects. It is available in several forms, such as capsules, tinctures, and teas, making it accessible for those seeking a natural remedy for insomnia and anxiety.

Detailed Uses of Valerian:

Sleep Enhancement:

- **Improves Sleep Quality:** Valerian is widely used to combat insomnia and improve the quality of sleep. It helps reduce the time it takes to fall asleep and increases the depth and restfulness of sleep.

- **Regulates Sleep Patterns:** Regular use of valerian can help regulate the sleep-wake cycle, making it beneficial for those with irregular sleep patterns or those experiencing jet lag.

Anxiety and Stress Reduction:

- **Calms the Nervous System:** Valerian has a soothing effect on the nervous system, helping to alleviate stress and reduce anxiety levels.

- **Supports Mental Health:** Its ability to promote relaxation aids in managing symptoms of mild to moderate anxiety and stress-related conditions.

Muscle Relaxation:

- **Eases Muscle Tension:** Valerian's antispasmodic properties help relax muscle tension and spasms, contributing to overall physical relaxation and pain relief.

- **Beneficial for Menstrual Cramps:** It can be particularly effective in relieving the discomfort of menstrual cramps by relaxing uterine muscles.

Tips for Enhancing the Use of Valerian:

- To aid in sleep, take valerian root 30 minutes to an hour before bedtime for the best results.

- Combine valerian with other calming herbs like chamomile, lavender, or lemon balm to enhance its relaxing effects.

- Start with a low dose to assess your body's response and gradually increase as needed, keeping in mind that the effects of valerian can accumulate over time.

Benefits:

Valerian's effectiveness as a natural sleep aid and its ability to reduce anxiety and muscle tension make it a valuable herb in holistic health practices. Its gentle sedative properties provide a safe and natural alternative to pharmaceutical sleep medications, supporting restful sleep and overall mental and physical well-being.

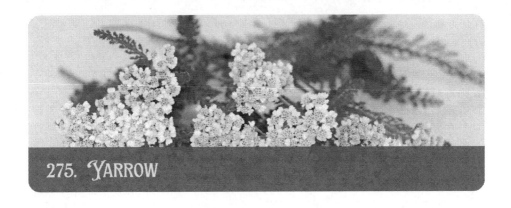

275. YARROW

Introduction:

Yarrow, scientifically known as Achillea millefolium, is a perennial herb with a long history of use in traditional medicine. It is recognized for its feathery leaves and clusters of small, usually white or pink flowers. Yarrow is esteemed for its ability to stop bleeding and reduce fevers, thanks to its astringent and antiseptic properties.

Basic Uses and Information:

Yarrow contains several active compounds, including flavonoids, tannins, and volatile oils, which contribute to its medicinal effects. It is used in various forms, such as fresh or dried herb for teas and tinctures, powders, and even as an essential oil.

Detailed Uses of Yarrow:

Hemostatic and Wound Healing:

- **Stops Bleeding:** Yarrow is effective in quickly stopping bleeding from minor cuts and wounds due to its astringent properties. Applying crushed yarrow leaves or a poultice can promote clot formation and healing.

- **Heals Wounds and Skin Injuries:** The antiseptic and anti-inflammatory properties of yarrow help prevent infection and support the healing process of wounds and skin irritations.

Fever Reduction:

- **Lowers Body Temperature:** Yarrow can induce sweating and help reduce fever. It works as a natural diaphoretic, increasing the body's heat dissipation, which is particularly useful in treating fevers associated with colds and flu.

- **Supports Immune Function:** By aiding in fever reduction, yarrow helps the body's natural immune response to infection.

Digestive Health:

Improves Digestion: Yarrow can stimulate the secretion of digestive enzymes and bile, aiding in the digestion of fats and overall gastrointestinal health.

Relieves Digestive Discomfort: Its antispasmodic properties help reduce cramping and bloating, soothing various gastrointestinal disorders.

Circulatory System Support:

- **Enhances Circulation:** Yarrow is known to improve circulation, helping to regulate blood flow and pressure, and is sometimes used to treat varicose veins and hemorrhoids.

- **Anti-inflammatory Effects:** The herb's anti-inflammatory actions can alleviate conditions like rheumatism and arthritis.

Tips for Enhancing the Use of Yarrow:

- To harness yarrow's hemostatic and healing properties, apply the fresh leaves directly to cuts or wounds, or use a yarrow tea or tincture as a wash.

- For fever reduction, drink yarrow tea at the onset of symptoms. Steep dried yarrow in hot water for 10-15 minutes and consume hot to induce sweating.

- Combine yarrow with other herbs like peppermint or elderflower to enhance its effectiveness in fever and cold treatments.

Benefits:

Yarrow's multifaceted healing properties make it a valuable herb in natural medicine, capable of addressing everything from bleeding and fevers to digestive and circulatory issues. Its widespread use across various cultures underscores its reliability and effectiveness as a healing agent.

PART 14

VIBRATIONAL HEALING AND ENERGY MEDICINE

(276-305)

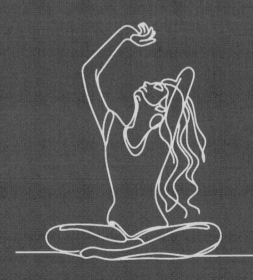

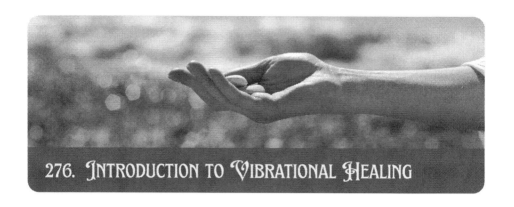

276. Introduction to Vibrational Healing

Introduction:

Vibrational healing is a holistic approach to wellness that focuses on the subtle energies within and around the body. By aligning these energies, vibrational healing aims to restore balance and promote overall health. This practice incorporates various techniques and natural elements to harmonize the body's vibrations and enhance well-being.

Basic Uses and Information:

Vibrational healing involves methods that use sound, light, touch, and natural substances to influence the body's energy fields. These techniques can help reduce stress, alleviate physical pain, and improve mental clarity. The underlying principle is that everything in the universe vibrates at specific frequencies, and maintaining a harmonious vibration is essential for optimal health.

Detailed Uses of Vibrational Healing:

Sound Healing with Natural Tones:

- **Improves Mental Clarity:** Using instruments like tuning forks, singing bowls, and chimes can help clear mental fog and improve focus.

- **Reduces Stress:** Natural tones can induce deep relaxation and reduce anxiety by aligning the body's vibrational frequencies with harmonious sounds.

Deep Breathing for Stress Relief:

- **Promotes Relaxation:** Practicing deep, mindful breathing can help calm the nervous system and reduce stress levels.

- **Enhances Oxygen Flow:** Deep breathing increases oxygen intake, which is essential for maintaining energy and reducing fatigue.

Relaxing Herbal Baths:

- **Soothes Muscles:** Adding herbs like lavender, chamomile, and rosemary to bathwater can relieve muscle tension and promote relaxation.

- **Cleanses Energy Fields:** Herbal baths can help clear negative energy from the body and restore a sense of balance.

Tips for Enhancing Vibrational Healing:

- **Consistency:** Practice vibrational healing techniques regularly to maintain and enhance their benefits.

- **Personalization:** Tailor the methods to your individual needs and preferences, as different techniques resonate differently with each person.

- **Mindfulness:** Incorporate mindfulness into your vibrational healing practices to deepen their effects and foster a greater sense of connection with your body and surroundings.

Benefits:

Vibrational healing offers a gentle, non-invasive approach to improving overall health. By aligning the body's energies, these practices can help reduce stress, enhance mental clarity, and promote physical and emotional well-being. This holistic approach supports the body's natural healing processes and encourages a balanced, harmonious life.

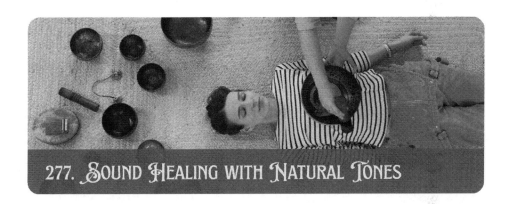

277. Sound Healing with Natural Tones

Introduction:

Sound healing with natural tones utilizes the vibrational frequencies of various instruments to promote physical and emotional well-being. Instruments like singing bowls, tuning forks, and chimes produce sounds that resonate with the body's energy fields, helping to restore balance and harmony.

Basic Uses and Information:

Sound healing works by using the principle that different sounds can influence our brainwaves and energy fields. These natural tones can help reduce stress, improve concentration, and support overall wellness. The vibrations produced by these instruments can penetrate deep into the body, facilitating healing at a cellular level.

Detailed Uses of Sound Healing with Natural Tones:

Mental Clarity and Focus:

- **Enhances Concentration:** Regular exposure to harmonious sounds can help improve mental clarity and focus, making it easier to concentrate on tasks.

- **Reduces Mental Fog:** The vibrational frequencies of natural tones can help clear mental fog and enhance cognitive function.

Stress Reduction:

- **Promotes Relaxation:** The calming sounds of instruments like singing bowls and chimes can induce deep relaxation, reducing anxiety and stress.

- **Balances Energy:** Sound healing helps align the body's energy fields, promoting a sense of peace and balance.

Physical Healing:

- **Alleviates Pain:** The vibrations from sound healing instruments can help relieve physical pain by stimulating cellular repair and reducing inflammation.

- **Enhances Sleep Quality:** Regular sound healing sessions can improve sleep quality by promoting relaxation and reducing insomnia.

Tips for Enhancing Sound Healing with Natural Tones:

- **Choose the Right Instrument:** Select an instrument that resonates with you, whether it's a singing bowl, tuning fork, or chime, to enhance your sound healing experience.

- **Create a Peaceful Environment:** Conduct sound healing sessions in a quiet, comfortable space to maximize the benefits.

- **Regular Practice:** Integrate sound healing into your routine to maintain and enhance its effects on your well-being.

Benefits:

Sound healing with natural tones offers a holistic way to improve mental clarity, reduce stress, and promote physical healing. By aligning the body's vibrations with harmonious sounds, this practice supports overall health and well-being, making it a valuable addition to a holistic wellness routine.

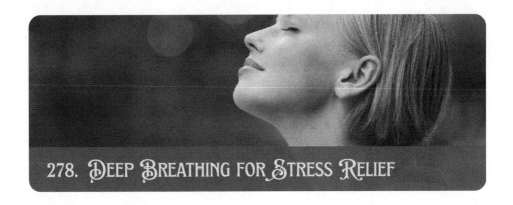

278. Deep Breathing for Stress Relief

Introduction:

Deep breathing is a simple yet powerful technique that can significantly reduce stress and promote relaxation. By consciously controlling your breath, you can activate the body's natural relaxation response, leading to reduced anxiety, lower blood pressure, and a sense of calm.

Basic Uses and Information:

Deep breathing exercises involve inhaling slowly and deeply through the nose, allowing the lungs to fill with air, and then exhaling slowly through the mouth. This practice increases oxygen intake, slows the heartbeat, and helps release tension from the body, making it an effective method for stress relief.

Detailed Uses of Deep Breathing for Stress Relief:

Activating the Relaxation Response:

- **Reduces Anxiety:** Deep breathing stimulates the parasympathetic nervous system, which counteracts the stress response and induces a state of relaxation.

- **Lowers Blood Pressure:** By promoting relaxation, deep breathing can help lower blood pressure and reduce the risk of stress-related cardiovascular issues.

Enhancing Mental Clarity:

- **Improves Focus:** Deep breathing increases oxygen flow to the brain, which can enhance concentration and mental clarity.

- **Reduces Mental Fatigue:** Regular deep breathing exercises can help reduce mental fatigue and improve cognitive function.

Physical Benefits:

- **Relieves Muscle Tension:** Deep breathing helps relax muscles and reduce physical tension, which is often a byproduct of stress.

- **Boosts Immune Function:** By reducing stress, deep breathing can support a healthier immune system and overall physical well-being.

Tips for Enhancing Deep Breathing for Stress Relief:

- 💡 **Practice Regularly:** Set aside a few minutes each day for deep breathing exercises to maintain and enhance their stress-relieving benefits.

- 💡 **Find a Comfortable Position:** Sit or lie down in a comfortable position to fully relax your body and focus on your breath.

- 💡 **Incorporate Mindfulness:** Combine deep breathing with mindfulness practices, such as focusing on the present moment or using guided imagery, to deepen relaxation.

Benefits:

Deep breathing is an accessible and effective technique for managing stress and promoting relaxation. By regularly practicing deep breathing exercises, you can enhance mental clarity, reduce anxiety, and support overall physical health, making it a valuable tool for maintaining well-being in daily life.

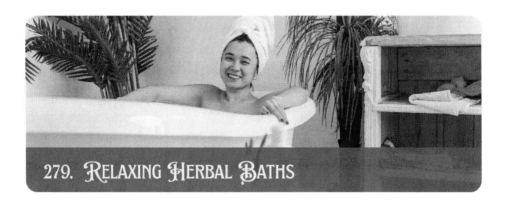

279. Relaxing Herbal Baths

Introduction:

Relaxing herbal baths combine the therapeutic benefits of warm water and healing herbs to promote relaxation, relieve stress, and soothe muscle tension. This ancient practice utilizes the natural properties of various herbs to enhance physical and mental well-being.

Basic Uses and Information:

Herbal baths involve adding fresh or dried herbs, essential oils, or herbal infusions to bathwater. The warm water helps release the essential oils and beneficial compounds from the herbs, allowing them to be absorbed through the skin and inhaled through steam, providing a holistic approach to relaxation and stress relief.

Detailed Uses of Relaxing Herbal Baths:

Stress Relief and Relaxation:

- **Calms the Mind:** Herbs like lavender, chamomile, and rose petals are known for their calming effects, helping to reduce anxiety and promote a sense of peace.

- **Improves Sleep:** Taking a warm herbal bath before bedtime can enhance sleep quality by relaxing the body and mind.

Soothes Muscle Tension:

- **Eases Soreness:** Herbs such as rosemary, eucalyptus, and arnica have anti-inflammatory properties that can help soothe sore muscles and reduce pain.

- **Enhances Circulation:** The warmth of the bath combined with the therapeutic properties of herbs can improve blood circulation, aiding in muscle recovery and overall relaxation.

Skin Care:

- **Nourishes the Skin:** Herbs like calendula, oat straw, and aloe vera can help moisturize and nourish the skin, leaving it soft and rejuvenated.

- **Treats Skin Conditions:** Herbal baths can alleviate symptoms of skin conditions such as eczema, psoriasis, and dryness by reducing inflammation and providing soothing relief.

Tips for Enhancing Relaxing Herbal Baths:

- **Choose the Right Herbs:** Select herbs based on their specific properties and your desired outcome, whether it's relaxation, pain relief, or skin care.

- **Prepare Herbal Infusions:** For a more potent bath, prepare an herbal infusion by steeping herbs in boiling water for 15-20 minutes, then strain and add the liquid to your bathwater.

- **Combine with Essential Oils:** Enhance the benefits of your herbal bath by adding a few drops of complementary essential oils, such as lavender, eucalyptus, or chamomile, for added aromatherapy effects.

Benefits:

Relaxing herbal baths provide a holistic and enjoyable way to reduce stress, soothe muscle tension, and improve skin health. By incorporating this practice into your routine, you can create a calming and therapeutic environment that promotes overall well-being and relaxation.

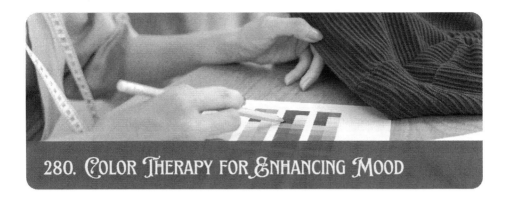

280. Color Therapy for Enhancing Mood

Introduction:

Color therapy, also known as chromotherapy, is a holistic healing practice that uses colors to affect mood and mental well-being. Each color has specific wavelengths and energy frequencies that can influence the body and mind, promoting balance and enhancing emotional health.

Basic Uses and Information:

Color therapy can be implemented in various ways, such as through colored lights, visualization, clothing, and decor. Different colors are believed to stimulate different responses in the body and mind, helping to improve mood, reduce stress, and promote overall emotional well-being.

Detailed Uses of Color Therapy for Enhancing Mood:

Red:

- **Boosts Energy:** Red is a stimulating color that can increase energy levels and enhance alertness.

- **Improves Mood:** This color can also help combat feelings of depression and lethargy by invigorating the mind and body.

Blue:

- **Promotes Calmness:** Blue is known for its calming and soothing effects, helping to reduce anxiety and promote relaxation.

- **Enhances Focus:** This color can also improve concentration and mental clarity.

Green:

- **Balances Emotions:** Green is associated with balance and harmony, making it ideal for reducing stress and promoting a sense of well-being.

- **Restores Energy:** This color can help restore depleted energy levels and encourage relaxation.

Yellow:

- **Increases Positivity:** Yellow is a cheerful and uplifting color that can enhance mood and promote feelings of happiness.

- **Stimulates Mental Activity:** This color is also associated with intellectual stimulation and creativity.

Purple:

- **Encourages Creativity:** Purple can stimulate the imagination and enhance creativity.

- **Promotes Inner Peace:** This color is often used to promote spiritual awareness and inner peace.

Tips for Enhancing Color Therapy:

- 💡 **Use Colored Lights:** Incorporate colored lights or light filters in your living or workspace to create an environment that supports your emotional needs.

- 💡 **Wear Colorful Clothing:** Choose clothing in colors that align with the mood you wish to achieve. For example, wear blue for calmness or yellow for positivity.

- 💡 **Decorate with Intent:** Use color in your home decor to influence the ambiance of different rooms. Soft blues and greens can create a calming bedroom, while vibrant reds and yellows can energize a living area.

Benefits:

Color therapy offers a simple yet effective way to influence mood and emotional well-being. By understanding the psychological and physiological effects of different colors, you can create environments and choose clothing that enhance your mood, reduce stress, and promote overall mental health.

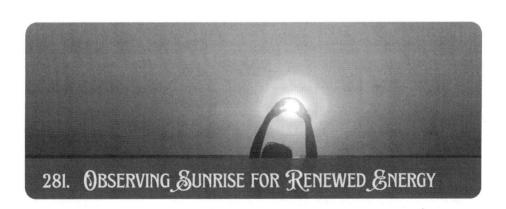

281. OBSERVING SUNRISE FOR RENEWED ENERGY

Introduction:

Observing the sunrise is a powerful practice that can rejuvenate the mind and body. The early morning light, rich in blue and red wavelengths, has unique properties that can enhance mood, boost energy levels, and set a positive tone for the day ahead.

Basic Uses and Information:

Sunlight exposure, particularly during sunrise, helps regulate the body's circadian rhythms, which control sleep-wake cycles and other physiological processes. The natural light triggers the release of hormones such as cortisol and serotonin, which are vital for energy, mood, and overall well-being.

Detailed Uses of Observing Sunrise for Renewed Energy:

Boosts Mood and Energy Levels:

- **Increases Serotonin Production:** Exposure to early morning sunlight stimulates the production of serotonin, a hormone that enhances mood and promotes feelings of well-being.

- **Enhances Alertness:** The blue light present during sunrise helps increase alertness and cognitive function, making it easier to start the day with energy and focus.

Regulates Sleep Patterns:

- **Sets Circadian Rhythms:** Observing the sunrise helps synchronize your internal clock with the natural day-night cycle, improving sleep quality and duration.

- **Reduces Insomnia:** Regular exposure to morning sunlight can help reduce symptoms of insomnia and other sleep disorders by promoting a healthy sleep-wake cycle.

Mental Clarity and Mindfulness:

- **Promotes Mindfulness:** Taking time to observe the sunrise encourages a mindful start to the day, fostering a sense of peace and presence.

- **Inspires Positivity:** The beauty and tranquility of the sunrise can inspire positive thoughts and a hopeful outlook for the day ahead.

Tips for Enhancing the Practice of Observing Sunrise:

- **Consistent Routine:** Make observing the sunrise a part of your daily routine to maximize its benefits. Aim to wake up early enough to spend at least 10-20 minutes outside during sunrise.

- **Choose a Peaceful Spot:** Find a quiet and comfortable location where you can fully experience the sunrise without distractions. This could be a balcony, garden, park, or beach.

- **Combine with Other Practices:** Enhance the experience by combining sunrise observation with other morning routines, such as deep breathing exercises, meditation, or gentle stretching.

Benefits:

Observing the sunrise offers a natural and uplifting way to boost energy levels, improve mood, and regulate sleep patterns. This simple practice can set a positive tone for the day, enhance mental clarity, and promote overall well-being, making it a valuable addition to your daily routine.

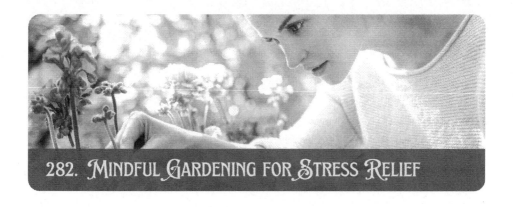

282. Mindful Gardening for Stress Relief

Introduction:

Mindful gardening is a practice that combines the benefits of gardening with mindfulness techniques to promote relaxation and reduce stress. By focusing on the present moment and engaging all the senses, mindful gardening helps create a deeper connection with nature, fostering a sense of calm and well-being.

Basic Uses and Information:

Mindful gardening involves being fully present while tending to plants, paying attention to the sights, sounds, smells, and textures of the garden. This practice encourages you to slow down, breathe deeply, and appreciate the simple pleasures of gardening, helping to alleviate stress and improve mental clarity.

Detailed Uses of Mindful Gardening for Stress Relief:

Reduces Anxiety and Promotes Relaxation:

- **Focus on the Present:** Mindful gardening encourages you to concentrate on the task at hand, whether it's planting, weeding, or watering. This focus can help quiet the mind and reduce anxiety.

- **Engages the Senses:** Paying attention to the colors, scents, and sounds of the garden can provide a sensory-rich experience that promotes relaxation and reduces stress.

Enhances Mental Clarity and Mindfulness:

- **Improves Concentration:** Gardening tasks that require attention to detail, such as pruning or arranging plants, can enhance concentration and mindfulness.

- **Encourages Reflection:** Spending time in the garden allows for quiet reflection and introspection, helping to clear the mind and improve mental clarity.

Promotes Physical Well-Being:

- **Encourages Physical Activity:** Gardening involves physical activities like digging, planting, and weeding, which can improve physical fitness and overall health.

- **Boosts Mood:** Exposure to natural sunlight and fresh air while gardening can boost mood and energy levels, thanks to increased vitamin D production and improved circulation.

Tips for Enhancing Mindful Gardening for Stress Relief:

- **Set Intentions:** Begin your gardening session by setting a positive intention, such as cultivating calm or appreciating nature's beauty. This can help guide your focus and enhance the mindfulness aspect of gardening.

- **Take Your Time:** Avoid rushing through gardening tasks. Instead, take your time to fully engage with each activity, paying close attention to your actions and the environment around you.

- **Use All Your Senses:** Engage all your senses by noticing the textures of leaves, the sounds of birds, the smell of flowers, and the sight of growing plants. This sensory awareness can deepen your connection with the garden and enhance the stress-relieving benefits.

Benefits:

Mindful gardening offers a holistic approach to stress relief, combining the therapeutic effects of nature with the mental health benefits of mindfulness. By engaging fully with the gardening process, you can reduce anxiety, enhance mental clarity, and promote physical well-being, making it a rewarding practice for overall health and happiness.

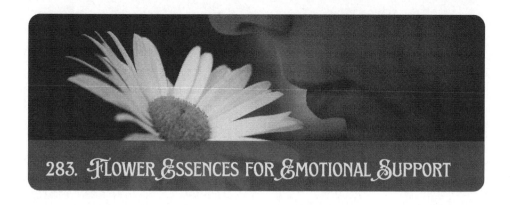

283. FLOWER ESSENCES FOR EMOTIONAL SUPPORT

Introduction:

Flower essences are natural remedies made from the extracts of various flowers, designed to address emotional and psychological imbalances. Unlike essential oils, flower essences do not carry the fragrance of the flowers but their energetic imprint, which is believed to help balance emotions and support mental well-being.

Basic Uses and Information:

Flower essences are typically taken orally by placing drops under the tongue or adding them to water. They can also be applied topically or added to bathwater. Each flower essence is associated with specific emotional states and can be used to address a wide range of issues, from anxiety and stress to lack of confidence and grief.

Detailed Uses of Flower Essences for Emotional Support:

Anxiety and Stress Relief:

- **Calming the Mind:** Essences like Bach's Rescue Remedy, which combines five different flower essences, are known for their ability to reduce anxiety and promote a sense of calm.

- **Managing Everyday Stress:** Lavender and chamomile flower essences can help manage everyday stress by promoting relaxation and mental clarity.

Enhancing Mood and Emotional Balance:

- **Lifting Depression:** St. John's Wort and mustard flower essences are used to alleviate symptoms of depression and bring light to dark moods.

- **Balancing Emotions:** Essences such as yarrow and rose help to balance emotions and support overall emotional health, providing stability during challenging times.

Building Confidence and Self-Esteem:

- **Boosting Self-Confidence:** Larch flower essence is often used to boost self-confidence and encourage a positive self-image.

- **Enhancing Inner Strength:** Oak and elm flower essences can help build inner strength and resilience, making it easier to cope with life's demands.

Supporting Grief and Loss:

- **Healing from Loss:** Star of Bethlehem and honeysuckle flower essences are effective in supporting individuals through grief and loss, helping to soothe emotional pain and promote healing.

- **Letting Go:** Willow and pine flower essences aid in releasing past traumas and negative emotions, facilitating the process of letting go and moving forward.

Tips for Enhancing the Use of Flower Essences:

- **Choose the Right Essence:** Select flower essences based on your specific emotional needs. You can use a single essence or a combination tailored to address multiple issues.

- **Regular Use:** For best results, use flower essences consistently over a period of time. Follow the recommended dosage instructions on the product label.

- **Combine with Other Practices:** Enhance the effects of flower essences by combining them with other supportive practices, such as meditation, journaling, or mindfulness exercises.

Benefits:

Flower essences provide a gentle, natural way to support emotional well-being and address various psychological challenges. By working on an energetic level, they help balance emotions, reduce stress, and enhance overall mental health, making them a valuable addition to holistic health practices.

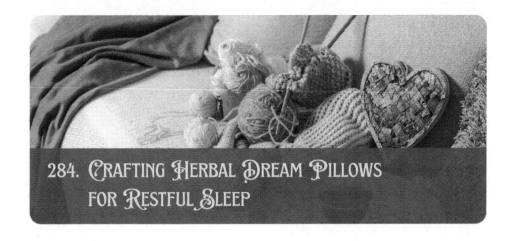

284. Crafting Herbal Dream Pillows for Restful Sleep

Introduction:

Herbal dream pillows are small sachets filled with a blend of dried herbs known for their calming and sleep-inducing properties. Placed under your pillow or beside your bed, these pillows release subtle, soothing aromas that can help improve sleep quality and promote restful dreams.

Basic Uses and Information:

Herbal dream pillows harness the power of aromatherapy to support restful sleep. Common ingredients include lavender, chamomile, and hops, which are known for their relaxing effects. Creating these pillows is a simple and enjoyable craft that combines the therapeutic benefits of herbs with the comfort of a handmade item.

Detailed Uses of Herbal Dream Pillows for Restful Sleep:

Improving Sleep Quality:

- **Induces Relaxation:** The calming scent of herbs like lavender and chamomile can help relax the mind and body, making it easier to fall asleep.

- **Enhances Sleep Depth:** Certain herbs, such as valerian root and hops, are known to improve the depth and quality of sleep, promoting more restful and rejuvenating slumber.

Promoting Restful Dreams:

- **Encourages Peaceful Sleep:** Herbs like mugwort and rose petals are believed to encourage vivid and peaceful dreams, enhancing the overall sleep experience.

- **Reduces Nightmares:** The soothing properties of these herbal blends can help reduce the occurrence of nightmares and night disturbances.

Relieving Stress and Anxiety:

- **Calms the Nervous System:** The gentle aromas released by the dream pillow help calm the nervous system, reducing stress and anxiety that can interfere with sleep.

- **Balances Emotions:** Herbs such as lemon balm and mint can help balance emotions and promote a sense of well-being, contributing to better sleep.

Tips for Crafting and Using Herbal Dream Pillows:

- **Select High-Quality Herbs:** Use high-quality, dried herbs for the best aromatic and therapeutic effects. Organic herbs are preferred to avoid exposure to pesticides.

- **Blend Your Herbs:** Create a blend of herbs tailored to your specific sleep needs. For example, combine lavender, chamomile, and hops for a relaxing mix, or add mugwort for dream enhancement.

- **Sewing the Pillow:** Use a small, breathable fabric pouch or sew your own pillow from soft, natural fabric. Fill the pouch with your herbal blend and close it securely.

- **Placement:** Place the herbal dream pillow under your regular pillow or near your head on the bed to inhale the soothing aromas throughout the night.

Benefits:

Herbal dream pillows provide a natural and gentle way to improve sleep quality and promote restful dreams. By combining the therapeutic properties of herbs with the comforting presence of a handmade item, these pillows offer a holistic approach to achieving better sleep and reducing nighttime anxiety.

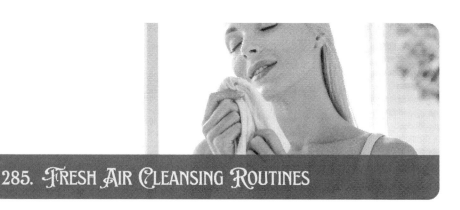

285. FRESH AIR CLEANSING ROUTINES

Introduction:

Fresh air cleansing routines involve practices that utilize the natural purifying properties of outdoor air to cleanse the body and mind. Spending time in fresh air can help reduce stress, improve mental clarity, and enhance overall well-being by providing a break from indoor pollutants and creating a connection with nature.

Basic Uses and Information:

These routines often include activities such as outdoor walks, deep breathing exercises, and simply spending time in natural settings. Fresh air is essential for respiratory health and mental rejuvenation, making it a vital component of holistic health practices.

- **Promotes Mindfulness:** Engaging in outdoor activities encourages mindfulness and a deeper connection with the natural world, enhancing overall emotional well-being.

Detailed Uses of Fresh Air Cleansing Routines:

Mental Clarity and Stress Reduction:

- **Improves Focus:** Exposure to fresh air and natural environments can help clear the mind, improve concentration, and enhance cognitive function.

- **Reduces Stress:** Being outdoors and breathing in fresh air can lower stress levels by reducing cortisol, the stress hormone, and promoting relaxation.

Physical Health Benefits:

- **Enhances Respiratory Health:** Fresh air can improve lung function by increasing oxygen intake and expelling indoor pollutants and toxins.

- **Boosts Immune System:** Regular exposure to fresh air and natural environments can strengthen the immune system by reducing inflammation and increasing the production of white blood cells.

Emotional and Psychological Well-Being:

- **Elevates Mood:** Spending time outdoors can elevate mood and reduce symptoms of depression and anxiety, thanks to the combination of physical activity, natural light, and fresh air.

Tips for Enhancing Fresh Air Cleansing Routines:

- **Daily Outdoor Time:** Aim to spend at least 20-30 minutes outside each day, whether through a walk, sitting in a garden, or practicing outdoor yoga or meditation.

- **Deep Breathing Exercises:** Incorporate deep breathing exercises while outside to maximize the intake of fresh air and enhance relaxation.

- **Explore Natural Settings:** Visit parks, forests, beaches, or mountains to experience the diverse benefits of different natural environments.

- **Open Windows:** Even when indoors, opening windows to allow fresh air to circulate can help improve indoor air quality and bring some of the benefits of fresh air inside.

Benefits:

Fresh air cleansing routines offer a simple yet powerful way to improve mental clarity, reduce stress, and enhance overall physical and emotional health. By making fresh air a regular part of your routine, you can harness the natural healing properties of the outdoors to support a balanced and healthy lifestyle.

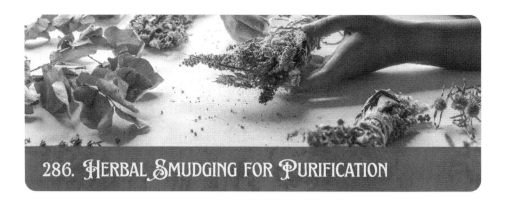

286. Herbal Smudging for Purification

Introduction:

Herbal smudging is a traditional practice used to cleanse and purify spaces, objects, and individuals by burning specific herbs and allowing the smoke to carry away negative energy. Commonly used in various cultural rituals, smudging with herbs like sage, cedar, and sweetgrass can help create a positive, harmonious environment.

Basic Uses and Information:

Smudging involves lighting a bundle of dried herbs and then blowing out the flame, allowing the herbs to smolder and produce smoke. This smoke is then directed around the area or object to be cleansed. The practice is believed to remove negative energy, promote healing, and invite positive energy.

Detailed Uses of Herbal Smudging for Purification:

Cleansing Spaces:

- **Home and Office:** Smudging can cleanse homes, offices, and other spaces of negative energy,

promoting a calm and peaceful environment.

- **New Locations:** It is particularly beneficial to smudge new homes or workspaces to remove any residual energy from previous occupants.

Purifying Objects:

- **Crystals and Jewelry:** Smudging is used to cleanse crystals, jewelry, and other personal items, removing negative energies they may have absorbed.

- **Sacred Items:** It is also common to smudge sacred objects, such as altars or meditation tools, to maintain their purity and enhance their spiritual significance.

Personal Cleansing:

- **Energy Clearing:** Individuals can be smudged to cleanse their personal energy field, promoting emotional balance and spiritual well-being.

- **Ritual Preparation:** Smudging is often used before rituals, ceremonies, or meditation to prepare and purify participants.

Tips for Enhancing Herbal Smudging for Purification:

- **Choose Appropriate Herbs:** Select herbs based on their traditional uses and desired effects. Common choices include white sage for purification, cedar for protection, and sweetgrass for attracting positive energy.

- **Safe Practices:** Use a fireproof bowl or abalone shell to catch ashes and embers. Ensure proper ventilation to avoid excessive smoke inhalation.

- **Set Intentions:** Before beginning the smudging process, set a clear intention for what you wish to achieve, whether it is cleansing, healing, or protection.

- **Direct the Smoke:** Use a feather, fan, or your hand to gently direct the smoke around the space, object, or person being cleansed.

Benefits:

Herbal smudging offers a simple and effective way to purify spaces, objects, and individuals, promoting a harmonious and balanced environment. By incorporating this practice into your routine, you can enhance spiritual well-being, remove negative energy, and invite positivity into your life.

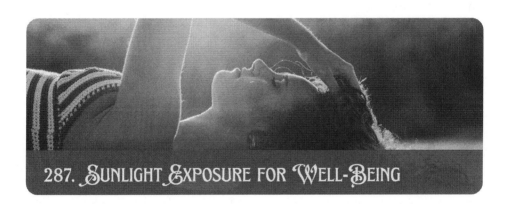

287. SUNLIGHT EXPOSURE FOR WELL-BEING

Introduction:

Sunlight exposure is essential for maintaining physical and mental health. Natural sunlight not only helps regulate the body's circadian rhythms but also stimulates the production of vital hormones and vitamins that support overall well-being. Spending time in the sun can boost mood, enhance sleep quality, and improve immune function.

Basic Uses and Information:

Exposure to sunlight triggers the production of vitamin D in the skin, which is crucial for bone health, immune function, and mood regulation. Sunlight also helps balance serotonin and melatonin levels, which are important for mood and sleep. Regular, moderate sun exposure can provide numerous health benefits while promoting a positive and energetic lifestyle.

Detailed Uses of Sunlight Exposure for Well-Being:

Boosts Mood and Energy Levels:

- **Increases Serotonin Production:** Sunlight exposure stimulates the production of serotonin, a hormone that enhances mood and promotes feelings of well-being and happiness.

- **Combats Depression:** Regular sunlight exposure can help alleviate symptoms of seasonal affective disorder (SAD) and other forms of depression by improving mood and energy levels.

Improves Sleep Quality:

- **Regulates Circadian Rhythms:** Sunlight helps regulate the body's internal clock, promoting healthy sleep-wake cycles and improving overall sleep quality.

- **Increases Melatonin Production:** Exposure to natural light during the day helps boost melatonin production at night, aiding in better sleep.

Supports Immune Function:

- **Boosts Vitamin D Production:** Sunlight triggers the synthesis of vitamin D in the skin, which is essential for a strong immune system and bone health.

- **Reduces Inflammation:** Sunlight exposure can help reduce inflammation and support the body's natural defense mechanisms.

Tips for Enhancing Sunlight Exposure for Well-Being:

- **Moderate Exposure:** Aim for 15-30 minutes of sunlight exposure several times a week, preferably in the morning or late afternoon when the sun is less intense.

- **Protect Your Skin:** Use sunscreen to protect against harmful UV rays if you plan to be in the sun for extended periods, and wear protective clothing as needed.

- **Combine with Outdoor Activities:** Engage in outdoor activities such as walking, gardening, or exercising to maximize the benefits of sunlight exposure and enhance physical fitness.

- **Indoor Light:** If outdoor sunlight is limited, consider using light therapy lamps to mimic natural sunlight and support your circadian rhythms and mood.

Benefits:

Sunlight exposure offers a natural and effective way to boost mood, improve sleep quality, and support overall well-being. By incorporating regular sun exposure into your routine, you can enhance your physical and mental health, increase your energy levels, and promote a positive and balanced lifestyle.

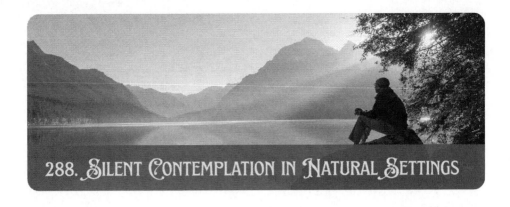

288. Silent Contemplation in Natural Settings

Introduction:

Silent contemplation in natural settings involves spending quiet, uninterrupted time in nature to reflect, meditate, and connect with the natural world. This practice can help reduce stress, improve mental clarity, and foster a sense of peace and well-being. The tranquility of natural environments provides the perfect backdrop for deep contemplation and self-discovery.

Basic Uses and Information:

Engaging in silent contemplation in nature allows you to disconnect from the distractions and noise of daily life, creating space for introspection and mindfulness. This practice can be done in various settings, such as forests, beaches, mountains, or parks, and can involve activities like sitting quietly, walking mindfully, or simply observing the natural surroundings.

Detailed Uses of Silent Contemplation in Natural Settings:

Reduces Stress and Anxiety:

- **Promotes Relaxation:** The calming effect of nature helps to lower cortisol levels, reducing stress and anxiety.

- **Enhances Emotional Balance:** Silent contemplation provides an opportunity to process emotions and thoughts, promoting emotional stability and resilience.

Improves Mental Clarity and Focus:

- **Clears the Mind:** Spending time in nature without distractions allows the mind to rest and rejuvenate, improving concentration and mental clarity.

- **Encourages Mindfulness:** The practice of being fully present in a natural setting fosters mindfulness, helping you stay focused on the present moment.

Fosters a Deeper Connection with Nature:

- **Heightens Awareness:** Silent contemplation enhances your awareness of the natural world, deepening your appreciation and connection to the environment.

- **Promotes Environmental Stewardship:** Developing a deeper connection with nature can inspire a greater sense of responsibility for its preservation and care.

Tips for Enhancing Silent Contemplation in Natural Settings:

- 💡 **Choose a Quiet Location:** Select a natural setting that is free from urban noise and disturbances to maximize the benefits of silent contemplation.
- 💡 **Set Aside Time:** Dedicate a specific time for silent contemplation, whether it's a few minutes each day or a longer period on weekends.

- 💡 **Comfortable Position:** Find a comfortable position, whether sitting or walking, that allows you to relax and focus on your surroundings.
- 💡 **Be Present:** Focus on the sights, sounds, smells, and sensations of the natural environment, letting go of any distracting thoughts or worries.

Benefits:

Silent contemplation in natural settings provides a powerful way to reduce stress, enhance mental clarity, and foster a deep sense of peace and well-being. By regularly practicing this form of mindfulness, you can improve your emotional balance, connect more deeply with nature, and gain greater insight and clarity in your life.

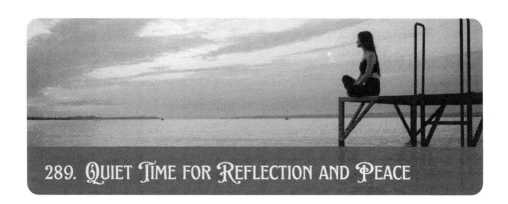

289. QUIET TIME FOR REFLECTION AND PEACE

Introduction:

Quiet time for reflection and peace involves setting aside dedicated moments in your day to pause, reflect, and find inner tranquility. This practice helps reduce stress, improve mental

clarity, and foster a deeper sense of self-awareness. In a fast-paced world, taking quiet time is essential for maintaining emotional and mental well-being.

Basic Uses and Information:

Quiet time can be spent in various ways, such as meditating, journaling, praying, or simply sitting in silence. The key is to create a calm, uninterrupted environment where you can focus on your thoughts and feelings without distractions. This practice encourages mindfulness and helps cultivate a peaceful state of mind.

Detailed Uses of Quiet Time for Reflection and Peace:

Reduces Stress and Anxiety:

- **Promotes Relaxation:** Taking time to sit quietly and reflect can activate the body's relaxation response, lowering cortisol levels and reducing stress.

- **Alleviates Anxiety:** Quiet reflection helps manage anxiety by allowing you to process your thoughts and emotions calmly.

Enhances Mental Clarity and Self-Awareness:

- **Improves Focus:** Regular quiet time can enhance your ability to concentrate and stay focused throughout the day.

- **Encourages Self-Reflection:** Reflecting on your thoughts, actions, and experiences fosters greater self-awareness and personal growth.

Fosters Emotional Balance:

- **Processes Emotions:** Quiet time provides a safe space to explore and understand your emotions, promoting emotional healing and stability.

- **Builds Resilience:** Regular periods of reflection can help build emotional resilience, making it easier to cope with life's challenges.

Tips for Enhancing Quiet Time for Reflection and Peace:

- **Create a Peaceful Environment:** Choose a quiet, comfortable space where you won't be disturbed. Consider adding calming elements like soft lighting, cushions, or soothing music.

- **Set a Routine:** Establish a regular time each day for your quiet reflection, whether it's in the morning, during a lunch break, or before bed.

- **Use Journaling:** Writing down your thoughts and feelings can enhance the reflective process and provide valuable insights into your inner world.

- **Practice Mindfulness:** Focus on your breath, body sensations, or a particular thought to stay present and deepen your reflective experience.

Benefits:

Quiet time for reflection and peace offers a sanctuary from the stresses of daily life, helping to restore mental clarity, emotional balance, and inner peace. By integrating this practice into your routine, you can enhance your overall well-being, gain greater self-awareness, and develop a resilient, mindful approach to life's challenges.

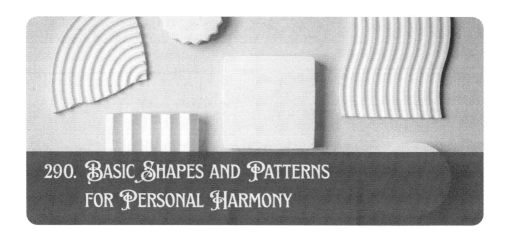

290. BASIC SHAPES AND PATTERNS FOR PERSONAL HARMONY

Introduction:

The use of basic shapes and patterns in daily life can promote personal harmony and well-being. This concept, rooted in both ancient wisdom and modern design principles, suggests that certain shapes and patterns can influence our mood, energy levels, and overall sense of balance.

Basic Uses and Information:

Shapes and patterns are present in everything from nature to architecture, and they impact our subconscious mind. By consciously incorporating harmonious shapes and patterns into our surroundings, clothing, and even our daily practices, we can enhance our mental and emotional state.

Detailed Uses of Basic Shapes and Patterns for Personal Harmony:

Circles:

- **Symbol of Unity and Wholeness:** Circles represent unity, completeness, and infinity. They can promote a sense of inclusiveness and balance.

- **Calming Effect:** Incorporating circular patterns in your environment, such as in rugs, tables, or artwork, can create a calming and harmonious atmosphere.

Squares and Rectangles:

- **Stability and Order:** Squares and rectangles symbolize stability, order, and reliability. They are often used in architecture and interior design to create a sense of groundedness.

- **Practicality:** Use square and rectangular shapes in furniture and layout to promote a sense of structure and practicality in your living or working space.

Triangles:

- **Dynamic Energy:** Triangles are associated with direction, movement, and progress. They can introduce a dynamic and energizing element to your environment.

- **Focus and Intent:** Incorporating triangular shapes in decor or design can help focus energy and intentions, promoting clarity and purpose.

Spirals:

- **Growth and Evolution:** Spirals symbolize growth, evolution, and transformation. They are found abundantly in nature and can inspire personal growth and change.

- **Meditative Quality:** Spiral patterns can be used in artwork or meditation tools to enhance focus and promote a meditative state.

Natural Patterns:

- **Organic Harmony:** Patterns found in nature, such as leaves, waves, and honeycombs, promote a sense of organic harmony and connection to the natural world.

- **Inspiration and Creativity:** Using natural patterns in your surroundings can stimulate creativity and a deeper connection to the environment.

Tips for Enhancing Personal Harmony with Shapes and Patterns:

- ⚲ **Decorate Thoughtfully:** Choose home decor items with shapes and patterns that resonate with you and promote the feelings you wish to cultivate, such as calmness, stability, or energy.

- ⚲ **Wear Patterns Mindfully:** Select clothing and accessories with shapes and patterns that reflect your personal intentions and desired state of mind.

- ⚲ **Create Art:** Engage in artistic activities that incorporate these shapes and patterns, such as drawing mandalas or creating nature-inspired designs, to enhance mindfulness and personal expression.

- ⚲ **Practice Visualization:** Use visualization techniques to imagine being surrounded by harmonious shapes and patterns, enhancing your mental and emotional state.

Benefits:

Incorporating basic shapes and patterns into your daily life can promote personal harmony by influencing your mood and energy levels. Whether through home decor, clothing, or personal practices, these elements can help create a balanced and harmonious environment, supporting overall well-being and emotional health.

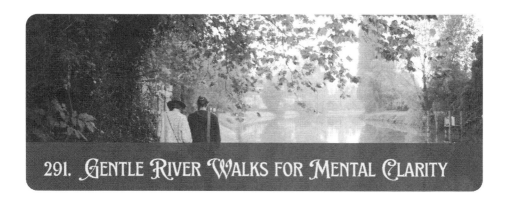

291. GENTLE RIVER WALKS FOR MENTAL CLARITY

Introduction:

Gentle river walks combine the soothing presence of flowing water with the benefits of physical activity to enhance mental clarity and promote relaxation. Walking along a riverbank can provide a peaceful and restorative experience, helping to clear the mind and reduce stress.

Basic Uses and Information:

Engaging in gentle walks along a river allows you to connect with nature, enjoy the rhythmic sounds of water, and benefit from fresh air and light exercise. This practice can improve cognitive function, elevate mood, and offer a break from the demands of daily life.

Detailed Uses of Gentle River Walks for Mental Clarity:

Reduces Stress and Anxiety:

- **Natural Calm:** The sound of flowing water and the tranquility of a river setting can reduce cortisol levels, helping to alleviate stress and anxiety.

- **Promotes Relaxation:** Walking in a serene environment encourages relaxation and provides a natural escape from daily pressures.

Enhances Cognitive Function:

- **Improves Focus:** The combination of physical activity and natural surroundings can enhance concentration and mental clarity.

- **Boosts Creativity:** The peaceful ambiance and natural beauty of a river walk can stimulate creative thinking and problem-solving.

Supports Physical Health:

- **Light Exercise:** Gentle walking is a low-impact exercise that improves cardiovascular health, boosts energy levels, and enhances overall physical fitness.

- **Increases Endorphins:** Physical activity triggers the release of endorphins, which can elevate mood and promote a sense of well-being.

Encourages Mindfulness:

- **Presence in Nature:** Walking along a river encourages mindfulness and a deeper connection with the natural environment, helping you stay present and grounded.

- **Meditative Experience:** The repetitive nature of walking combined with the rhythmic flow of the river can create a meditative experience, enhancing inner peace and mental clarity.

Tips for Enhancing Gentle River Walks for Mental Clarity:

- ☙ **Choose the Right Time:** Select a time of day when the river path is less crowded to fully immerse yourself in the tranquility of the setting.

- ☙ **Walk Mindfully:** Focus on your breath, the sounds of the river, and the sights around you. Let go of distracting thoughts and be fully present in the moment.

- ☙ **Combine with Other Practices:** Integrate deep breathing exercises or simple stretching during your walk to enhance relaxation and physical well-being.

- ☙ **Regular Routine:** Make river walks a regular part of your routine to consistently benefit from the mental and physical health advantages.

Benefits:

Gentle river walks offer a holistic approach to improving mental clarity and reducing stress. By combining the therapeutic effects of nature with light exercise, these walks can enhance cognitive function, promote relaxation, and support overall well-being. Incorporating regular river walks into your routine can provide a refreshing and restorative break from daily life, fostering mental and emotional health.

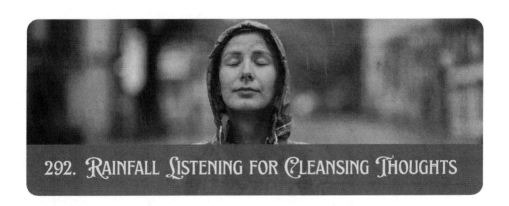

292. RAINFALL LISTENING FOR CLEANSING THOUGHTS

Introduction:

Listening to the sound of rainfall is a soothing and therapeutic practice that can help cleanse the mind and promote mental clarity. The natural, rhythmic sound of rain can create a calming atmosphere, reducing stress and encouraging a sense of peace and tranquility.

Basic Uses and Information:

Rainfall listening involves focusing on the sound of rain, whether it's a gentle drizzle or a heavy downpour. This practice can be done indoors by listening to recorded rain sounds or outdoors during actual rain. It can help clear mental clutter, reduce anxiety, and enhance relaxation.

Detailed Uses of Rainfall Listening for Cleansing Thoughts:

Reduces Stress and Anxiety:

- **Calming Effect:** The steady, rhythmic sound of rain can calm the nervous system, lowering cortisol levels and reducing stress and anxiety.

- **Promotes Relaxation:** The natural white noise of rainfall can create a peaceful environment, promoting relaxation and reducing mental tension.

Enhances Mental Clarity:

- **Clears Mental Clutter:** Focusing on the sound of rain can help clear away distracting thoughts and mental clutter, improving concentration and mental clarity.

- **Encourages Mindfulness:** Rainfall listening encourages mindfulness by helping you stay present in the moment, enhancing overall mental focus.

Improves Sleep Quality:

- **Promotes Deep Sleep:** The soothing sound of rain can help improve sleep quality by creating a relaxing auditory environment that promotes deeper and more restful sleep.

- **Reduces Insomnia:** Listening to rainfall can help reduce symptoms of insomnia by calming the mind and preparing the body for sleep.

Supports Emotional Well-Being:

- **Elevates Mood:** The therapeutic effects of rainfall listening can elevate mood and promote emotional balance, helping to alleviate feelings of sadness or depression.

- **Provides Comfort:** The familiar and gentle sound of rain can provide a sense of comfort and security, enhancing emotional well-being.

Tips for Enhancing Rainfall Listening for Cleansing Thoughts:

- **Find a Comfortable Space:** Choose a quiet and comfortable place where you can sit or lie down without distractions, whether it's indoors or outside under a shelter.

- **Use Quality Audio:** If natural rain is not available, use high-quality recordings of rainfall sounds. Many apps and online platforms offer various types of rain sounds.

- **Combine with Other Practices:** Enhance the experience by combining rainfall listening with deep breathing exercises, meditation, or visualization techniques.

Regular Practice: Incorporate rainfall listening into your regular routine, especially during times of high stress or before bed, to consistently benefit from its calming effects.

Benefits:

Rainfall listening provides a natural and effective way to cleanse the mind and promote mental clarity. By focusing on the soothing sounds of rain, you can reduce stress, enhance mindfulness, and improve emotional well-being. This simple yet powerful practice can be a valuable addition to your holistic wellness routine, helping to create a peaceful and balanced mental state.

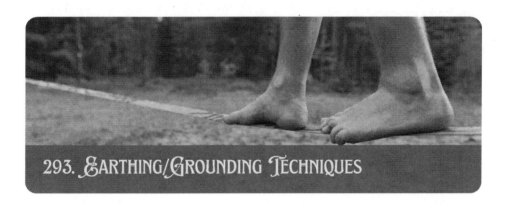

293. EARTHING/GROUNDING TECHNIQUES

Introduction:

Earthing, also known as grounding, is a practice that involves direct physical contact with the Earth's surface to balance the body's electrical energy and promote overall health. This technique is based on the idea that the Earth's electrons can neutralize free radicals and reduce inflammation in the body. By reconnecting with the Earth, you can enhance mental clarity, reduce stress, and improve physical well-being.

Basic Uses and Information:

Earthing can be practiced by walking barefoot on natural surfaces like grass, sand, or soil, or by using grounding products such as mats and sheets that connect to the Earth. This practice helps synchronize the body with the Earth's natural rhythms, providing a sense of stability and calm.

Detailed Uses of Earthing/ Grounding Techniques:

Reduces Stress and Anxiety:

- **Calms the Nervous System:** Direct contact with the Earth can reduce cortisol levels, helping to alleviate stress and anxiety.

- **Promotes Relaxation:** The grounding effect of earthing can create a deep sense of relaxation and emotional balance.

Enhances Physical Health:

- **Reduces Inflammation:** Grounding can help neutralize free radicals, reducing chronic inflammation and pain in the body.

- **Improves Sleep:** Regular earthing can regulate sleep patterns and improve the quality of sleep by balancing the body's natural circadian rhythms.

Boosts Immune System:

- **Enhances Immunity:** Contact with the Earth's electrons can support the immune system, making the body more resilient against illnesses.

- **Accelerates Healing:** Grounding can speed up the healing process by reducing inflammation and improving circulation.

Increases Energy Levels:

- **Enhances Vitality:** Connecting with the Earth can boost energy levels and reduce feelings of fatigue by aligning the body's electrical energy.

- **Improves Mood:** Regular grounding can elevate mood and enhance overall mental clarity and focus.

Tips for Enhancing Earthing/Grounding Techniques:

- **Spend Time Outdoors:** Aim to spend at least 20-30 minutes a day walking barefoot on natural surfaces like grass, sand, or soil to maximize the benefits of earthing.

- **Use Grounding Products:** If access to natural surfaces is limited, consider using grounding products like mats, sheets, or footwear that can connect you to the Earth's energy.

- **Combine with Mindfulness:** Enhance your grounding practice by incorporating mindfulness or meditation techniques while you are in contact with the Earth.

- **Regular Practice:** Make earthing a regular part of your daily routine to consistently benefit from its stress-reducing and health-enhancing effects.

Benefits:

Earthing or grounding offers a simple and natural way to enhance physical and mental well-being. By reconnecting with the Earth's energy, you can reduce stress, improve sleep, boost immunity, and increase energy levels. This practice promotes a sense of balance and harmony, supporting overall health and vitality.

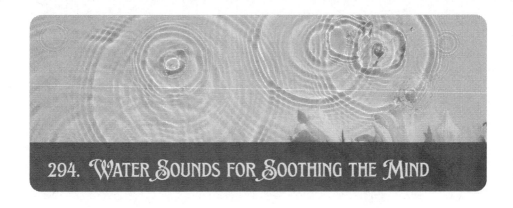

Introduction:

Listening to water sounds, such as flowing rivers, ocean waves, or gentle rain, is a natural and effective way to soothe the mind and promote relaxation. The rhythmic and calming nature of water sounds can help reduce stress, enhance mental clarity, and improve overall emotional well-being.

Basic Uses and Information:

Water sounds can be experienced in natural settings or through recordings. This practice involves focusing on the auditory experience of water to create a tranquil environment that supports mental relaxation and mindfulness. Incorporating water sounds into your daily routine can provide a peaceful escape from the noise and demands of everyday life.

Detailed Uses of Water Sounds for Soothing the Mind:

Reduces Stress and Anxiety:

- **Calms the Nervous System:** The steady, rhythmic sounds of water can help lower cortisol levels, reducing stress and anxiety.

- **Promotes Relaxation:** Listening to water sounds can induce a state of deep relaxation, making it easier to unwind and let go of tension.

Enhances Mental Clarity and Focus:

- **Clears Mental Clutter:** Focusing on the soothing sounds of water can help clear away distracting thoughts and mental clutter, improving concentration and mental clarity.

- **Encourages Mindfulness:** Water sounds encourage mindfulness by helping you stay present in the moment and fully engage with your surroundings.

Improves Sleep Quality:

- **Promotes Deep Sleep:** The calming effect of water sounds can help improve sleep quality by creating a relaxing auditory environment that promotes deeper and more restful sleep.

- **Reduces Insomnia:** Listening to water sounds before bed can help reduce symptoms of insomnia by calming the mind and preparing the body for sleep.

Supports Emotional Well-Being:

- **Elevates Mood:** The therapeutic effects of water sounds can elevate mood and promote emotional balance, helping to alleviate feelings of sadness or depression.

- **Provides Comfort:** The familiar and gentle sound of water can provide a sense of comfort and security, enhancing emotional well-being.

Tips for Enhancing the Use of Water Sounds:

- **Find Natural Water Sources:** Whenever possible, spend time near natural water sources such as rivers, lakes, or the ocean to fully experience the benefits of water sounds.

- **Use Quality Recordings:** If natural water sources are not accessible, use high-quality recordings of water sounds. Many apps and online platforms offer a variety of water soundscapes.

- **Combine with Relaxation Techniques:** Enhance the calming effects of water sounds by combining them with deep breathing exercises, meditation, or gentle stretching.

- **Regular Practice:** Incorporate water sounds into your regular routine, especially during times of high stress or before bed, to consistently benefit from their soothing effects.

Benefits:

Listening to water sounds offers a natural and effective way to soothe the mind and promote relaxation. By focusing on the calming auditory experience of water, you can reduce stress, enhance mental clarity, improve sleep quality, and support overall emotional well-being. Incorporating water sounds into your daily routine can help create a peaceful and balanced mental state.

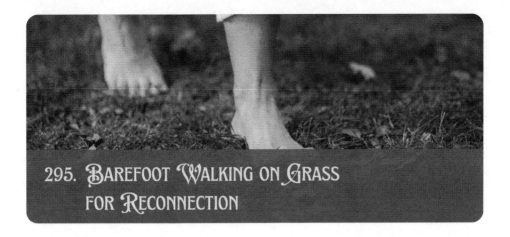

295. Barefoot Walking on Grass for Reconnection

Introduction:

Walking barefoot on grass, also known as grounding or earthing, is a practice that involves direct physical contact with the Earth's surface to reconnect with nature and balance the body's energy. This simple yet powerful activity can enhance mental clarity, reduce stress, and promote overall well-being by aligning the body with the Earth's natural rhythms.

Basic Uses and Information:

Barefoot walking on grass allows you to absorb the Earth's electrons through your feet, which can help neutralize free radicals and reduce inflammation. This practice can improve physical health, emotional balance, and a sense of connection to the natural world.

Detailed Uses of Barefoot Walking on Grass for Reconnection:

Reduces Stress and Anxiety:

- **Calms the Nervous System:** Direct contact with the Earth can lower cortisol levels, helping to alleviate stress and anxiety.

- **Promotes Relaxation:** Walking barefoot on grass can create a deep sense of relaxation and peace, reducing mental tension and promoting emotional balance.

Enhances Physical Health:

- **Improves Circulation:** The physical activity of walking combined with the grounding effect of the grass can enhance blood flow and circulation.

- **Reduces Inflammation:** Grounding can help neutralize free radicals, reducing chronic inflammation and pain in the body.

Boosts Mental Clarity and Focus:

- **Clears the Mind:** Spending time in nature and walking barefoot can help clear mental clutter, enhancing concentration and mental clarity.

- **Encourages Mindfulness:** This practice encourages mindfulness by helping you stay present and fully engage with the natural environment.

Promotes Emotional Well-Being:

- **Elevates Mood:** The grounding effect of walking barefoot on grass can boost mood and promote a sense of happiness and well-being.

- **Enhances Connection to Nature:** This practice fosters a deeper connection to the natural world, enhancing feelings of grounding and centeredness.

Tips for Enhancing Barefoot Walking on Grass for Reconnection:

- **Choose a Safe Location:** Find a clean, safe area with soft grass free of sharp objects and debris to walk barefoot.

- **Take Your Time:** Walk slowly and mindfully, paying attention to the sensations under your feet and the natural surroundings.

- **Combine with Deep Breathing:** Enhance the benefits by incorporating deep breathing exercises as you walk, further promoting relaxation and mindfulness.

- **Regular Practice:** Aim to spend at least 15-30 minutes a day walking barefoot on grass to consistently benefit from its grounding effects.

Benefits:

Barefoot walking on grass offers a natural and effective way to reconnect with the Earth, enhancing mental clarity, reducing stress, and promoting overall well-being. By integrating this simple practice into your daily routine, you can foster a deeper connection to nature, improve physical and emotional health, and achieve a greater sense of balance and harmony.

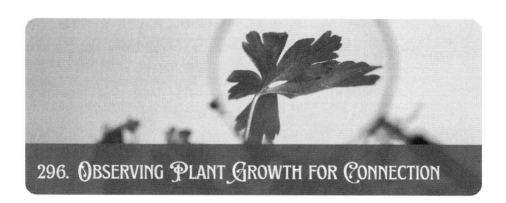

296. Observing Plant Growth for Connection

Introduction:

Observing plant growth is a mindful practice that fosters a deep connection with nature and promotes a sense of tranquility and wonder. By taking time to watch plants grow and develop, you can enhance your awareness of natural cycles, reduce stress, and cultivate patience and mindfulness.

Basic Uses and Information:

This practice involves regularly spending time with plants, whether in a garden, home, or natural setting, to observe their growth and changes. It can be a solitary activity or shared with others, and it helps deepen your connection to the environment, promoting emotional and mental well-being.

Detailed Uses of Observing Plant Growth for Connection:

Reduces Stress and Anxiety:

- **Calms the Mind:** Watching plants grow can be a calming activity that helps to lower stress levels and reduce anxiety by encouraging a slower, more mindful pace.

- **Promotes Relaxation:** The act of observing the natural growth process can induce a state of relaxation and mental peace.

Enhances Mindfulness and Patience:

- **Encourages Presence:** Focusing on the slow, steady growth of plants fosters mindfulness, helping you stay present and attentive to the moment.

- **Cultivates Patience:** Observing plants over time teaches patience and appreciation for gradual progress and natural cycles.

Improves Mental Clarity and Focus:

- **Clears the Mind:** Spending time with plants can clear mental clutter, enhancing concentration and cognitive function.

- **Inspires Creativity:** The natural beauty and intricate details of plant growth can stimulate creative thinking and problem-solving.

Fosters Emotional Well-Being:

- **Elevates Mood:** Engaging with nature and observing plant life can boost mood and promote feelings of happiness and well-being.

- **Builds Connection:** Developing a relationship with the plants you observe enhances your sense of connection to nature and the environment.

Tips for Enhancing the Practice of Observing Plant Growth for Connection:

- **Choose a Variety of Plants:** Select a range of plants with different growth rates and characteristics to observe, from fast-growing annuals to slow-growing perennials.

- **Create a Regular Routine:** Dedicate specific times each day or week to spend with your plants, observing their growth and changes.

- **Keep a Journal:** Document your observations, noting changes in the plants and your reflections on the process. This can deepen your understanding and appreciation of plant growth.

- **Engage with All Senses:** Use sight, touch, and smell to fully engage with the plants, enhancing your sensory experience and connection to nature.

Benefits:

Observing plant growth is a rewarding practice that enhances mindfulness, reduces stress, and fosters a deep connection with nature. By regularly engaging in this activity, you can improve mental clarity, promote emotional well-being, and develop a greater appreciation for the natural world and its cycles.

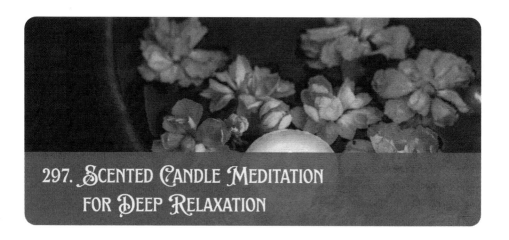

297. SCENTED CANDLE MEDITATION FOR DEEP RELAXATION

Introduction:

Scented candle meditation combines the calming effects of candlelight with the soothing aromas of essential oils to create a deeply relaxing experience. This practice helps to reduce stress, improve focus, and promote a sense of peace and well-being by engaging multiple senses.

Basic Uses and Information:

Scented candle meditation involves lighting a candle infused with essential oils, focusing on the flickering flame, and breathing in the therapeutic scents. This practice can be done at any time of day to create a serene environment, enhance mindfulness, and support emotional balance.

Detailed Uses of Scented Candle Meditation for Deep Relaxation:

Reduces Stress and Anxiety:

- **Calming Aromas:** The essential oils in scented candles, such as lavender, chamomile, or sandalwood, help to calm the mind and reduce anxiety.

- **Soothing Candlelight:** The gentle flicker of candlelight creates a tranquil atmosphere that promotes relaxation and stress relief.

Enhances Mindfulness and Focus:

- **Promotes Presence:** Focusing on the candle flame encourages mindfulness, helping you stay present and attentive to the moment.

- **Improves Concentration:** The combined sensory experience of sight and smell can enhance concentration and mental clarity.

Supports Emotional Well-Being:

- **Elevates Mood:** The pleasant scents and calming visuals can boost mood and create a sense of emotional balance and well-being.

- **Provides Comfort:** The warm glow of the candle and familiar scents can provide a sense of comfort and security, enhancing emotional stability.

Facilitates Deep Relaxation:

- **Induces Relaxation:** The overall sensory experience helps to induce a state of deep relaxation, promoting physical and mental rest.

- **Improves Sleep Quality:** Practicing candle meditation before bed can help prepare the mind and body for restful sleep by reducing stress and tension.

Tips for Enhancing Scented Candle Meditation for Deep Relaxation:

- **Choose High-Quality Candles:** Select candles made with natural essential oils and non-toxic materials to ensure a safe and effective meditation experience.

- **Create a Peaceful Space:** Set up a comfortable and quiet area for your meditation, free from distractions and disturbances.

- **Focus on the Flame:** Sit comfortably and focus your gaze on the candle flame, allowing your mind to settle and your breathing to slow.

- **Incorporate Deep Breathing:** Enhance the relaxation effects by incorporating deep breathing exercises, inhaling the soothing scents deeply and exhaling slowly.

- **Regular Practice:** Make scented candle meditation a regular part of your routine to consistently benefit from its calming and relaxing effects.

Benefits:

Scented candle meditation offers a simple yet powerful way to achieve deep relaxation and mental clarity. By combining the calming effects of candlelight and aromatherapy, this practice can reduce stress, enhance mindfulness, and promote emotional well-being. Incorporating scented candle meditation into your daily routine can create a peaceful and balanced mental state, supporting overall health and happiness.

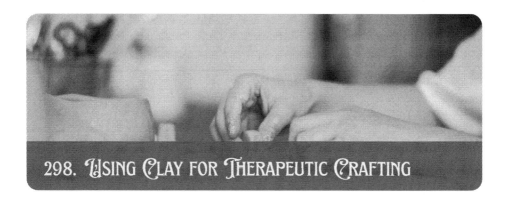

298. USING CLAY FOR THERAPEUTIC CRAFTING

Introduction:

Using clay for therapeutic crafting is a hands-on activity that promotes relaxation, creativity, and emotional expression. Working with clay can help reduce stress, improve focus, and foster a sense of accomplishment and well-being. This tactile and immersive practice allows individuals to connect with their inner selves and find calm through the creative process.

Basic Uses and Information:

Therapeutic crafting with clay involves shaping, molding, and creating objects from natural clay. This practice can be done individually or in group settings and is suitable for all ages. The tactile experience of working with clay can be soothing and meditative, providing both mental and physical benefits.

Detailed Uses of Using Clay for Therapeutic Crafting:

Reduces Stress and Anxiety:

- **Tactile Soothing:** The physical act of manipulating clay can be deeply calming, helping to lower stress levels and reduce anxiety.

- **Focus and Distraction:** Engaging in a creative task like clay crafting can distract from negative thoughts and provide a mental break from stressors.

Enhances Mindfulness and Focus:

- **Promotes Presence:** The immersive nature of clay crafting encourages mindfulness, helping you stay focused on the present moment.

- **Improves Concentration:** The detailed and repetitive actions involved in shaping clay can enhance concentration and mental clarity.

Supports Emotional Expression and Healing:

- **Expressive Outlet:** Clay crafting provides a non-verbal outlet for expressing emotions, helping to process feelings and experiences creatively.

- **Emotional Release:** The act of creating can be therapeutic, allowing for the release of pent-up emotions and promoting emotional balance.

Boosts Creativity and Self-Esteem:

- **Stimulates Creativity:** Working with clay encourages creative thinking and problem-solving, enhancing overall creativity.

- **Sense of Accomplishment:** Completing a clay project can boost self-esteem and provide a sense of achievement and satisfaction.

Tips for Enhancing the Use of Clay for Therapeutic Crafting:

- ◊ **Choose the Right Clay:** Select a type of clay that is easy to work with and suitable for your skill level, such as air-dry clay or polymer clay.

- ◊ **Create a Comfortable Workspace:** Set up a comfortable and quiet area for your crafting, with all necessary tools and materials within reach.

- ◊ **Set Intentions:** Begin your crafting session with a clear intention, whether it's relaxation, emotional expression, or simply enjoying the creative process.

- ◊ **Be Patient and Open:** Allow yourself to experiment and make mistakes, focusing on the process rather than the final product.

- ◊ **Regular Practice:** Incorporate clay crafting into your routine to regularly benefit from its therapeutic effects.

Benefits:

Using clay for therapeutic crafting offers a hands-on approach to reducing stress, enhancing mindfulness, and promoting emotional well-being. This creative practice can improve mental clarity, boost self-esteem, and provide a meaningful outlet for self-expression. By integrating clay crafting into your routine, you can enjoy a calming and fulfilling activity that supports overall mental and emotional health.

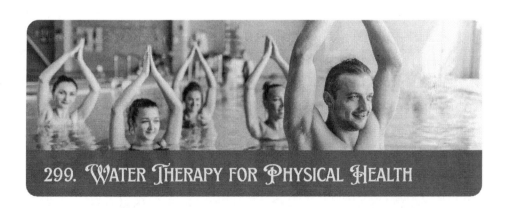

299. WATER THERAPY FOR PHYSICAL HEALTH

Introduction:

Water therapy, also known as hydrotherapy, utilizes the healing properties of water to improve physical health and well-being. This therapeutic practice involves various techniques such as immersion, contrast baths, and aquatic exercises to alleviate pain, enhance circulation, and promote overall health.

Water's unique properties, including buoyancy, resistance, and thermal effects, make it an effective medium for physical therapy and rehabilitation.

Basic Uses and Information:

Water therapy can be conducted in different settings, including pools, hot tubs, and bathtubs. The practice can be tailored to individual needs and conditions, making it suitable for a wide range of health issues. Water therapy leverages water's supportive and therapeutic qualities to aid in physical recovery and improve bodily functions.

Detailed Uses of Water Therapy for Physical Health:

Pain Relief and Management:

- **Reduces Joint Pain:** The buoyancy of water reduces the impact on joints, making it ideal for individuals with arthritis or joint pain.

- **Alleviates Muscle Soreness:** Warm water helps relax muscles and alleviate soreness, providing relief from conditions like fibromyalgia and chronic pain.

Enhances Circulation and Cardiovascular Health:

- **Improves Blood Flow:** The warmth of the water can dilate blood vessels, enhancing circulation and promoting cardiovascular health.

- **Reduces Swelling:** Hydrostatic pressure from water immersion helps reduce swelling and improve lymphatic drainage.

Supports Physical Rehabilitation:

- **Facilitates Movement:** Water's buoyancy supports the body, reducing strain and allowing for greater range of motion during physical therapy exercises.

- **Builds Strength:** Water resistance provides a gentle yet effective way to strengthen muscles without the risk of injury.

Promotes Relaxation and Stress Relief:

- **Eases Tension:** Immersion in warm water can reduce muscle tension and promote relaxation, reducing stress and anxiety levels.

- **Improves Sleep:** Regular water therapy can improve sleep quality by promoting relaxation and reducing physical discomfort.

Tips for Enhancing Water Therapy for Physical Health:

- **Choose the Right Temperature:** Use warm water for relaxation and pain relief, and cool water for reducing inflammation and invigorating the body.

- **Incorporate Aquatic Exercises:** Engage in gentle exercises such as walking, stretching, or resistance movements in water to enhance physical fitness and rehabilitation.

- **Use Contrast Baths:** Alternate between hot and cold water to stimulate circulation and reduce muscle soreness. Start with hot water for 3-4 minutes, followed by cold water for 1-2 minutes, and repeat.
- **Hydrate Properly:** Ensure you drink plenty of water before and after water therapy sessions to stay hydrated and support overall health.

Benefits:

Water therapy offers a versatile and effective way to enhance physical health through pain relief, improved circulation, and support for physical rehabilitation. By incorporating water therapy into your health routine, you can benefit from its soothing and therapeutic effects, promoting overall physical well-being and quality of life.

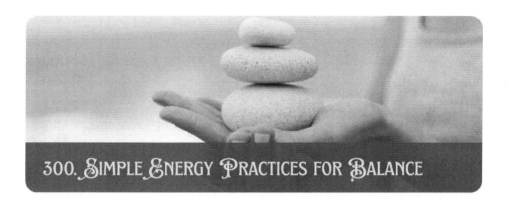

300. Simple Energy Practices for Balance

Introduction:

Simple energy practices focus on balancing and harmonizing the body's natural energy flow to promote overall well-being. These practices can help reduce stress, increase vitality, and enhance emotional and mental clarity. By incorporating easy and accessible techniques into your daily routine, you can maintain energetic balance and support your health.

Basic Uses and Information:

Energy practices often draw from ancient traditions and modern wellness methods, including techniques like breathwork, visualization, and gentle movements. These practices can be performed anywhere and require no special equipment, making them ideal for integrating into everyday life.

Detailed Uses of Simple Energy Practices for Balance:

Breathwork:

- **Deep Breathing:** Simple deep breathing exercises help calm the nervous system, reduce stress, and increase oxygen flow to the brain and body.

- **Alternate Nostril Breathing:** This practice balances the left and right hemispheres of the brain, promoting mental clarity and emotional balance. Close one nostril and inhale deeply, then switch and exhale through the other nostril, repeating the cycle.

Visualization:

- **Energy Cleansing Visualization:** Imagine a bright light entering your body with each inhale, cleansing and revitalizing your energy. With each exhale, visualize releasing any negative energy or tension.

- **Grounding Visualization:** Picture roots extending from your feet into the earth, grounding and stabilizing your energy. This can help you feel centered and connected.

Gentle Movements:

- **Qi Gong:** This ancient Chinese practice involves gentle, flowing movements combined with breathwork to enhance energy flow and balance within the body. Simple routines can be practiced daily to improve overall energy.

- **Tai Chi:** Known for its slow, deliberate movements, Tai Chi helps harmonize energy, improve balance, and reduce stress.

Energy Points Stimulation:

- **Acupressure:** Applying gentle pressure to specific points on the body can stimulate energy flow and alleviate various ailments. Common points include the temples, wrists, and the base of the skull.

- **Tapping (EFT):** This technique involves tapping on energy meridian points while focusing on specific issues or affirmations to balance energy and reduce emotional distress.

Tips for Enhancing Simple Energy Practices for Balance:

Consistency: Practice energy balancing techniques regularly, even if only for a few minutes each day, to maintain and enhance their benefits.

Mindfulness: Be present and fully engaged during your practice, paying attention to how your body and energy feel.

Create a Routine: Establish a routine that incorporates energy practices at specific times of day, such as morning breathwork or evening visualization, to create a habit.

- **Stay Hydrated:** Drink plenty of water to support energy flow and overall health.

Benefits:

Simple energy practices for balance offer a holistic approach to improving mental, emotional, and physical well-being. By incorporating these techniques into your daily routine, you can reduce stress, increase vitality, and maintain a harmonious balance of energy, supporting overall health and enhancing quality of life.

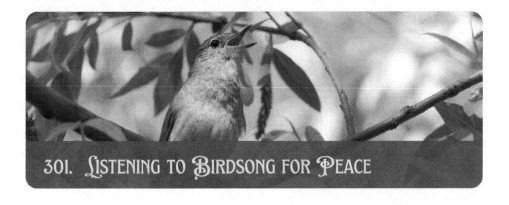

301. LISTENING TO BIRDSONG FOR PEACE

Introduction:

Listening to birdsong is a natural and effective way to cultivate a sense of peace and tranquility. The melodic sounds of birds can soothe the mind, reduce stress, and promote overall well-being. Integrating this practice into your daily routine can enhance mental clarity, improve mood, and create a deeper connection with nature.

Basic Uses and Information:

Birdsong can be enjoyed by spending time in natural settings, such as parks, forests, or gardens, or by listening to recordings of bird sounds. This practice leverages the calming and rhythmic nature of birdsong to create a peaceful environment conducive to relaxation and mindfulness.

Detailed Uses of Listening to Birdsong for Peace:

Reduces Stress and Anxiety:

- **Calming Effect:** The natural melodies of birdsong have a calming effect on the nervous system, helping to lower cortisol levels and reduce stress.

- **Promotes Relaxation:** Listening to birds can create a serene atmosphere that encourages relaxation and mental calmness.

Enhances Mental Clarity and Focus:

Clears the Mind: The gentle and repetitive nature of birdsong can help clear mental clutter, improving concentration and mental clarity. .

Encourages Mindfulness: Focusing on the sounds of birds can enhance mindfulness, helping you stay present and attentive to the moment.

Improves Mood and Emotional Well-Being:

- **Elevates Mood:** The cheerful and harmonious sounds of birdsong can boost mood and promote feelings of happiness and well-being.

- **Provides Comfort:** The familiarity and beauty of bird sounds can provide a sense of comfort and security, enhancing emotional stability.

Fosters Connection with Nature:

- **Increases Appreciation:** Regularly listening to birdsong can deepen your appreciation for nature and its beauty, fostering a greater sense of connection to the environment.

- **Encourages Outdoor Activity:** This practice can motivate you to spend more time outdoors, benefiting both your physical and mental health.

Tips for Enhancing the Practice of Listening to Birdsong for Peace:

- 💡 **Find Natural Settings:** Whenever possible, spend time in areas where birds are present, such as parks, gardens, or nature reserves, to fully experience the calming effects of birdsong.

- 💡 **Use Recordings:** If natural settings are not accessible, use high-quality recordings of birdsong to create a peaceful atmosphere at home or work.

- 💡 **Combine with Meditation:** Enhance the practice by combining birdsong listening with meditation or deep breathing exercises to further promote relaxation and mindfulness.

- 💡 **Regular Practice:** Integrate listening to birdsong into your daily routine, especially during times of high stress or before bed, to consistently benefit from its soothing effects.

Benefits:

Listening to birdsong provides a natural and accessible way to reduce stress, enhance mental clarity, and promote emotional well-being. By incorporating this practice into your daily life, you can create a peaceful and harmonious environment that supports overall mental and emotional health. Regular exposure to the calming sounds of birds can foster a deeper connection with nature and enhance your quality of life.

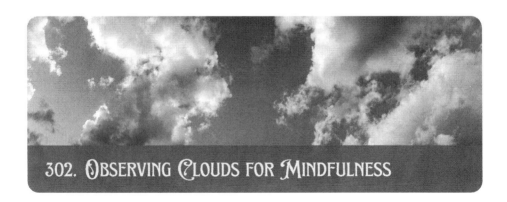

302. OBSERVING CLOUDS FOR MINDFULNESS

Introduction:

Observing clouds is a simple yet profound practice that encourages mindfulness and a deep sense of presence. By watching the ever-changing shapes and movements of clouds, you can cultivate a calm and focused mind, reduce stress, and enhance your connection to the natural world. This meditative activity is accessible to anyone and can be done almost anywhere.

Basic Uses and Information:

Cloud watching involves sitting or lying down in an open area with a clear view of the sky and observing the clouds without any specific agenda or goal. This practice encourages you to slow down, breathe deeply, and fully engage with the present moment, fostering a sense of peace and tranquility.

Detailed Uses of Observing Clouds for Mindfulness:

Reduces Stress and Anxiety:

- **Calming Effect:** The gentle, slow movement of clouds can have a soothing effect on the mind, helping to lower cortisol levels and reduce stress.

- **Promotes Relaxation:** Cloud watching creates a serene environment that encourages relaxation and mental calmness.

Enhances Mental Clarity and Focus:

- **Clears the Mind:** Focusing on the natural and dynamic patterns of clouds can help clear mental clutter, improving concentration and mental clarity.

- **Encourages Mindfulness:** Observing clouds enhances mindfulness by helping you stay present and attentive to the moment, fostering a deeper sense of awareness.

Improves Mood and Emotional Well-Being:

- **Elevates Mood:** The beauty and tranquility of the sky can uplift your spirits and promote feelings of happiness and well-being.

- **Provides Perspective:** Watching clouds drift across the sky can provide a sense of perspective, helping you feel more connected to the larger world.

Fosters Connection with Nature:

- **Increases Appreciation:** Regularly observing clouds can deepen your appreciation for the natural world and its rhythms, fostering a greater sense of connection to the environment.

- **Encourages Outdoor Activity:** This practice can motivate you to spend more time outdoors, benefiting both your physical and mental health.

Tips for Enhancing the Practice of Observing Clouds for Mindfulness:

- Find a Comfortable Spot: Choose a quiet and comfortable place to sit or lie down where you have a clear view of the sky, such as a park, garden, or open field.

- Breathe Deeply: Incorporate deep breathing exercises to enhance relaxation and mindfulness while observing the clouds.

- Stay Present: Focus solely on the clouds, letting go of any distracting thoughts or worries, and simply observe their shapes, movements, and colors.

- 💡 Combine with Other Practices: Enhance the experience by combining cloud watching with other mindfulness practices, such as meditation or journaling.

- 💡 Regular Practice: Integrate cloud watching into your regular routine, especially during times of high stress or when you need a mental break, to consistently benefit from its calming effects.

Benefits:

Observing clouds for mindfulness offers a natural and effective way to reduce stress, enhance mental clarity, and promote emotional well-being. By incorporating this practice into your daily life, you can create a peaceful and balanced mental state, foster a deeper connection with nature, and enjoy a simple yet profound sense of tranquility and presence. Regularly taking time to watch the clouds can enrich your life, providing a moment of calm and reflection amidst the busyness of daily life.

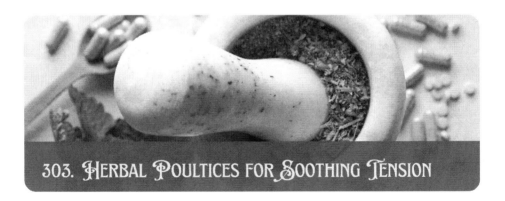

303. HERBAL POULTICES FOR SOOTHING TENSION

Introduction:

Herbal poultices are natural remedies that involve applying a mixture of herbs directly to the skin to alleviate tension, reduce pain, and promote healing. This traditional practice harnesses the therapeutic properties of herbs to provide relief from muscle tension, inflammation, and various skin conditions. Poultices can be made easily at home and are a gentle yet effective way to soothe the body.

Basic Uses and Information:

A poultice is created by mixing fresh or dried herbs with a small amount of hot water to form a paste, which is then applied to the affected area. The herbs are typically wrapped in a cloth or directly applied and covered with a warm, damp cloth to keep the herbs in place and enhance their effects. Herbal poultices can be used to treat a variety of conditions, including sore muscles, joint pain, bruises, and skin irritations.

Detailed Uses of Herbal Poultices for Soothing Tension:

Muscle and Joint Pain Relief:

- **Eases Muscle Tension:** Herbs such as arnica, ginger, and cayenne pepper have anti-inflammatory and warming properties that help relax tense muscles and reduce pain.

- **Reduces Joint Pain:** Poultices made from herbs like comfrey, turmeric, and eucalyptus can alleviate joint pain and inflammation, providing relief from conditions such as arthritis.

Soothes Inflammation and Bruises:

- **Anti-Inflammatory Effects:** Herbs such as chamomile, calendula, and plantain have anti-inflammatory properties that can reduce swelling and soothe inflamed tissues.

- **Promotes Healing:** Applying a poultice to bruises can speed up the healing process by increasing blood flow and reducing discoloration.

Treats Skin Conditions:

- **Heals Wounds and Infections:** Antiseptic and healing herbs like thyme, garlic, and lavender can be used in poultices to treat minor wounds, cuts, and infections.

- **Relieves Skin Irritations:** Poultices made from herbs such as aloe vera, marshmallow root, and chamomile can soothe and heal skin irritations, rashes, and burns.

Tips for Enhancing the Use of Herbal Poultices for Soothing Tension:

- **Select Appropriate Herbs:** Choose herbs based on their specific properties and your particular needs. Fresh herbs are often more potent, but dried herbs can also be effective.

- **Prepare Properly:** Mix the herbs with warm water to form a paste. Ensure the mixture is not too hot to avoid burns. Apply the paste to a clean cloth before placing it on the skin.

- **Secure the Poultice:** Use a bandage or cloth to secure the poultice in place. Cover with a warm, damp cloth to enhance the herbal effects and keep the poultice moist.

- **Leave on for Sufficient Time:** Allow the poultice to remain on the affected area for at least 20-30 minutes, or longer if needed, to maximize its benefits.

- **Regular Use:** For chronic conditions, apply poultices regularly to achieve the best results. Adjust the frequency based on the severity of the symptoms and the body's response.

Benefits:

Herbal poultices provide a natural and effective way to soothe muscle tension, reduce inflammation, and treat various skin conditions. By incorporating this practice into your health routine, you can benefit from the healing properties of herbs, promote relaxation, and support overall well-being. Using herbal poultices is a gentle and holistic approach to managing pain and discomfort, offering a therapeutic alternative to conventional treatments.

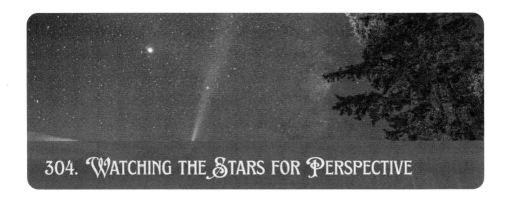

304. Watching the Stars for Perspective

Introduction:

Watching the stars is a timeless practice that fosters a sense of wonder and perspective. By observing the vastness of the night sky, you can gain a deeper appreciation for the universe and your place within it. This meditative activity can reduce stress, enhance mental clarity, and promote a sense of peace and connection to the larger cosmos.

Basic Uses and Information:

Star gazing involves finding a dark, clear spot away from city lights, lying down or sitting comfortably, and simply observing the stars. This practice can be done alone or with others, and it encourages mindfulness, reflection, and a sense of awe. It can be enhanced with the use of telescopes or star charts, but these tools are not necessary to enjoy the experience.

Detailed Uses of Watching the Stars for Perspective:

Reduces Stress and Anxiety:

- **Calming Effect:** The stillness and beauty of the night sky can have a calming effect on the mind, helping to lower stress levels and reduce anxiety.

- **Promotes Relaxation:** Watching the stars creates a serene environment that encourages relaxation and mental peace.

Enhances Mental Clarity and Focus:

- **Clears the Mind:** The vastness of the universe can help clear mental clutter, allowing for better concentration and mental clarity.

- **Encourages Mindfulness:** Focusing on the stars enhances mindfulness, helping you stay present and fully engaged with the moment.

Improves Mood and Emotional Well-Being:

- **Elevates Mood:** The awe-inspiring view of the night sky can uplift your spirits and promote feelings of happiness and well-being.

- **Provides Perspective:** Contemplating the enormity of the universe can help put personal problems into perspective, fostering a sense of humility and acceptance.

Fosters Connection with Nature and the Universe:

- **Increases Appreciation:** Regularly watching the stars can deepen your appreciation for the natural world and the mysteries of the cosmos.

- **Encourages Reflection:** The quiet and contemplative nature of star gazing can inspire introspection and a deeper connection to your own inner thoughts and feelings.

Tips for Enhancing the Practice of Watching the Stars for Perspective:

- 💡 **Find a Dark Spot:** Choose a location away from city lights and pollution to get the clearest view of the stars. Parks, beaches, or rural areas are ideal.

- 💡 **Use Comfortable Seating:** Bring a blanket, chair, or mat to sit or lie on comfortably while you observe the sky.

- 💡 **Check the Weather:** Ensure the sky is clear and free of clouds for optimal star gazing conditions.

- 💡 **Allow Your Eyes to Adjust:** Give your eyes 10-20 minutes to adjust to the darkness for the best visibility of stars.

- 💡 **Combine with Reflection:** Use the time to reflect on your life, goals, and the bigger picture, enhancing the sense of perspective and tranquility.

Benefits:

Watching the stars provides a natural and profound way to reduce stress, enhance mental clarity, and gain a greater perspective on life. By incorporating this practice into your routine, you can foster a sense of peace, connection, and awe, enriching your mental and emotional well-being. Regular star gazing can offer a moment of calm and reflection, helping you navigate the complexities of daily life with a renewed sense of perspective and tranquility.

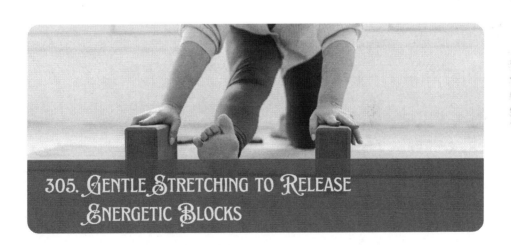

305. GENTLE STRETCHING TO RELEASE ENERGETIC BLOCKS

Introduction:

Gentle stretching is an effective way to release energetic blocks, improve flexibility, and enhance overall well-being. This practice involves slow, mindful movements that help to open up the body's energy pathways, promoting the free flow of energy and reducing physical and emotional tension.

Basic Uses and Information:

Gentle stretching can be done at any time of the day and requires no special equipment. The key is to move slowly and with intention, focusing on the sensations in your body and your breath. This practice can help to release stored tension, improve circulation, and support mental clarity and emotional balance.

Detailed Uses of Gentle Stretching to Release Energetic Blocks:

Reduces Physical Tension:

- **Relieves Muscle Tightness:** Gentle stretching helps to lengthen and relax muscles, reducing tightness and discomfort.

- **Improves Flexibility:** Regular stretching can increase the flexibility of muscles and joints, enhancing overall physical function and reducing the risk of injury.

Promotes Energy Flow:

- **Opens Energy Pathways:** Stretching can help to open up the body's energy pathways, promoting the free flow of energy and reducing energetic blockages.

- **Enhances Vitality:** By improving energy flow, stretching can boost overall vitality and reduce feelings of fatigue.

Supports Emotional Well-Being:

- **Reduces Stress:** The mindful, slow movements of gentle stretching can help to calm the nervous system, reducing stress and anxiety.

- **Balances Emotions:** Stretching can help to release stored emotional tension, promoting a sense of balance and emotional well-being.

Improves Mental Clarity:

- **Enhances Focus:** The meditative nature of gentle stretching can improve concentration and mental clarity.

- **Promotes Mindfulness:** Focusing on your breath and body during stretching can enhance mindfulness and help you stay present in the moment.

Tips for Enhancing Gentle Stretching to Release Energetic Blocks:

- **Move Slowly and Mindfully:** Focus on slow, controlled movements and pay attention to how your body feels with each stretch.

- **Breathe Deeply:** Use deep, rhythmic breathing to enhance relaxation and support the release of tension.

- **Incorporate Regular Breaks:** Integrate gentle stretching into your daily routine, taking breaks to stretch and move throughout the day.

- **Focus on Key Areas:** Pay special attention to areas where tension tends to build up, such as the neck, shoulders, back, and hips.

☀ **Create a Relaxing Environment:** Stretch in a calm, quiet space where you can fully focus on your practice without distractions.

Benefits:

Gentle stretching offers a holistic approach to releasing energetic blocks and promoting overall well-being. By incorporating this practice into your daily routine, you can reduce physical and emotional tension, enhance flexibility, and support mental clarity and emotional balance. Gentle stretching is a simple yet powerful tool for maintaining a healthy, vibrant body and mind.

PART 15

Addressing Common Ailments

(306-325)

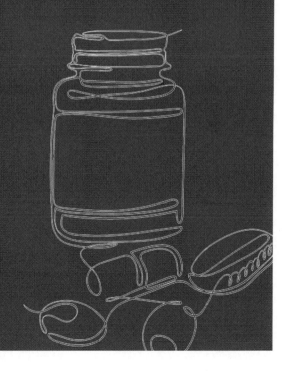

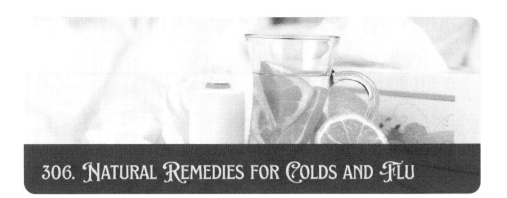

Introduction:

Colds and flu are common respiratory illnesses caused by viruses. While they often resolve on their own, natural remedies can help alleviate symptoms, boost the immune system, and speed up recovery. These remedies focus on using herbs, foods, and practices that support the body's natural healing processes.

Basic Uses and Information:

Natural remedies for colds and flu include herbal teas, supplements, essential oils, and lifestyle practices. These remedies can help reduce symptoms such as congestion, sore throat, cough, and fever, while also enhancing the body's ability to fight off infections.

Detailed Uses of Natural Remedies for Colds and Flu:

Herbal Teas and Infusions:

- **Elderberry:** Rich in antioxidants and vitamins, elderberry syrup or tea can help boost the immune system and reduce the duration of colds and flu.

- **Ginger:** Ginger tea can soothe sore throats, reduce inflammation, and help clear nasal congestion.

- **Echinacea:** Echinacea tea or supplements can enhance immune function and help the body fight off viral infections.

Essential Oils:

- **Eucalyptus:** Inhaling eucalyptus oil can help relieve congestion and improve respiratory function.

- **Peppermint:** Peppermint oil has antiviral and decongestant properties that can ease symptoms of colds and flu.

- **Tea Tree Oil:** Known for its antimicrobial properties, tea tree oil can help combat respiratory infections when used in steam inhalation.

Immune-Boosting Foods:

- **Garlic:** Garlic has antiviral and antibacterial properties that can help fight off colds and flu. Add raw or cooked garlic to your meals.

- **Honey:** Honey has natural antibacterial properties and can soothe sore throats and coughs. Mix honey with warm water or herbal tea.

- **Citrus Fruits:** High in vitamin C, citrus fruits like oranges, lemons, and grapefruits can boost the immune system and reduce symptoms.

Hydration and Rest:

- **Stay Hydrated:** Drink plenty of fluids such as water, herbal teas, and broths to stay hydrated and help thin mucus.

- **Rest:** Ensure you get adequate rest to allow your body to recover and fight off the infection.

Warm Compresses and Baths:

- **Warm Compresses:** Apply warm compresses to the sinuses to relieve congestion and sinus pressure.

- **Warm Baths:** Taking a warm bath with Epsom salts and essential oils can help reduce muscle aches and promote relaxation.

Tips for Using Natural Remedies for Colds and Flu:

- **Consistency:** Use these remedies consistently at the first sign of symptoms to maximize their effectiveness.

- **Combine Remedies:** Combine different natural remedies for a synergistic effect. For example, drink herbal teas while using essential oils in a diffuser.

- **Avoid Overexertion:** Rest and avoid strenuous activities to give your body the best chance to heal.

- **Monitor Symptoms:** If symptoms persist for more than a week or worsen, seek medical advice to rule out more serious conditions.

Benefits:

Natural remedies for colds and flu offer a gentle and effective way to alleviate symptoms, boost the immune system, and support the body's natural healing processes. By incorporating these remedies into your routine, you can reduce the severity and duration of colds and flu, enhance overall well-being, and maintain a healthier lifestyle.

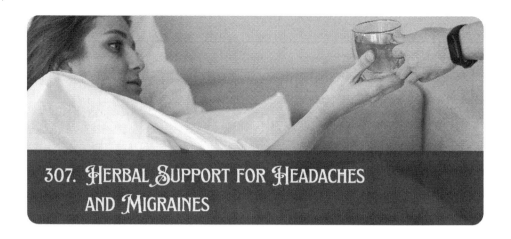

307. Herbal Support for Headaches and Migraines

Introduction:

Headaches and migraines can be debilitating, affecting daily activities and overall well-being. Herbal remedies provide a natural and effective way to alleviate the pain and discomfort associated with headaches and migraines. These remedies focus on using herbs with anti-inflammatory, analgesic, and calming properties to reduce symptoms and promote relief.

Basic Uses and Information:

Herbal support for headaches and migraines includes teas, tinctures, essential oils, and supplements. These natural treatments can help reduce the frequency, severity, and duration of headaches and migraines by addressing underlying causes such as inflammation, stress, and muscle tension.

Detailed Uses of Herbal Support for Headaches and Migraines:

Herbal Teas and Infusions:

- **Peppermint:** Peppermint tea has menthol, which can help relieve tension headaches by relaxing muscles and improving blood flow.

- **Ginger:** Ginger tea can reduce inflammation and pain associated with headaches and migraines. It also helps with nausea, which often accompanies migraines.

- **Feverfew:** Feverfew tea or supplements can help prevent and reduce the severity of migraines by inhibiting the release of inflammatory substances in the brain.

Essential Oils:

- **Lavender:** Inhaling lavender oil or applying it to the temples can reduce the intensity of migraines and promote relaxation.

- **Peppermint:** Peppermint oil applied to the temples and neck can provide a cooling effect and reduce headache pain.

- **Eucalyptus:** Eucalyptus oil can help relieve sinus headaches by reducing inflammation and clearing nasal passages.

Supplements:

- **Magnesium:** Magnesium supplements can help prevent migraines by relaxing blood vessels and reducing muscle tension.

- **Riboflavin (Vitamin B2):** Taking riboflavin supplements daily can reduce the frequency and severity of migraines.

- **Butterbur:** Butterbur supplements have been shown to reduce the frequency of migraine attacks by reducing inflammation and stabilizing blood flow in the brain.

Lifestyle Practices:

- **Stay Hydrated:** Dehydration can trigger headaches and migraines. Drink plenty of water throughout the day to stay hydrated.

- **Regular Sleep:** Maintain a regular sleep schedule to reduce the risk of headaches and migraines triggered by sleep disturbances.

- **Stress Management:** Practice stress-reducing techniques such as meditation, yoga, or deep breathing exercises to prevent tension headaches and migraines.

Topical Applications:

- **Cold Compresses:** Applying a cold compress to the forehead or back of the neck can help constrict blood vessels and reduce headache pain.

- **Herbal Balms:** Use balms containing menthol or camphor on the temples and neck to relieve tension and provide pain relief.

Tips for Using Herbal Support for Headaches and Migraines:

- Identify Triggers: Keep a headache diary to identify and avoid triggers such as certain foods, stress, or lack of sleep.

- Start Early: Use herbal remedies at the first sign of a headache or migraine to prevent it from worsening.

- Combine Remedies: Combine different herbal treatments and lifestyle practices for a comprehensive approach to managing headaches and migraines.

- Consult a Healthcare Provider: If you have chronic or severe headaches and migraines, consult a healthcare provider to rule out underlying conditions and discuss appropriate treatments.

Benefits:

Herbal support for headaches and migraines provides a natural, holistic approach to managing pain and discomfort. By incorporating these remedies into your routine, you can reduce the frequency and severity of headaches and migraines, improve your quality of life, and maintain overall well-being. These natural treatments offer a gentle and effective way to address headaches and migraines without the side effects associated with many conventional medications.

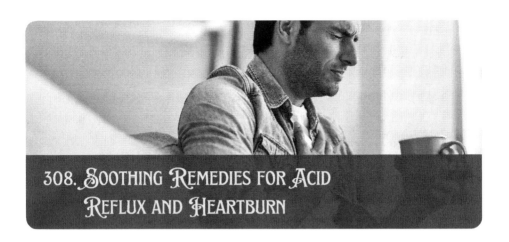

308. Soothing Remedies for Acid Reflux and Heartburn

Introduction:

Acid reflux and heartburn are common digestive issues that can cause discomfort and pain. Natural remedies can provide relief by soothing the digestive tract, reducing stomach acid, and promoting healthy digestion. These remedies focus on using herbs, foods, and lifestyle practices to alleviate symptoms and support gastrointestinal health.

Basic Uses and Information:

Natural remedies for acid reflux and heartburn include herbal teas, supplements, dietary adjustments, and lifestyle changes. These remedies aim to neutralize stomach acid, soothe the esophagus, and improve overall digestion.

Detailed Uses of Soothing Remedies for Acid Reflux and Heartburn:

Herbal Teas and Infusions:

- **Chamomile:** Chamomile tea can reduce inflammation and soothe the esophagus, providing relief from acid reflux and heartburn.

- **Ginger:** Ginger tea can help improve digestion and reduce stomach acid, easing symptoms of acid reflux.

- **Licorice Root:** Deglycyrrhizinated licorice (DGL) can help protect the lining of the esophagus and stomach, reducing irritation and discomfort.

Dietary Adjustments:

- **Alkaline Foods:** Incorporating alkaline foods such as bananas, melons, and leafy greens can help neutralize stomach acid and reduce symptoms.

- **Avoid Trigger Foods:** Avoid foods that can trigger acid reflux, such as spicy foods, fatty foods, chocolate, caffeine, and citrus fruits.

- **Smaller, Frequent Meals:** Eating smaller, more frequent meals can prevent the stomach from becoming too full and reduce the risk of acid reflux.

Supplements:

- **Aloe Vera:** Aloe vera juice can help soothe the digestive tract and reduce inflammation, providing relief from acid reflux.

- **Probiotics:** Taking probiotic supplements can improve gut health and digestion, reducing the likelihood of acid reflux and heartburn.

- **Apple Cider Vinegar:** A small amount of apple cider vinegar mixed with water before meals can help balance stomach acid levels and improve digestion.

Lifestyle Practices:

- **Elevate the Head:** Elevating the head of your bed by 6-8 inches can prevent stomach acid from flowing back into the esophagus during sleep.

- **Maintain a Healthy Weight:** Excess weight can put pressure on the stomach, leading to acid reflux. Maintaining a healthy weight can reduce symptoms.

- **Avoid Lying Down After Eating:** Wait at least 2-3 hours after eating before lying down to prevent acid reflux.

Topical Applications and Natural Remedies:

- **Baking Soda:** A small amount of baking soda mixed with water can neutralize stomach acid and provide quick relief from heartburn.

- **Slippery Elm:** Slippery elm supplements or tea can coat the lining of the esophagus and stomach, reducing irritation and soothing discomfort.

Tips for Using Soothing Remedies for Acid Reflux and Heartburn:

- Identify Triggers: Keep a food diary to identify and avoid foods that trigger acid reflux and heartburn.

- Stay Hydrated: Drink plenty of water throughout the day to aid digestion and prevent acid reflux.

- Chew Food Thoroughly: Chewing food thoroughly can improve digestion and reduce the risk of acid reflux.

- Practice Mindful Eating: Eat slowly and mindfully to prevent overeating and reduce the risk of acid reflux.

Benefits:

Soothing remedies for acid reflux and heartburn offer a natural and effective way to manage these common digestive issues. By incorporating these remedies into your routine, you can reduce symptoms, improve digestion, and support overall gastrointestinal health. These natural treatments provide a gentle and holistic approach to alleviating acid reflux and heartburn, promoting long-term digestive well-being.

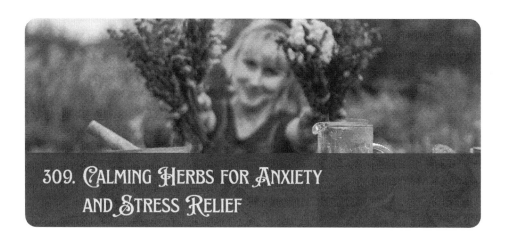

309. CALMING HERBS FOR ANXIETY AND STRESS RELIEF

Introduction:

Anxiety and stress are common issues that can significantly impact daily life and overall well-being. Calming herbs offer a natural and effective way to alleviate these feelings by promoting relaxation, reducing tension, and supporting mental clarity. These herbs have been used for centuries to help manage stress and anxiety through their soothing properties.

Basic Uses and Information:

Calming herbs can be used in various forms, including teas, tinctures, capsules, and essential oils. These herbs work by interacting with the nervous system to promote a sense of calm and relaxation, making them a valuable addition to stress and anxiety management routines.

Detailed Uses of Calming Herbs for Anxiety and Stress Relief:

Herbal Teas and Infusions:

- **Chamomile:** Chamomile tea is renowned for its calming effects, helping to reduce anxiety and promote restful sleep. It works by binding to receptors in the brain that help relax the nervous system.

- **Lavender:** Lavender tea can help reduce anxiety and improve mood through its natural sedative properties. The aroma of lavender is also effective in calming the mind.

- **Lemon Balm:** Lemon balm tea has mild sedative effects that can help reduce stress and anxiety. It also improves mood and cognitive function.

Tinctures and Extracts:

- **Valerian Root:** Valerian root tinctures are commonly used to alleviate anxiety and promote relaxation without causing drowsiness. It works by increasing levels of gamma-aminobutyric acid (GABA) in the brain, which has a calming effect.

- **Passionflower:** Passionflower tinctures can help reduce anxiety and improve sleep quality by increasing GABA levels in the brain.

- **Ashwagandha:** Ashwagandha tinctures or capsules are adaptogenic, helping the body adapt to stress and reduce anxiety by lowering cortisol levels.

Essential Oils:

- **Lavender Oil:** Inhaling lavender essential oil or using it in a diffuser can reduce anxiety and promote relaxation. It can also be applied topically when diluted with a carrier oil.

- **Frankincense Oil:** Frankincense essential oil has grounding properties that can help reduce stress and anxiety when inhaled or used in aromatherapy.

- **Bergamot Oil:** Bergamot essential oil is known for its uplifting and calming effects, making it useful for reducing anxiety and improving mood.

Capsules and Supplements:

- **Rhodiola Rosea:** Rhodiola capsules can help reduce fatigue and anxiety by balancing stress hormones and supporting the nervous system.

- **L-Theanine:** This amino acid, found in green tea, promotes relaxation and reduces stress without causing drowsiness. It can be taken as a supplement.

- **Magnesium:** Magnesium supplements can help reduce anxiety by relaxing muscles and calming the nervous system.

Lifestyle Practices:

- **Herbal Baths:** Adding calming herbs like lavender, chamomile, or rose petals to a warm bath can promote relaxation and reduce stress.

- **Herbal Pillows:** Sleeping with an herbal pillow filled with calming herbs such as lavender and hops can improve sleep quality and reduce nighttime anxiety.

- **Mindfulness Practices:** Combining herbal remedies with mindfulness techniques like meditation, deep breathing, or yoga can enhance their calming effects.

Tips for Using Calming Herbs for Anxiety and Stress Relief:

- **Start Slowly:** Begin with small doses to see how your body responds, especially if you are new to using herbs for anxiety and stress relief.

- **Consistency:** Use these herbs regularly as part of your daily routine for the best results.

- **Combine Methods:** Use a combination of teas, tinctures, essential oils, and supplements to create a comprehensive approach to managing anxiety and stress.

- **Consult a Healthcare Provider:** If you have any underlying health conditions or are taking other medications, consult with a healthcare provider before starting any new herbal regimen.

Benefits:

Calming herbs provide a natural and holistic approach to managing anxiety and stress. By incorporating these herbs into your daily routine, you can reduce symptoms, promote relaxation, and support overall mental and emotional well-being. These natural remedies offer a gentle and effective alternative to conventional treatments, helping to maintain a balanced and peaceful state of mind.

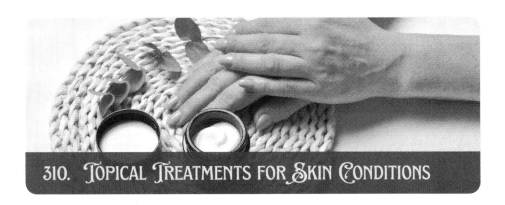

310. TOPICAL TREATMENTS FOR SKIN CONDITIONS

Introduction:

Skin conditions such as eczema, psoriasis, acne, and dermatitis can cause discomfort and affect overall well-being. Natural topical treatments using herbs and other natural ingredients can provide relief, promote healing, and improve skin health. These treatments focus on soothing inflammation, reducing irritation, and supporting the skin's natural healing processes.

Basic Uses and Information:

Topical treatments for skin conditions include herbal salves, creams, oils, and poultices. These remedies utilize the healing properties of natural ingredients to address specific skin issues and improve skin health. They are applied directly to the affected area for targeted relief.

Detailed Uses of Topical Treatments for Skin Conditions:

Herbal Salves and Creams:

- **Calendula:** Calendula salve or cream is highly effective for soothing irritated skin, reducing inflammation, and promoting healing in conditions like eczema and dermatitis.

- **Chamomile:** Chamomile cream can calm irritated skin and reduce redness and itching associated with eczema and other inflammatory skin conditions.

- **Comfrey:** Comfrey salve promotes skin cell regeneration and is useful for treating wounds, burns, and skin ulcers.

Essential Oils:

- **Tea Tree Oil:** Tea tree oil has antibacterial and anti-inflammatory properties, making it effective for treating acne and preventing infections in minor cuts and scrapes. Dilute with a carrier oil before applying to the skin.

- **Lavender Oil:** Lavender essential oil can soothe and heal skin irritations, burns, and insect bites. It also has antiseptic properties.

- **Frankincense Oil:** This oil helps reduce inflammation and can be beneficial for conditions like psoriasis and eczema. Mix with a carrier oil for topical use.

Carrier Oils:

- **Coconut Oil:** Coconut oil has antimicrobial properties and is deeply moisturizing, making it ideal for dry skin conditions such as eczema.

- **Jojoba Oil:** Jojoba oil mimics the skin's natural sebum, making it effective for balancing oily skin and treating acne.

- **Rosehip Oil:** Rich in vitamins and antioxidants, rosehip oil can help reduce scarring and promote healing in damaged skin.

Herbal Poultices:

- **Plantain:** Plantain leaves can be made into a poultice to soothe insect bites, rashes, and minor wounds. The herb has anti-inflammatory and antimicrobial properties.

- **Aloe Vera:** Fresh aloe vera gel can be applied directly to the skin to soothe burns, rashes, and irritation. It promotes healing and reduces inflammation.

- **Turmeric:** A turmeric poultice can reduce inflammation and speed up the healing of minor cuts and skin infections.

Natural Remedies:

- **Oatmeal:** Oatmeal baths or poultices can soothe itchy and inflamed skin, making it beneficial for eczema and dermatitis.

- **Honey:** Raw honey has antibacterial and healing properties. It can be applied to wounds, burns, and acne to promote healing and reduce infection.

- **Apple Cider Vinegar:** Diluted apple cider vinegar can be used as a toner to balance the skin's pH and treat acne.

Tips for Using Topical Treatments for Skin Conditions:

- ♀ **Patch Test:** Always perform a patch test before applying any new topical treatment to a larger area to ensure there is no allergic reaction.
- ♀ **Clean Skin:** Apply treatments to clean skin to ensure better absorption and effectiveness.
- ♀ **Regular Application:** Consistently apply the treatments as recommended to achieve the best results.

- ♀ **Combine Treatments:** Use a combination of treatments, such as herbal salves and essential oils, to address different aspects of the skin condition.
- ♀ **Consult a Healthcare Provider:** If you have persistent or severe skin conditions, consult a healthcare provider to rule out underlying issues and discuss appropriate treatments.

Benefits:

Natural topical treatments for skin conditions provide a gentle and effective way to soothe, heal, and improve skin health. By incorporating these remedies into your skincare routine, you can alleviate symptoms, promote healing, and support overall skin wellness. These treatments offer a holistic approach to managing skin conditions, utilizing the healing properties of natural ingredients to enhance skin health and comfort.

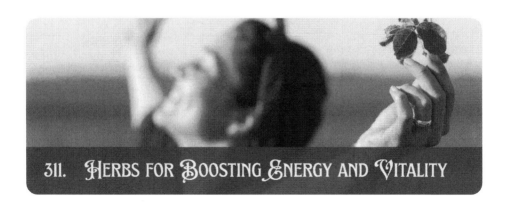

311. ℋERBS FOR ℬOOSTING ℰNERGY AND 𝒱ITALITY

Introduction:

Maintaining energy and vitality is crucial for overall well-being and productivity. Herbs can provide a natural and

effective way to enhance energy levels, improve stamina, and support physical and mental vitality. These herbs work by nourishing the body, supporting the adrenal glands, and improving circulation and oxygen flow.

Basic Uses and Information:

Herbs for boosting energy and vitality can be used in various forms, including teas, tinctures, capsules, and powders. These herbs help to reduce fatigue, enhance physical performance, and promote mental clarity without the jittery effects of caffeine.

Detailed Uses of Herbs for Boosting Energy and Vitality:

Adaptogenic Herbs:

- **Ashwagandha:** Ashwagandha is an adaptogen that helps the body cope with stress and fatigue, improving overall energy levels and stamina.

- **Rhodiola Rosea:** Rhodiola enhances physical performance and reduces mental fatigue by improving oxygen utilization and reducing stress.

- **Ginseng:** Ginseng, particularly Panax ginseng, is known for its ability to boost energy, enhance physical endurance, and improve mental clarity.

Herbal Teas and Infusions:

- **Yerba Mate:** Yerba mate tea provides a balanced energy boost, improves focus, and supports overall vitality due to its caffeine and antioxidant content.

- **Green Tea:** Green tea contains a moderate amount of caffeine and L-theanine, which together promote alertness and a calm focus.

- **Peppermint:** Peppermint tea can invigorate the senses and enhance mental clarity, making it a refreshing energy booster.

Nutrient-Rich Herbs:

- **Maca Root:** Maca root powder is rich in vitamins and minerals that support energy production and hormonal balance, enhancing overall vitality.

- **Spirulina:** Spirulina is a nutrient-dense algae that provides protein, vitamins, and minerals, boosting energy and supporting overall health.

- **Eleuthero (Siberian Ginseng):** Eleuthero is known for its ability to improve endurance, reduce fatigue, and enhance physical and mental performance.

Circulation-Enhancing Herbs:

- **Ginkgo Biloba:** Ginkgo biloba improves blood flow and oxygen supply to the brain, enhancing mental clarity and reducing fatigue.

- **Gotu Kola:** Gotu kola supports circulation and cognitive function, promoting energy and vitality.

- **Cayenne Pepper:** Cayenne pepper stimulates circulation and boosts metabolism, providing a natural energy lift.

Herbal Supplements:

- **Cordyceps:** Cordyceps mushrooms enhance energy levels and physical performance by improving oxygen utilization and increasing ATP production.

- **Bee Pollen:** Bee pollen is a superfood rich in nutrients that support energy, stamina, and overall vitality.

- **Licorice Root:** Licorice root supports adrenal health and helps maintain energy levels by modulating cortisol production.

Tips for Using Herbs for Boosting Energy and Vitality:

- Start with Small Doses: Begin with small doses to see how your body responds and gradually increase as needed.

- Consistency: Use these herbs regularly as part of your daily routine to maintain steady energy levels and vitality.

- Combine with a Balanced Diet: Complement herbal use with a balanced diet rich in whole foods to support overall health and energy.

- Stay Hydrated: Drink plenty of water throughout the day to support energy production and overall well-being.

- Consult a Healthcare Provider: If you have any underlying health conditions or are taking other medications, consult with a healthcare provider before starting any new herbal regimen.

Benefits:

Using herbs to boost energy and vitality offers a natural and holistic approach to maintaining physical and mental well-being. By incorporating these herbs into your daily routine, you can reduce fatigue, enhance stamina, and improve overall vitality without the negative side effects associated with stimulants. These natural remedies support a balanced and energetic lifestyle, promoting long-term health and productivity.

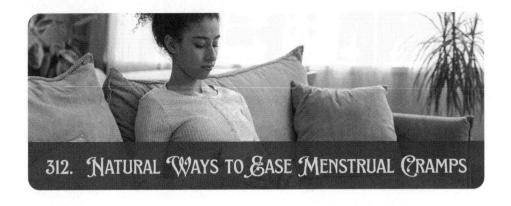

312. Natural Ways to Ease Menstrual Cramps

Introduction:

Menstrual cramps, also known as dysmenorrhea, can cause significant discomfort and affect daily activities for many women. Natural remedies offer effective ways to alleviate pain and discomfort without the side effects of medication. These methods focus on using herbs, lifestyle practices, and dietary changes to reduce inflammation, improve circulation, and relax muscles.

Basic Uses and Information:

Natural ways to ease menstrual cramps include herbal teas, essential oils, supplements, and physical practices. These remedies help to soothe the muscles of the uterus, reduce inflammation, and balance hormones, providing relief from menstrual pain.

Detailed Uses of Natural Ways to Ease Menstrual Cramps:

Herbal Teas and Infusions:

- **Chamomile:** Chamomile tea has anti-inflammatory and antispasmodic properties that help relax the uterus and reduce menstrual cramps.

- **Ginger:** Ginger tea can alleviate pain and reduce inflammation associated with menstrual cramps. It also helps with nausea.

- **Peppermint:** Peppermint tea has muscle-relaxing properties that can help soothe menstrual cramps and reduce bloating.

Essential Oils:

- **Lavender Oil:** Applying diluted lavender oil to the lower abdomen can relieve pain and promote relaxation through its calming properties.

- **Clary Sage Oil:** Clary sage oil can be massaged into the lower abdomen to reduce cramps and balance hormones.

- **Eucalyptus Oil:** Eucalyptus oil has anti-inflammatory properties that can help reduce menstrual pain when used in a massage oil blend.

Supplements:

- **Magnesium:** Magnesium supplements can help relax muscles and reduce the severity of menstrual cramps.

- **Omega-3 Fatty Acids:** Omega-3 supplements, such as fish oil, can reduce inflammation and alleviate menstrual pain.

- **Vitamin E:** Vitamin E supplements can help reduce the intensity and duration of menstrual cramps.

Dietary Adjustments:

- **Hydration:** Drinking plenty of water can help reduce bloating and alleviate menstrual cramps.

- **Anti-Inflammatory Foods:** Incorporate anti-inflammatory foods such as berries, leafy greens, nuts, and fatty fish to reduce inflammation and menstrual pain.

- **Avoid Caffeine and Alcohol:** Limiting caffeine and alcohol can help reduce cramps and bloating.

Physical Practices:

- **Heat Therapy:** Applying a heating pad or hot water bottle to the lower abdomen can relax muscles and alleviate menstrual cramps.

- **Exercise:** Regular physical activity, such as walking, yoga, or stretching, can improve blood flow and reduce menstrual pain.

- **Acupressure:** Applying gentle pressure to specific points, such as the webbing between the thumb and index finger or the area just above the ankle, can help relieve menstrual cramps.

Tips for Using Natural Remedies to Ease Menstrual Cramps:

- Regular Practice: Incorporate these remedies into your routine consistently, especially in the days leading up to and during your period.

- Listen to Your Body: Pay attention to how your body responds to different remedies and adjust your approach as needed.

- Create a Relaxing Environment: Use these remedies in a calm, comfortable setting to enhance their effectiveness.

- Stay Active: Regular exercise and movement can help prevent and alleviate menstrual cramps.

- Consult a Healthcare Provider: If menstrual cramps are severe or persistent, consult a healthcare provider to rule out underlying conditions and discuss appropriate treatments.

Benefits:

Natural remedies for easing menstrual cramps offer a holistic and gentle approach to managing pain and discomfort. By incorporating these methods into your routine, you can reduce the severity of cramps, improve overall well-being, and maintain a more comfortable and balanced menstrual cycle. These natural treatments provide a safe and effective alternative to medication, supporting long-term health and comfort.

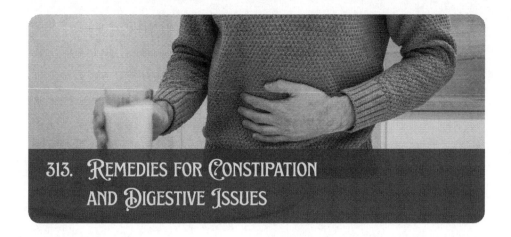

313. Remedies for Constipation and Digestive Issues

Introduction:

Constipation and digestive issues are common problems that can cause discomfort and affect overall health. Natural remedies can help alleviate these conditions by promoting healthy digestion, improving bowel movements, and soothing the digestive tract. These remedies focus on using herbs, dietary changes, and lifestyle practices to support digestive health.

Basic Uses and Information:

Remedies for constipation and digestive issues include herbal teas, supplements, dietary adjustments, and lifestyle changes. These natural treatments can help stimulate digestion, relieve constipation, and promote regular bowel movements.

Detailed Uses of Remedies for Constipation and Digestive Issues:

Herbal Teas and Infusions:

- **Peppermint:** Peppermint tea can help relax the digestive tract, relieve gas, and improve digestion.

- **Ginger:** Ginger tea can stimulate digestive enzymes, reduce inflammation, and alleviate nausea and bloating.

- **Fennel:** Fennel tea can help relieve gas, bloating, and constipation by promoting healthy digestion and relaxing the digestive muscles.

Supplements:

- **Psyllium Husk:** Psyllium husk is a natural fiber supplement that can help soften stools and promote regular bowel movements.

- **Probiotics:** Probiotic supplements can improve gut health and digestion by balancing the beneficial bacteria in the digestive tract.

- **Magnesium:** Magnesium supplements can help relax the

intestines and promote regular bowel movements.

Dietary Adjustments:

- **Increase Fiber Intake:** Consuming more fiber-rich foods such as fruits, vegetables, whole grains, and legumes can help prevent constipation and promote healthy digestion.

- **Stay Hydrated:** Drinking plenty of water throughout the day can help soften stools and prevent constipation.

- **Avoid Processed Foods:** Limiting processed foods and those high in sugar and unhealthy fats can improve digestive health.

Lifestyle Practices:

- **Regular Exercise:** Physical activity can stimulate digestion and help prevent constipation. Aim for at least 30 minutes of moderate exercise most days of the week.

- **Establish a Routine:** Try to eat meals at the same times each day and establish a regular bathroom routine to promote healthy bowel movements.

- **Mindful Eating:** Chew food thoroughly and eat slowly to improve digestion and prevent overeating.

Natural Remedies:

- **Aloe Vera:** Aloe vera juice can help soothe the digestive tract and promote regular bowel movements.

- **Flaxseeds:** Ground flaxseeds can be added to meals to increase fiber intake and promote healthy digestion.

- **Olive Oil:** A tablespoon of olive oil on an empty stomach can help stimulate the digestive system and relieve constipation.

Tips for Using Remedies for Constipation and Digestive Issues:

- Consistency: Use these remedies regularly to maintain digestive health and prevent constipation.

- Monitor Your Diet: Pay attention to how different foods affect your digestion and make adjustments as needed.

- Stay Active: Regular physical activity is essential for maintaining healthy digestion and preventing constipation.

- Stay Hydrated: Ensure you are drinking enough water throughout the day to support digestive health.

- Consult a Healthcare Provider: If you experience chronic constipation or digestive issues, consult a healthcare provider to rule out underlying conditions and discuss appropriate treatments.

Benefits:

Natural remedies for constipation and digestive issues provide a gentle and effective way to improve digestive health and promote regular bowel movements. By incorporating these methods into your routine, you can alleviate discomfort, support healthy digestion, and maintain overall well-being. These natural treatments offer a safe alternative to conventional medications, promoting long-term digestive health and comfort.

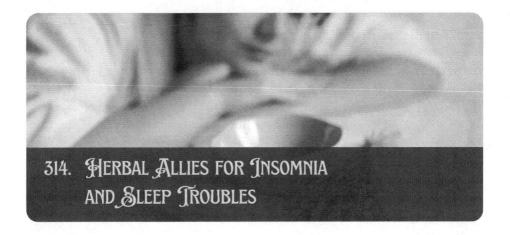

Introduction:

Insomnia and sleep troubles can significantly impact overall health and well-being. Herbal remedies offer a natural and effective way to improve sleep quality, reduce insomnia, and promote restful sleep. These herbs work by calming the nervous system, reducing anxiety, and supporting the body's natural sleep cycles.

Basic Uses and Information:

Herbal allies for insomnia and sleep troubles can be used in various forms, including teas, tinctures, capsules, and essential oils. These remedies help to relax the mind and body, making it easier to fall asleep and stay asleep.

Detailed Uses of Herbal Allies for Insomnia and Sleep Troubles:

Herbal Teas and Infusions:

- **Chamomile:** Chamomile tea is well-known for its calming and sedative properties, helping to relax the body and promote sleep.

- **Valerian Root:** Valerian root tea or tincture can improve sleep quality by reducing the time it takes to fall asleep and enhancing deep sleep.

- **Passionflower:** Passionflower tea can help reduce anxiety and improve sleep quality by increasing GABA levels in the brain, which promotes relaxation.

Tinctures and Extracts:

- **Lemon Balm:** Lemon balm tinctures can help ease anxiety and promote restful sleep. It is especially effective when combined with other calming herbs.

- **Lavender:** Lavender tincture or essential oil can be used to reduce stress and anxiety, helping to improve sleep quality.

- **Ashwagandha:** Ashwagandha tinctures can help balance stress hormones and promote relaxation, aiding in better sleep.

Essential Oils:

- **Lavender Oil:** Inhaling lavender essential oil or using it in a diffuser can create a calming atmosphere that promotes sleep. It can also be applied topically when diluted with a carrier oil.

- **Cedarwood Oil:** Cedarwood oil has sedative properties that can help induce sleep and improve sleep quality.

- **Roman Chamomile Oil:** Roman chamomile essential oil can be used in aromatherapy to relax the mind and body, making it easier to fall asleep.

Capsules and Supplements:

- **Melatonin:** Melatonin supplements can help regulate the sleep-wake cycle and are especially useful for people with disrupted sleep patterns.

- **Magnesium:** Magnesium supplements can help relax muscles and calm the nervous system, promoting better sleep.

- **5-HTP:** 5-HTP supplements can increase serotonin levels, which can improve mood and promote sleep.

Lifestyle Practices:

- **Consistent Sleep Schedule:** Establish a regular sleep routine by going to bed and waking up at the same time each day to regulate your internal clock.

- **Relaxation Techniques:** Practice relaxation techniques such as deep breathing, meditation, or gentle yoga before bedtime to prepare your body for sleep.

- **Sleep Environment:** Create a sleep-friendly environment by keeping your bedroom cool, dark,

and quiet, and avoid using electronic devices before bed.

Tips for Using Herbal Allies for Insomnia and Sleep Troubles:

- **Start with Small Doses:** Begin with small doses to see how your body responds and gradually increase as needed.

- **Consistency:** Use these herbs regularly as part of your nightly routine to maintain steady sleep patterns.

- **Combine Methods:** Use a combination of teas, tinctures, essential oils, and supplements to create a comprehensive approach to improving sleep.

- **Monitor Your Response:** Pay attention to how different remedies affect your sleep and adjust your approach accordingly.

- **Consult a Healthcare Provider:** If sleep troubles persist, consult a healthcare provider to rule out underlying conditions and discuss appropriate treatments.

Benefits:

Herbal allies for insomnia and sleep troubles provide a natural and holistic approach to improving sleep quality and reducing insomnia. By incorporating these herbs into your nightly routine, you can promote relaxation, reduce anxiety, and support a healthy sleep cycle. These natural remedies offer a gentle and effective alternative to conventional sleep aids, helping you achieve restful and rejuvenating sleep.

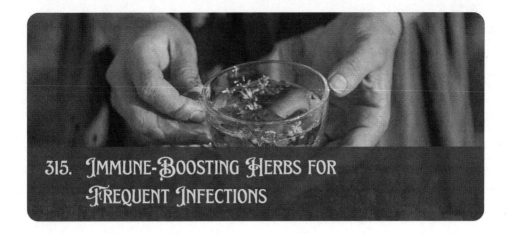

315. Immune-Boosting Herbs for Frequent Infections

Introduction:

Frequent infections can weaken the body and disrupt daily life. Immune-boosting herbs offer a natural way to strengthen the immune system and increase the body's resistance to infections. These herbs help enhance the body's natural defense mechanisms, making it more capable of fighting off viruses, bacteria, and other pathogens.

Basic Uses and Information:

Herbs that boost the immune system can be used in various forms, including teas, tinctures, capsules, and powders. These remedies work by stimulating immune activity, providing antioxidants, and supporting overall health to reduce the frequency and severity of infections.

Detailed Uses of Immune-Boosting Herbs for Frequent Infections:

Herbal Teas and Infusions:

- **Echinacea:** Echinacea tea can stimulate the immune system,

helping to ward off infections and reduce their duration.

- **Elderberry:** Elderberry tea or syrup is rich in antioxidants and vitamins that boost immune function and protect against colds and flu.

- **Astragalus:** Astragalus tea helps enhance immune activity and improve the body's resistance to infections.

Tinctures and Extracts:

- **Olive Leaf:** Olive leaf tincture has antiviral and antibacterial properties, making it effective in boosting the immune system and fighting infections.

- **Goldenseal:** Goldenseal tincture can help combat bacterial infections and support overall immune health.

- **Propolis:** Propolis tincture has powerful antimicrobial properties that can help prevent and treat infections.

Capsules and Supplements:

- **Garlic:** Garlic capsules can boost immune function due to its antiviral and antibacterial properties. Fresh garlic can also be added to meals for additional benefits.

- **Turmeric:** Turmeric supplements contain curcumin, which has anti-inflammatory and antioxidant properties that support immune health.

- **Reishi Mushroom:** Reishi mushroom capsules or powder can enhance immune function and increase the body's resistance to infections.

Essential Oils:

- **Oregano Oil:** Oregano essential oil has potent antimicrobial properties that can help fight infections. It can be taken internally in diluted form or used in aromatherapy.

- **Thyme Oil:** Thyme essential oil can support the immune system and help fight respiratory infections when inhaled or applied topically.

- **Tea Tree Oil:** Tea tree oil can be used topically to prevent infections in cuts and wounds and can also be used in a diffuser to purify the air.

Lifestyle Practices:

- **Balanced Diet:** Eating a diet rich in fruits, vegetables, lean proteins, and whole grains can provide essential nutrients that support immune function.

- **Regular Exercise:** Engaging in regular physical activity can boost the immune system and improve overall health.

- **Adequate Sleep:** Ensuring sufficient rest and quality sleep is crucial for maintaining a strong immune system.

Tips for Using Immune-Boosting Herbs for Frequent Infections:

- **Start with Small Doses:** Begin with small doses to see how your body responds and gradually increase as needed.

- **Consistency:** Use these herbs regularly as part of your daily routine to maintain strong immune function.

- **Combine Methods:** Use a combination of teas, tinctures, capsules, and essential oils to create a comprehensive approach to immune support.

- **Monitor Your Response:** Pay attention to how different remedies affect your immune health and adjust your approach accordingly.

- **Consult a Healthcare Provider:** If you have any underlying health conditions or are taking other medications, consult with a healthcare provider before starting any new herbal regimen.

Benefits:

Immune-boosting herbs provide a natural and effective way to strengthen the body's defenses against frequent infections. By incorporating these herbs into your routine, you can enhance immune function, reduce the incidence of infections, and support overall health. These natural remedies offer a holistic approach to maintaining a robust immune system and improving resilience against illness.

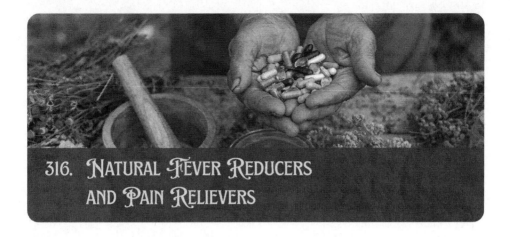

316. Natural Fever Reducers and Pain Relievers

Introduction:

Fevers and pain are common symptoms of various illnesses and conditions. Natural remedies can provide effective relief by reducing fever, alleviating pain, and promoting overall comfort without the side effects of conventional medications. These remedies utilize the healing properties of herbs and other natural substances to support the body's natural healing processes.

Basic Uses and Information:

Natural fever reducers and pain relievers can be used in various forms, including teas, tinctures, essential oils, and compresses. These remedies help to lower body temperature, reduce inflammation, and alleviate discomfort.

Detailed Uses of Natural Fever Reducers and Pain Relievers:

Herbal Teas and Infusions:

- **Willow Bark:** Willow bark tea contains salicin, a natural compound similar to aspirin, which can reduce fever and alleviate pain.

- **Ginger:** Ginger tea can reduce fever by promoting sweating and has anti-inflammatory properties that help relieve pain.

- **Peppermint:** Peppermint tea can help reduce fever by cooling the body and relieve pain through its muscle-relaxing effects.

Tinctures and Extracts:

- **Turmeric:** Turmeric tinctures contain curcumin, which has strong anti-inflammatory and pain-relieving properties.

- **Elderflower:** Elderflower tincture can help reduce fever by promoting sweating and has anti-inflammatory properties.

- **Feverfew:** Feverfew tincture can help reduce fever and alleviate pain, particularly headaches and migraines.

Essential Oils:

- **Lavender Oil:** Lavender essential oil can be used to relieve pain and reduce fever through its calming and analgesic properties. It can be applied topically when diluted or used in aromatherapy.

- **Peppermint Oil:** Peppermint essential oil can reduce fever and relieve pain when applied topically with a carrier oil or inhaled.

- **Eucalyptus Oil:** Eucalyptus essential oil can help reduce fever and alleviate pain, especially when used in steam inhalation or diluted for topical application.

Compresses and Baths:

- **Cool Compress:** Applying a cool compress to the forehead, wrists, and ankles can help reduce fever and provide relief from discomfort.

- **Epsom Salt Bath:** Taking a bath with Epsom salts can reduce inflammation and relieve muscle pain.

- **Herbal Poultices:** Applying a poultice made from anti-inflammatory herbs such as chamomile or comfrey can help reduce pain and swelling.

Dietary Adjustments:

- **Hydration:** Drinking plenty of fluids, such as water, herbal teas, and broths, can help reduce fever and alleviate pain by keeping the body hydrated.

- **Anti-Inflammatory Foods:** Incorporating foods rich in anti-inflammatory compounds, such as berries, leafy greens, and fatty fish, can help reduce pain and support overall health.

Tips for Using Natural Fever Reducers and Pain Relievers:

- **Start with Small Doses:** Begin with small doses to see how your body responds and gradually increase as needed.

- **Consistency:** Use these remedies regularly, as needed, to maintain comfort and support healing.

- **Combine Methods:** Use a combination of teas, tinctures, essential oils, and compresses to create a comprehensive approach to reducing fever and alleviating pain.

- **Monitor Your Response:** Pay attention to how different remedies affect your symptoms and adjust your approach accordingly.

- **Consult a Healthcare Provider:** If fever or pain persists or is severe, consult a healthcare provider to rule out underlying conditions and discuss appropriate treatments.

Benefits:

Natural fever reducers and pain relievers offer a holistic approach to managing these common symptoms, supporting the body's natural healing processes. By incorporating these remedies into your routine, you can reduce discomfort, promote healing, and improve overall well-being. These natural treatments provide a gentle and effective alternative to conventional medications, enhancing comfort and health naturally.

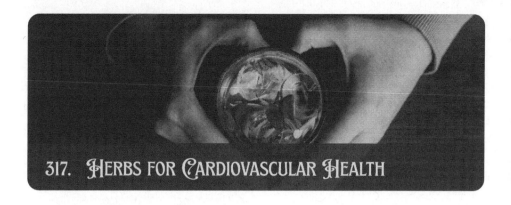

317. Herbs for Cardiovascular Health

Introduction:

Maintaining cardiovascular health is essential for overall well-being and longevity. Herbs can provide a natural and effective way to support heart health, improve circulation, and reduce the risk of cardiovascular diseases. These herbs work by promoting healthy blood pressure, reducing cholesterol levels, and enhancing blood vessel function.

Basic Uses and Information:

Herbs for cardiovascular health can be used in various forms, including teas, tinctures, capsules, and powders. These remedies help to strengthen the heart, improve blood flow, and support the overall health of the cardiovascular system.

Detailed Uses of Herbs for Cardiovascular Health:

Herbal Teas and Infusions:

- **Hawthorn:** Hawthorn tea can strengthen the heart muscle, improve blood flow, and reduce blood pressure.

It is also rich in antioxidants that protect the cardiovascular system.

- **Green Tea:** Green tea is high in catechins, which can reduce cholesterol levels and improve blood vessel function.

- **Hibiscus:** Hibiscus tea has been shown to lower blood pressure and reduce cholesterol levels, supporting overall heart health.

Tinctures and Extracts:

- **Garlic:** Garlic tincture can help reduce cholesterol levels, lower blood pressure, and improve overall cardiovascular health.

- **Ginkgo Biloba:** Ginkgo biloba tincture improves circulation and blood flow, which can benefit cardiovascular health and reduce the risk of clots.

- **Turmeric:** Turmeric tincture contains curcumin, which has anti-inflammatory and antioxidant properties that support heart health.

Capsules and Supplements:

- **Omega-3 Fatty Acids:** Omega-3 supplements, such as fish oil or flaxseed oil, can reduce inflammation, lower triglycerides, and improve heart health.

- **Coenzyme Q10 (CoQ10):** CoQ10 supplements support heart function and energy production, particularly in individuals with heart conditions.

- **Magnesium:** Magnesium supplements can help regulate blood pressure and support overall cardiovascular health.

Essential Oils:

- **Lavender Oil:** Lavender essential oil can reduce stress and anxiety, which are risk factors for heart disease. It can be used in aromatherapy or applied topically when diluted.

- **Rosemary Oil:** Rosemary essential oil can improve circulation and has antioxidant properties that support heart health.

- **Frankincense Oil:** Frankincense essential oil can reduce inflammation and support overall cardiovascular health.

Lifestyle Practices:

- **Balanced Diet:** Eating a diet rich in fruits, vegetables, whole grains, lean proteins, and healthy fats can support heart health.

- **Regular Exercise:** Engaging in regular physical activity can improve cardiovascular function, reduce blood pressure, and lower cholesterol levels.

- **Stress Management:** Practicing stress-reducing techniques such as meditation, yoga, or deep breathing can benefit heart health by lowering stress levels.

Tips for Using Herbs for Cardiovascular Health:

- **Start with Small Doses:** Begin with small doses to see how your body responds and gradually increase as needed.

- **Consistency:** Use these herbs regularly as part of your daily routine to maintain cardiovascular health.

- **Combine Methods:** Use a combination of teas, tinctures, capsules, and lifestyle practices to create a comprehensive approach to heart health.

- **Monitor Your Response:** Pay attention to how different remedies affect your cardiovascular health and adjust your approach accordingly.

- **Consult a Healthcare Provider:** If you have any underlying heart conditions or are taking other medications, consult with a healthcare provider before starting any new herbal regimen.

Benefits:

Herbs for cardiovascular health offer a natural and holistic approach to maintaining a healthy heart and circulatory system. By incorporating these herbs into your daily routine, you can support heart function, improve blood flow, and reduce the risk of cardiovascular diseases. These natural remedies provide a gentle and effective way to enhance cardiovascular health and promote overall well-being.

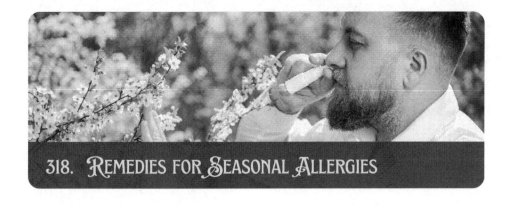

318. Remedies for Seasonal Allergies

Introduction:

Seasonal allergies, also known as hay fever or allergic rhinitis, can cause a range of symptoms such as sneezing, runny nose, itchy eyes, and congestion. Natural remedies can provide effective relief from these symptoms by reducing inflammation, supporting the immune system, and alleviating discomfort. These remedies focus on using herbs, dietary changes, and lifestyle practices to manage and reduce allergy symptoms.

Basic Uses and Information:

Remedies for seasonal allergies include herbal teas, supplements, essential oils, and dietary adjustments. These natural treatments help to minimize allergic reactions, soothe irritated tissues, and support overall respiratory health.

Detailed Uses of Remedies for Seasonal Allergies:

Herbal Teas and Infusions:

- **Nettle:** Nettle tea acts as a natural antihistamine, reducing inflammation and alleviating allergy symptoms.

- **Butterbur:** Butterbur tea can help reduce nasal congestion and relieve symptoms of hay fever by blocking histamines and leukotrienes.

- **Peppermint:** Peppermint tea has anti-inflammatory and decongestant properties that can help open up the nasal passages and ease breathing.

Supplements:

- **Quercetin:** Quercetin is a natural flavonoid that can reduce histamine production and alleviate allergy symptoms. It can be taken as a supplement or found in foods such as apples, onions, and berries.

- **Bromelain:** Bromelain, an enzyme found in pineapples, can reduce nasal swelling and mucus production. It is often used in combination with quercetin.

- **Probiotics:** Probiotic supplements can improve gut health and modulate the immune system, potentially reducing the severity of allergic reactions.

Essential Oils:

- **Eucalyptus Oil:** Eucalyptus essential oil can help clear nasal congestion and improve respiratory function when used in steam inhalation or diffused in the air.

- **Lavender Oil:** Lavender essential oil has anti-inflammatory and calming properties that can help soothe allergy symptoms. It can be inhaled or applied topically when diluted.

- **Tea Tree Oil:** Tea tree essential oil can reduce inflammation and fight off airborne allergens when used in a diffuser.

Dietary Adjustments:

- **Anti-Inflammatory Foods:** Incorporate anti-inflammatory foods such as turmeric, ginger, leafy greens, and fatty fish to reduce inflammation and support the immune system.

- **Local Honey:** Consuming local honey may help your body adapt to local pollen, potentially reducing allergic reactions over time.

- **Hydration:** Drinking plenty of water can help thin mucus and reduce congestion.

Lifestyle Practices:

- **Nasal Irrigation:** Using a neti pot with saline solution can help flush out allergens and reduce nasal congestion.

- **Air Purifiers:** Using an air purifier with a HEPA filter can reduce indoor allergens such as pollen, dust mites, and pet dander.

- **Regular Cleaning:** Keep windows closed during high pollen seasons, and regularly clean your home to reduce dust and allergens.

Tips for Using Remedies for Seasonal Allergies:

- Start Early: Begin using these remedies before allergy season starts to build up your body's defenses.

- Consistency: Use these remedies regularly throughout the allergy season to maintain relief from symptoms.

- Combine Methods: Use a combination of teas, supplements, essential oils, and lifestyle practices to create a comprehensive approach to managing allergies.

- Monitor Your Response: Pay attention to how different remedies affect your symptoms and adjust your approach accordingly.

- Consult a Healthcare Provider: If your allergy symptoms are severe or persistent, consult a healthcare provider to discuss appropriate treatments and rule out other conditions.

Benefits:

Natural remedies for seasonal allergies offer a gentle and effective way to manage and reduce allergy symptoms. By incorporating these remedies into your routine, you can alleviate discomfort, support your immune system, and maintain respiratory health. These natural treatments provide a holistic approach to managing seasonal allergies, promoting overall well-being and comfort.

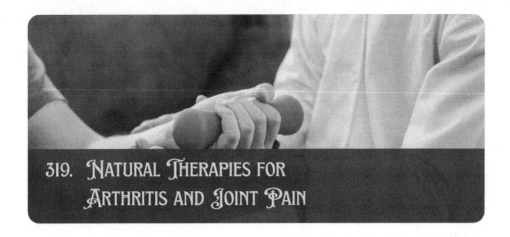

319. Natural Therapies for Arthritis and Joint Pain

Introduction:

Arthritis and joint pain can significantly impact daily life and mobility. Natural therapies can provide relief by reducing inflammation, alleviating pain, and improving joint function. These therapies focus on using herbs, dietary changes, and lifestyle practices to support joint health and manage arthritis symptoms.

Basic Uses and Information:

Natural therapies for arthritis and joint pain include herbal teas, supplements, essential oils, topical applications, and physical practices. These remedies help to reduce inflammation, support cartilage health, and enhance overall joint mobility.

Detailed Uses of Natural Therapies for Arthritis and Joint Pain:

Herbal Teas and Infusions:

- **Turmeric:** Turmeric tea contains curcumin, which has powerful anti-inflammatory and antioxidant properties that can help reduce joint pain and swelling.

- **Ginger:** Ginger tea can reduce inflammation and improve circulation, alleviating pain associated with arthritis.

- **Green Tea:** Green tea is rich in antioxidants that can reduce inflammation and protect joint health.

Supplements:

- **Glucosamine and Chondroitin:** These supplements can help maintain cartilage health, reduce joint pain, and improve mobility in individuals with arthritis.

- **Boswellia:** Boswellia (also known as frankincense) supplements have anti-inflammatory properties that can help reduce arthritis symptoms.

- **Omega-3 Fatty Acids:** Omega-3 supplements, such as fish oil or flaxseed oil, can reduce inflammation and alleviate joint pain.

Essential Oils:

- **Eucalyptus Oil:** Eucalyptus essential oil can be used topically to reduce inflammation and pain in the joints. Dilute with a carrier oil and apply to affected areas.

- **Peppermint Oil:** Peppermint essential oil has cooling and analgesic properties that can help relieve joint pain when applied topically with a carrier oil.

- **Lavender Oil:** Lavender essential oil can reduce inflammation and promote relaxation, helping to alleviate joint pain.

Topical Applications:

- **Capsaicin Cream:** Capsaicin cream, derived from chili peppers, can reduce pain by depleting substance P, a compound that transmits pain signals.

- **Arnica Gel:** Arnica gel can be applied to the skin to reduce inflammation and pain associated with arthritis.

- **Comfrey Salve:** Comfrey salve can promote healing and reduce pain and inflammation in joints.

Dietary Adjustments:

- **Anti-Inflammatory Foods:** Incorporate anti-inflammatory foods such as berries, leafy greens, nuts, and fatty fish to reduce inflammation and support joint health.

- **Avoid Trigger Foods:** Limit foods that can trigger inflammation, such as processed foods, sugar, and trans fats.

- **Hydration:** Drink plenty of water to keep joints lubricated and maintain overall health.

Physical Practices:

- **Exercise:** Regular exercise, such as swimming, walking, and yoga, can improve joint mobility, reduce pain, and strengthen muscles around the joints.

- **Stretching:** Gentle stretching can improve flexibility and reduce stiffness in the joints.

- **Heat and Cold Therapy:** Applying heat can relax muscles and improve circulation, while cold therapy can reduce inflammation and numb pain.

Tips for Using Natural Therapies for Arthritis and Joint Pain:

- **Start with Small Doses:** Begin with small doses to see how your body responds and gradually increase as needed.

- **Consistency:** Use these therapies regularly to maintain joint health and reduce pain.

- **Combine Methods:** Use a combination of teas, supplements, essential oils, and physical practices to create a comprehensive approach to managing arthritis and joint pain.

- **Monitor Your Response:** Pay attention to how different therapies affect your symptoms and adjust your approach accordingly.

- **Consult a Healthcare Provider:** If you have severe or persistent joint pain, consult a healthcare provider to discuss appropriate treatments and rule out other conditions.

Benefits:

Natural therapies for arthritis and joint pain provide a holistic approach to managing these conditions. By incorporating these remedies into your routine, you can reduce inflammation, alleviate pain, and improve joint mobility. These natural treatments offer a gentle and effective alternative to conventional medications, promoting long-term joint health and overall well-being.

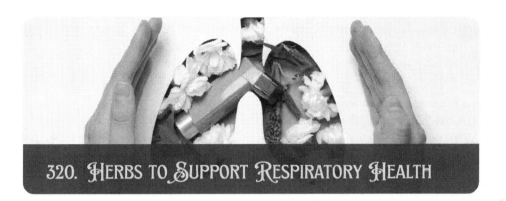

320. Herbs to Support Respiratory Health

Introduction:

Respiratory health is essential for overall well-being, especially in managing conditions such as asthma, bronchitis, and colds. Herbs can provide natural support for the respiratory system by reducing inflammation, clearing mucus, and improving lung function. These herbs work by soothing the airways, enhancing immune function, and promoting healthy breathing.

Basic Uses and Information:

Herbs for respiratory health can be used in various forms, including teas, tinctures, capsules, and essential oils. These remedies help to alleviate respiratory symptoms, support lung health, and boost overall respiratory function.

Detailed Uses of Herbs to Support Respiratory Health:

Herbal Teas and Infusions:

- **Peppermint:** Peppermint tea has menthol, which acts as a natural decongestant, helping to clear the respiratory tract and ease breathing.

- **Ginger:** Ginger tea can reduce inflammation in the respiratory system and help to clear mucus from the lungs.

- **Mullein:** Mullein tea is known for its soothing effects on the respiratory tract, helping to relieve coughs and clear congestion.

Tinctures and Extracts:

- **Licorice Root:** Licorice root tincture can soothe irritated airways, reduce inflammation, and act as an expectorant to help clear mucus.

- **Elderberry:** Elderberry tincture boosts the immune system and has antiviral properties that can help manage colds and respiratory infections.

- **Elecampane:** Elecampane tincture helps clear mucus and supports overall lung health, making it beneficial for chronic respiratory conditions.

Capsules and Supplements:

- **N-Acetyl Cysteine (NAC):** NAC supplements help to thin mucus and support lung health by increasing levels of the antioxidant glutathione.

- **Quercetin:** Quercetin has anti-inflammatory and antihistamine properties that can help reduce respiratory inflammation and improve breathing.

- **Astragalus:** Astragalus supplements can boost immune function and support the respiratory system by reducing inflammation and improving lung function.

Essential Oils:

- **Eucalyptus Oil:** Eucalyptus essential oil can help clear nasal congestion and improve respiratory function when used in steam inhalation or a diffuser.

- **Thyme Oil:** Thyme essential oil has antimicrobial properties and can support respiratory health by clearing congestion and reducing inflammation.

- **Tea Tree Oil:** Tea tree essential oil can help fight respiratory infections and clear congestion when used in a diffuser.

Lifestyle Practices:

- **Steam Inhalation:** Inhaling steam with added essential oils, such as eucalyptus or peppermint, can help clear congestion and soothe the respiratory tract.

- **Hydration:** Drinking plenty of fluids, including herbal teas and water, can help thin mucus and support respiratory health.

- **Avoiding Irritants:** Reducing exposure to smoke, pollution, and allergens can help maintain respiratory health and prevent irritation.

Tips for Using Herbs to Support Respiratory Health:

- Start with Small Doses: Begin with small doses to see how your body responds and gradually increase as needed.

- Consistency: Use these herbs regularly to maintain respiratory health and prevent respiratory issues.

- Combine Methods: Use a combination of teas, tinctures, capsules, and essential oils to create a comprehensive approach to supporting respiratory health.

- Monitor Your Response: Pay attention to how different herbs affect your respiratory symptoms and adjust your approach accordingly.

- Consult a Healthcare Provider: If you have chronic respiratory conditions or severe symptoms, consult a healthcare provider to discuss appropriate treatments and ensure the safe use of herbal remedies.

Benefits:

Herbs to support respiratory health offer a natural and holistic approach to maintaining healthy lungs and airways. By incorporating these herbs into your daily routine, you can alleviate respiratory symptoms, boost immune function, and promote overall respiratory well-being. These natural remedies provide a gentle and effective alternative to conventional medications, supporting long-term respiratory health and comfort.

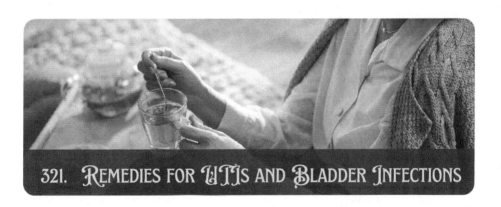

321. REMEDIES FOR UTIs AND BLADDER INFECTIONS

Introduction:

Urinary tract infections (UTIs) and bladder infections can cause discomfort and inconvenience. Natural remedies can provide effective relief by reducing inflammation, fighting infection, and promoting overall urinary tract health. These remedies focus on using herbs, dietary changes, and lifestyle practices to alleviate symptoms and prevent recurrence.

Basic Uses and Information:

Remedies for UTIs and bladder infections include herbal teas, supplements, essential oils, and dietary adjustments. These natural treatments help to eliminate bacteria, soothe the urinary tract, and support healthy bladder function.

Detailed Uses of Remedies for UTIs and Bladder Infections:

Herbal Teas and Infusions:

- **Cranberry:** Cranberry juice or tea can help prevent bacteria from adhering to the walls of the urinary tract, reducing the risk of infection.

- **Dandelion:** Dandelion tea acts as a diuretic, increasing urine production and helping to flush out bacteria.

- **Marshmallow Root:** Marshmallow root tea can soothe the urinary tract and reduce inflammation, providing relief from UTI symptoms.

Supplements:

- **D-Mannose:** D-Mannose is a sugar that can prevent E. coli bacteria from sticking to the urinary tract walls, helping to prevent and treat UTIs.

- **Probiotics:** Probiotic supplements can improve gut health and support the immune system, reducing the risk of UTIs and promoting urinary tract health.

- **Garlic:** Garlic supplements have antimicrobial properties that can help fight urinary tract infections.

Essential Oils:

- **Tea Tree Oil:** Tea tree essential oil has antibacterial properties that can help fight infections when used in a warm bath or diluted for topical application.

- **Lavender Oil:** Lavender essential oil can reduce inflammation and soothe the urinary tract when used in aromatherapy or diluted for topical application.

- **Oregano Oil:** Oregano essential oil has strong antibacterial properties that can help combat UTIs. It can be taken in capsule form or diluted for topical application.

Dietary Adjustments:

- **Increase Hydration:** Drinking plenty of water helps flush out bacteria and toxins from the urinary tract.

- **Avoid Irritants:** Reduce consumption of irritants such as caffeine, alcohol, spicy foods, and artificial sweeteners, which can exacerbate UTI symptoms.

- **Alkaline Foods:** Incorporate alkaline foods such as fruits and vegetables to balance the pH of the urine and create an inhospitable environment for bacteria.

Lifestyle Practices:

- **Good Hygiene:** Practice good hygiene by wiping from front to back after using the toilet and urinating after sexual intercourse to prevent bacterial transfer.

- **Frequent Urination:** Urinate regularly to flush out bacteria and reduce the risk of infection.

- **Loose Clothing:** Wear loose-fitting clothing and breathable fabrics to reduce moisture and prevent bacterial growth.

Tips for Using Remedies for UTIs and Bladder Infections:

- **Start with Small Doses:** Begin with small doses to see how your body responds and gradually increase as needed.
- **Consistency:** Use these remedies regularly to maintain urinary tract health and prevent infections.
- **Combine Methods:** Use a combination of teas, supplements, essential oils, and lifestyle practices to create a comprehensive approach to managing UTIs and bladder infections.
- **Monitor Your Response:** Pay attention to how different remedies affect your symptoms and adjust your approach accordingly.
- **Consult a Healthcare Provider:** If UTI symptoms persist or worsen, consult a healthcare provider to discuss appropriate treatments and rule out more serious conditions.

Benefits:

Natural remedies for UTIs and bladder infections offer a holistic and effective approach to managing these conditions. By incorporating these remedies into your routine, you can alleviate symptoms, promote urinary tract health, and reduce the risk of recurrent infections. These natural treatments provide a gentle and safe alternative to conventional medications, supporting overall urinary health and well-being.

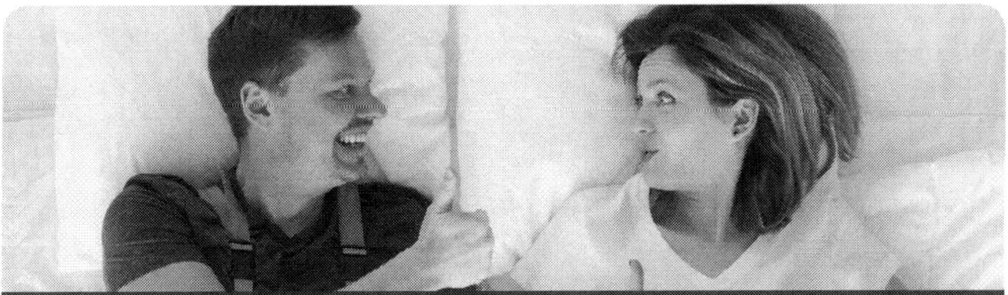

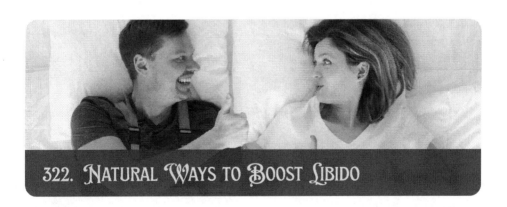

322. Natural Ways to Boost Libido

Introduction:

Low libido can affect quality of life and intimate relationships. Natural remedies can help enhance libido by balancing hormones, improving circulation, reducing stress, and boosting overall vitality. These remedies include herbs, dietary changes, and lifestyle practices that support sexual health and enhance desire.

Basic Uses and Information:

Natural ways to boost libido include herbal supplements, foods that enhance sexual health, essential oils, and lifestyle changes. These methods help to improve blood flow, balance hormones, and reduce stress, all of which can contribute to a healthy sex drive.

Detailed Uses of Natural Ways to Boost Libido:

Herbal Supplements:

- **Maca Root:** Maca root is known for its ability to balance hormones and increase sexual desire in both men and women. It can be taken as a powder or in capsule form.

- **Tribulus Terrestris:** This herb can enhance libido and improve sexual function by increasing testosterone levels and promoting blood flow.

- **Ginseng:** Ginseng can boost energy levels, reduce stress, and improve sexual performance and libido.

Foods that Enhance Sexual Health:

- **Dark Chocolate:** Dark chocolate contains phenylethylamine and serotonin, which can enhance mood and increase sexual desire.

- **Oysters:** Rich in zinc, oysters can boost testosterone levels and enhance libido.

- **Nuts and Seeds:** Nuts and seeds, such as almonds and flaxseeds, are rich in essential fatty acids that support hormone production and improve blood flow.

Essential Oils:

- **Ylang-Ylang:** Ylang-ylang essential oil has aphrodisiac properties that can enhance mood and sexual desire. It can be diffused or applied topically when diluted.

- **Rose:** Rose essential oil can boost libido by improving mood and reducing stress. It can be used in aromatherapy or as a massage oil.

- **Sandalwood:** Sandalwood essential oil can help balance hormones and enhance sexual arousal. It can be diffused or applied topically when diluted.

Lifestyle Practices:

- **Exercise:** Regular physical activity can improve circulation, boost energy levels, and enhance overall sexual health.

- **Stress Reduction:** Practices such as yoga, meditation, and deep breathing can reduce stress and anxiety, which can negatively impact libido.

- **Sleep:** Ensuring adequate rest and quality sleep is crucial for maintaining hormonal balance and sexual health.

Hydration and Diet:

- **Stay Hydrated:** Drinking plenty of water is essential for maintaining energy levels and overall health, which can positively affect libido.

- **Balanced Diet:** A diet rich in fruits, vegetables, lean proteins, and healthy fats supports overall health and hormone production, enhancing libido.

Tips for Using Natural Ways to Boost Libido:

- **Start with Small Doses:** Begin with small doses of herbs and supplements to see how your body responds and gradually increase as needed.

- **Consistency:** Use these natural remedies regularly to maintain libido and overall sexual health.

- **Combine Methods:** Use a combination of supplements, foods, essential oils, and lifestyle practices to create a comprehensive approach to boosting libido.

- **Monitor Your Response:** Pay attention to how different remedies affect your libido and adjust your approach accordingly.

- **Consult a Healthcare Provider:** If you have underlying health conditions or are taking other medications, consult a healthcare provider before starting any new herbal regimen.

Benefits:

Natural ways to boost libido provide a holistic approach to enhancing sexual desire and improving overall sexual health. By incorporating these remedies into your routine, you can balance hormones, reduce stress, improve circulation, and enhance your sex drive naturally. These treatments offer a safe and effective alternative to conventional medications, supporting long-term sexual vitality and well-being.

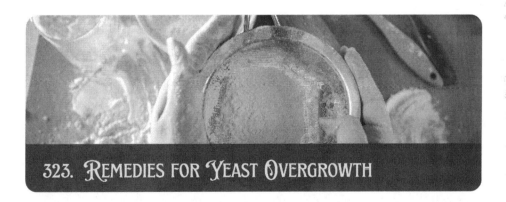

323. REMEDIES FOR YEAST OVERGROWTH

Introduction:

Yeast overgrowth, particularly of Candida species, can cause various health issues, including digestive discomfort, fatigue, and infections. Natural remedies can help manage and reduce yeast overgrowth by restoring balance to the microbiome, supporting immune function, and inhibiting the growth of yeast. These remedies include herbs, dietary changes, and lifestyle practices.

Basic Uses and Information:

Remedies for yeast overgrowth include herbal supplements, probiotic-rich foods, essential oils, and dietary adjustments. These natural treatments help to eliminate excess yeast, support gut health, and enhance the body's natural defenses.

Detailed Uses of Remedies for Yeast Overgrowth:

Herbal Teas and Infusions:

- **Pau D'Arco:** Pau d'arco tea has antifungal properties that can help inhibit the growth of Candida and other yeast.

- **Oregano:** Oregano tea or oil contains powerful antifungal compounds that can help reduce yeast overgrowth.

- **Ginger:** Ginger tea has anti-inflammatory and antifungal properties that support digestive health and reduce yeast levels.

Supplements:

- **Probiotics:** Probiotic supplements can help restore balance to the gut microbiome by promoting the growth of beneficial bacteria that inhibit yeast growth.

- **Caprylic Acid:** Caprylic acid supplements can penetrate yeast cell membranes, causing them to die off.

- **Berberine:** Berberine supplements have antimicrobial properties that can help reduce Candida and other yeast in the digestive tract.

Essential Oils:

- **Tea Tree Oil:** Tea tree essential oil has strong antifungal properties that can be used topically to treat skin infections caused by yeast.

- **Clove Oil:** Clove essential oil can be used in aromatherapy or diluted for topical application to inhibit yeast growth.

- **Thyme Oil:** Thyme essential oil has antifungal properties that can help manage yeast overgrowth when used in a diffuser or diluted for topical use.

Dietary Adjustments:

- **Reduce Sugar Intake:** Yeast feeds on sugar, so reducing or eliminating sugar from your diet can help starve the yeast and reduce overgrowth.

- **Increase Fiber Intake:** Fiber helps support a healthy gut microbiome and promotes the elimination of toxins and excess yeast from the body.

- **Consume Antifungal Foods:** Include foods with natural antifungal properties, such as garlic, coconut oil, and apple cider vinegar, in your diet.

Lifestyle Practices:

- **Good Hygiene:** Practice good hygiene, especially in areas prone to yeast infections, to prevent and manage overgrowth.

- **Stress Management:** Chronic stress can weaken the immune system, so incorporating stress-reducing practices such as meditation, yoga, and deep breathing can help manage yeast overgrowth.

- **Adequate Sleep:** Ensure you get sufficient rest to support immune function and overall health.

Tips for Using Remedies for Yeast Overgrowth:

- ♀ **Start with Small Doses:** Begin with small doses of herbs and supplements to see how your body responds and gradually increase as needed.

- ♀ **Consistency:** Use these remedies regularly to maintain balance and prevent yeast overgrowth.

- ♀ **Combine Methods:** Use a combination of teas, supplements, essential oils, and dietary adjustments to create a comprehensive approach to managing yeast overgrowth.

- ♀ **Monitor Your Response:** Pay attention to how different remedies affect your symptoms and adjust your approach accordingly.

- ♀ **Consult a Healthcare Provider:** If you have persistent or severe symptoms, consult a healthcare provider to discuss appropriate treatments and ensure safe use of herbal remedies.

Benefits:

Natural remedies for yeast overgrowth provide a holistic approach to managing and reducing excess yeast in the body. By incorporating these remedies into your routine, you can restore balance to your microbiome, support immune function, and improve overall health. These natural treatments offer a safe and effective alternative to conventional antifungal medications, promoting long-term well-being and comfort.

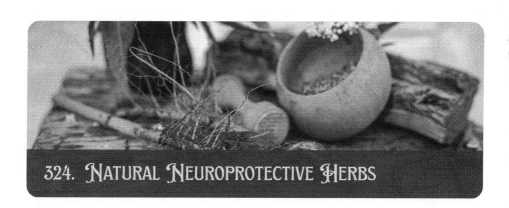

324. NATURAL NEUROPROTECTIVE HERBS

Introduction:

Neuroprotective herbs help protect the nervous system, enhance cognitive function, and prevent neurodegenerative conditions. These herbs support brain health by reducing inflammation, combating oxidative stress, and promoting the growth of new neurons. Incorporating these herbs into your routine can improve memory, focus, and overall brain function.

Basic Uses and Information:

Neuroprotective herbs can be used in various forms, including teas, tinctures, capsules, and powders. These remedies help to enhance cognitive function, protect against neurological diseases, and support overall brain health.

Detailed Uses of Natural Neuroprotective Herbs:

Herbal Teas and Infusions:

- **Ginkgo Biloba:** Ginkgo biloba tea can improve blood flow to the brain, enhance memory, and reduce the risk of cognitive decline.

- **Gotu Kola:** Gotu kola tea supports cognitive function, reduces anxiety, and promotes the regeneration of nerve cells.

- **Green Tea:** Green tea contains antioxidants, particularly EGCG, which protect brain cells from damage and improve cognitive function.

Tinctures and Extracts:

- **Lion's Mane Mushroom:** Lion's mane tincture stimulates the production of nerve growth factor (NGF), which supports the growth and maintenance of neurons.

- **Bacopa Monnieri:** Bacopa monnieri tincture enhances memory, learning, and overall cognitive

performance by reducing oxidative stress and inflammation.

- **Ashwagandha:** Ashwagandha tincture helps reduce stress and anxiety, supports brain function, and protects against neurodegenerative diseases.

Capsules and Supplements:

- **Rhodiola Rosea:** Rhodiola rosea capsules improve cognitive function, reduce mental fatigue, and protect the brain from stress-related damage.

- **Turmeric (Curcumin):** Curcumin supplements have strong anti-inflammatory and antioxidant properties that protect brain cells and improve cognitive function.

- **Phosphatidylserine:** This supplement supports brain health by maintaining the integrity of cell membranes and enhancing cognitive function.

Essential Oils:

- **Rosemary Oil:** Rosemary essential oil can enhance memory and concentration when used in aromatherapy or applied topically with a carrier oil.

- **Peppermint Oil:** Inhaling peppermint essential oil can improve focus, alertness, and overall cognitive function.

- **Lavender Oil:** Lavender essential oil has calming properties that can reduce stress and anxiety, supporting overall brain health.

Dietary Adjustments:

- **Omega-3 Fatty Acids:** Consuming foods rich in omega-3 fatty acids, such as fish, flaxseeds, and walnuts, supports brain health and cognitive `

- **Antioxidant-Rich Foods:** Include foods high in antioxidants, such as berries, dark chocolate, and leafy greens, to protect brain cells from oxidative stress.

- **Hydration:** Staying well-hydrated is essential for maintaining cognitive function and overall brain health.

Tips for Using Natural Neuroprotective Herbs:

- **Start with Small Doses:** Begin with small doses to see how your body responds and gradually increase as needed.

- **Consistency:** Use these herbs regularly to maintain and enhance cognitive function and brain health.

- **Combine Methods:** Use a combination of teas, tinctures, supplements, and dietary adjustments to create a comprehensive approach to neuroprotection.

- **Monitor Your Response:** Pay attention to how different herbs affect your cognitive function and adjust your approach accordingly.

- **Consult a Healthcare Provider:** If you have underlying health conditions or are taking other medications, consult a healthcare provider before starting any new herbal regimen.

Benefits:

Natural neuroprotective herbs provide a holistic approach to supporting brain health and cognitive function. By incorporating these herbs into your daily routine, you can protect against neurodegenerative diseases, enhance memory and focus, and maintain overall brain health. These natural remedies offer a safe and effective way to support long-term cognitive well-being and mental clarity.

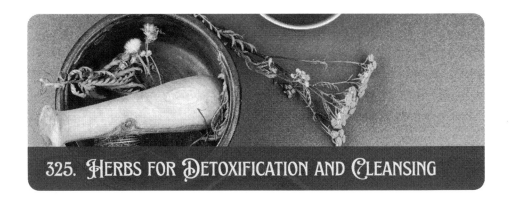

Introduction:

Detoxification and cleansing are essential for maintaining overall health and well-being. Herbs can provide a natural and effective way to support the body's detox processes, helping to eliminate toxins, improve digestion, and boost overall vitality. These herbs work by enhancing liver function, supporting kidney health, and promoting the elimination of waste from the body.

Basic Uses and Information:

Herbs for detoxification and cleansing can be used in various forms, including teas, tinctures, capsules, and powders. These remedies help to purify the blood, stimulate the liver and kidneys, and support the body's natural detoxification pathways.

Detailed Uses of Herbs for Detoxification and Cleansing:

Herbal Teas and Infusions:

- **Dandelion Root:** Dandelion root tea supports liver health by promoting bile production, which aids in the digestion and elimination of toxins.

- **Milk Thistle:** Milk thistle tea or tincture contains silymarin, a compound that protects liver cells and enhances liver function.

- **Nettle:** Nettle tea acts as a diuretic, helping to flush out toxins and support kidney health.

Tinctures and Extracts:

- **Burdock Root:** Burdock root tincture helps purify the blood and supports liver and kidney function, promoting overall detoxification.

- **Red Clover:** Red clover tincture aids in the elimination of toxins from the bloodstream and supports overall immune health.

- **Artichoke Leaf:** Artichoke leaf tincture supports liver function and bile production, aiding in digestion and detoxification.

Capsules and Supplements:

- **Chlorella:** Chlorella supplements are rich in chlorophyll and can help bind to heavy metals and other toxins, aiding in their elimination from the body.

- **Spirulina:** Spirulina supplements support detoxification by promoting liver health and enhancing the elimination of toxins.

- **Activated Charcoal:** Activated charcoal can bind to toxins in the digestive tract, helping to eliminate them from the body.

Essential Oils:

- **Lemon Oil:** Lemon essential oil can support detoxification by stimulating lymphatic drainage and promoting digestion. It can be added to water or used in aromatherapy.

- **Peppermint Oil:** Peppermint essential oil aids digestion and supports liver function, enhancing the body's detox processes. It can be used in aromatherapy or applied topically when diluted.

- **Ginger Oil:** Ginger essential oil can support digestion and reduce inflammation, aiding in detoxification. It can be used in a diffuser or applied topically when diluted.

Lifestyle Practices:

- **Hydration:** Drinking plenty of water helps flush out toxins and supports overall detoxification.

- **Regular Exercise:** Physical activity promotes circulation and lymphatic drainage, aiding in the elimination of toxins.

- **Balanced Diet:** Eating a diet rich in fruits, vegetables, lean proteins, and whole grains supports the body's natural detox processes.

Tips for Using Herbs for Detoxification and Cleansing:

- **Start with Small Doses:** Begin with small doses to see how your body responds and gradually increase as needed.

- **Consistency:** Use these herbs regularly as part of your daily routine to support ongoing detoxification and cleansing.

- **Combine Methods:** Use a combination of teas, tinctures, supplements, and lifestyle practices to create a comprehensive approach to detoxification.

- **Monitor Your Response:** Pay attention to how different herbs affect your detox process and adjust your approach accordingly.

- **Consult a Healthcare Provider:** If you have underlying health conditions or are taking other medications, consult a healthcare provider before starting any new herbal regimen.

Benefits:

Herbs for detoxification and cleansing offer a natural and holistic approach to supporting the body's detox processes. By incorporating these herbs into your routine, you can enhance liver and kidney function, purify the blood, and promote the elimination of toxins. These natural remedies provide a safe and effective way to maintain overall health and vitality, supporting long-term well-being.

Afterword:
Barbara O'Neill's Lasting Legacy

As we reach the end of this journey through Barbara O'Neill's inspired encyclopedia of herbal healing, it is natural to pause and reflect on the profound impact her life's work has had on the world of natural health.

Barbara's unwavering dedication to exploring and sharing the restorative powers of nature has touched countless lives. Her teachings have resonated with individuals from all walks of life, offering a gentle yet effective path towards holistic well-being.

Through her writings, lectures, and personal interactions, Barbara has ignited a flame of curiosity and empowerment within her students and followers. She has encouraged them to question conventional approaches and to embrace the wisdom of nature's pharmacy.

Barbara's approach to healing is rooted in the belief that true wellness stems from a harmonious balance of body, mind, and spirit. Her emphasis on wholesome nutrition, detoxification, and the judicious use of herbal remedies has provided a beacon of hope for those seeking alternatives to mainstream medical practices.

While her methods have faced scrutiny and criticism, Barbara's resilience and steadfast commitment to her principles have been unwavering. She has remained a humble student of nature, continuously seeking to deepen her understanding and share her knowledge with others.

One of Barbara's greatest gifts has been her ability to make complex concepts accessible to all. Her warm, nurturing presence and relatable storytelling have created a sense of comfort and trust, inviting individuals to embark on their own journeys of self-discovery and healing.

As we turn the final pages of this book, we are reminded that Barbara's legacy extends far beyond the written word. Her teachings have inspired a movement, a community of individuals who are passionate about reclaiming their health and embracing a more natural way of living.

In the years to come, Barbara's influence will continue to ripple outward, touching the lives of generations yet to come. Her wisdom will be passed down, her recipes shared, and her belief in the body's innate healing potential will continue to inspire and empower.

Let us carry Barbara's teachings forward, honoring her dedication to natural healing and her unwavering belief in the transformative power of nature's gifts. May her legacy serve as a reminder that true well-being is within our reach, and that the path to healing often begins with a simple step towards embracing the wisdom of the natural world.

₵AST ₩ORDS

As we reach the conclusion of this journey through the world of herbal remedies, I want to extend my heartfelt congratulations and gratitude to you, the reader, for embarking on this path of natural healing and holistic wellness. Your commitment to exploring and embracing the wisdom encapsulated in these pages is not only commendable but a vital step towards a more harmonious and balanced way of life.

This book, inspired by the teachings of Barbara O'Neill and the timeless wisdom of herbal medicine, is more than just a collection of recipes; it is a testament to the power of nature in healing and nurturing our bodies and minds. Each remedy, carefully crafted and detailed, is a drop in the vast ocean of natural healing practices that humanity has cultivated over millennia.

As you close this book, remember that it is not meant to be tucked away and forgotten. Let it be a living resource, a companion in your ongoing journey towards wellness. Keep it within reach, for the wisdom it contains is meant to be revisited, whether to find a remedy for a specific ailment or to seek inspiration for maintaining daily health and vitality.

The world of herbal medicine is dynamic and ever evolving, and so should be your relationship with these remedies. Feel encouraged to adapt and tailor these recipes to suit your unique needs and circumstances. Listen to your body, for it speaks a language older than any text, guiding you towards the herbs and preparations that resonate most with your personal journey to health.

Remember, each step you take in incorporating these natural remedies into your life is a step towards a deeper connection with the natural world and a more profound understanding of your own body. The path to wellness is as much about nurturing the spirit and mind as it is about healing the body.

In closing, let this book serve as your gateway to an empowered and informed approach to health, where you are the steward of your own well-being, inspired by the enduring wisdom of nature. Congratulations on completing Volume 1 of your journey through the art of herbal remedies. I hope it has been both enriching and enlightening, filled with moments of health and happiness.

With warm regards and best wishes for your continued health and wellness,

Margaret Willowbrook.

References

1. "The Herbal Apothecary: 100 Medicinal Herbs and How to Use Them" by JJ Pursell (2015)

2. "The Herbal Medicine-Maker's Handbook: A Home Manual" by James Green (2000)

3. "Making Plant Medicine" by Richo Cech (2000)

4. "The Complete Herbal Tutor" by Anne McIntyre (2010)

5. "Rosemary Gladstar's Medicinal Herbs: A Beginner's Guide" by Rosemary Gladstar (2012)

6. "Back To Eden" by Jethro Kloss (1939)

7. "Common Herbs for Natural Health" by Juliette de Bairacli Levy (1974)

8. "Complete Earth Medicine Handbook" by Susanne Fischer-Rizzi (1996)

9. "Herbal: 100 Herbs from the World's Healing Traditions" by Mimi Prunella Hernandez (2021)

10. "The Way of Herbs" by Michael Tierra (1998)

11. "Alchemy of Herbs" by Rosalee de la Forêt (2017)

12. "Herbal Recipes for Vibrant Health" by Rosemary Gladstar (2008)

13. Books and lectures from Barbara O'Neill.

Bonus Page:
Video Short Tutorials By Barbara O'Neill

Thank you for joining us on this journey through the world of herbal healing and natural medicine. To enrich your learning experience, we're thrilled to offer you exclusive access to a collection of video short tutorials featuring Barbara O'Neil. These tutorials, extracted directly from her lectures, provide practical, visual guidance on implementing the natural health practices discussed in this book.

By subscribing, you'll not only gain instant access to our current video library but also be updated with new videos as we continue to add to our collection. This is a fantastic way to stay connected with the latest in herbal healing and natural medicine, ensuring you're always equipped with the knowledge to support your wellness journey.

How to Access:

Simply scan the QR code below or follow the provided link to subscribe and unlock your access. This is our way of saying thank you and enhancing your journey toward holistic health with the invaluable wisdom of Barbara O'Neill.

As new tutorials become available, you'll be the first to know, allowing you to continuously expand your understanding and application of natural health principles.

@INFINITEWELLNESSWAVE

https://www.instagram.com/infinitewellnesswave

We hope these video tutorials serve as a valuable resource in your quest for wellness, bringing the teachings of Barbara O'Neill to life in a new and engaging way. Your feedback and suggestions are always welcome as we grow this library together.

A Message From The Publisher

Are you enjoying the book?
We would love to hear your thoughts!

Many readers do not know how hard reviews are to come by and how much they help a publisher. We would be incredibly grateful if you could take just a few seconds to write a brief review on Amazon, even if it's just a few sentences!

Please be aware that this is an ongoing project, and we are continuously improving the book's content thanks to your feedback. While it may not be perfect yet, your support greatly helps us!

Please go here to leave a quick review:
https://amazon.com/ryp

We would greatly appreciate it if you could take the time to post your review of the book and share your thoughts with the community. If you have enjoyed the book, please let us know what you loved the most about it and if you would recommend it to others. Your feedback is valuable to us, and it helps us to improve our services and continue to offer high-quality literature to our readers.

🌐   www.abetteryoueveryday.com

✉   Email: info@abetteryoueveryday.co